D0463600

END-OF-LIFE DECISIONS

A Psychosocial Perspective

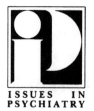

ISSUES IN PSYCHIATRY

Joseph D. Bloom, M.D.
Series Editor

END-OF-LIFE DECISIONS

A Psychosocial Perspective

Edited by
Maurice D. Steinberg, M.D.
Stuart J. Youngner, M.D.

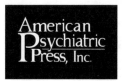

American Psychiatric Press, Inc.

Washington, DC
London, England

Note: The authors have worked to ensure that all information in this book concerning drug dosages, schedules, and routes of administration is accurate as of the time of publication and consistent with standards set by the U.S. Food and Drug Administration and the general medical community. As medical research and practice advance, however, therapeutic standards may change. For this reason and because human and mechanical errors sometimes occur, we recommend that readers follow the advice of a physician who is directly involved in their care or the care of a member of their family.

Books published by the American Psychiatric Press, Inc., represent the views and opinions of the individual authors and do not necessarily represent the policies and opinions of the Press or the American Psychiatric Association.

Copyright © 1998 American Psychiatric Press, Inc.
ALL RIGHTS RESERVED
Manufactured in the United States of America on acid-free paper
First Edition
01 00 99 98   4 3 2 1

American Psychiatric Press, Inc.
1400 K Street, N.W.
Washington, DC   20005
www.appi.org

Library of Congress Cataloging-in-Publication Data
End-of-life decisions : a psychosocial perspective / edited by Maurice D.
    Steinberg and Stuart J. Youngner.
        p.   cm.
    Includes bibliographical references and index.
    ISBN 0-88048-756-9
    1. Euthanasia—Psychological aspects. 2. Euthanasia—Social
aspects. 3. Right to die—Psychological aspects. 4. Right to die—
Social aspects. 5. Death—Psychological aspects. I. Steinberg,
Maurice D. II. Youngner, Stuart J.
    [DNLM: 1. Right to Die. 2. Decision Making. 3. Counseling.
4. Suicide, Assisted—psychology. 5. Euthanasia, Passive—
psychology. W 85.5 E56 1998]
R726.E49 1998
174'.24—dc21
DNLM/DLC
for Library of Congress   97-52636
                                                                                      CIP

British Library Cataloguing in Publication Data
A CIP record is available from the British Library.

To my wife, Sandy,
and children, Danny and Michael.
In memory of my father, Israel Steinberg.
M.D.S.

To my children,
Suzanne, Jonathan, and Matthew.
S.J.Y.

Contents

Contributors ix

Acknowledgments xi

Foreword xiii
Paul S. Appelbaum, M.D.

1   **Introduction** 1
Maurice D. Steinberg, M.D.
Stuart J. Youngner, M.D.

2   **Competence to Refuse Life-Sustaining
Treatment** 19
Stuart J. Youngner, M.D.

3   **Depression and the Refusal of Life-Saving
Medical Treatment** 55
Mark D. Sullivan, M.D., Ph.D.

4   **Family Dynamics in Decisions to
Withhold or Withdraw Treatment** 77
Ellen Rothchild, M.D.

5   **Obstacles to Doctor-Patient
Communication at the End of Life** 109
Mary F. Morrison, M.D.

6   **Consultation to End-of-Life Treatment
Decisions in Children** 137
Julie R. Van der Feen, M.D.C.M.
Michael S. Jellinek, M.D.

7   End-of-Life Decisions in AIDS **179**
  Alexandra Beckett, M.D.

**8   Evaluating Patient Requests for
  Euthanasia and Assisted Suicide
  in Terminal Illness:
  The Role of the Psychiatrist** **205**
  Susan D. Block, M.D.
  J. Andrew Billings, M.D.

**9   Legal Aspects of End-of-Life
  Decision Making** **235**
  Alan Meisel, J.D.

**10   Termination-of-Treatment Decisions:
  Ethical Underpinnings** **259**
  David Mayo, Ph.D.

**11   Physician-Assisted Suicide:
  Moral Questions** **283**
  Daniel Callahan, Ph.D.

Index **299**

Contributors

Paul S. Appelbaum, M.D.
Chairman, Department of Psychiatry; A. F. Zeleznik Professor of Psychiatry; Director, Law and Psychiatry Program, University of Massachusetts Medical Center, Worcester, Massachusetts

Alexandra Beckett, M.D.
Assistant Professor of Psychiatry, Harvard Medical School; Director, HIV/AIDS Program, Beth Israel Hospital, Boston, Massachusetts

J. Andrew Billings, M.D.
Assistant Clinical Professor of Medicine, Harvard Medical School; Director, Palliative Care Service, Massachusetts General Hospital, Boston, Massachusetts

Susan D. Block, M.D.
Assistant Professor of Psychiatry, Harvard Medical School, Boston, Massachusetts; National Program Director, Faculty Scholars Program, Project on Death in America, Open Society Institute, New York, New York

Daniel Callahan, Ph.D.
Director of International Programs, Hastings Center, Briarcliff Manor, New York

Michael S. Jellinek, M.D.
Professor of Psychiatry and Pediatrics, Harvard Medical School; Chief, Child Psychiatry Service; Senior Vice-President for Administration, Massachusetts General Hospital, Boston, Massachusetts

David Mayo, Ph.D.
Professor of Philosophy and Faculty Associate at Center for Biomedical Ethics, University of Minnesota, Duluth, Minnesota

Alan Meisel, J.D.
Dickie, McCamey and Chilcote Professor of Bioethics and Law,
University of Pittsburgh, Center for Medical Ethics, School of
Law, Pittsburgh, Pennsylvania

Mary F. Morrison, M.D.
Assistant Professor of Psychiatry and Medicine, University of
Pennsylvania, Philadelphia, Pennsylvania

Ellen Rothchild, M.D.
Clinical Professor of Child Psychiatry, Case Western Reserve University School of Medicine, Cleveland, Ohio

Maurice D. Steinberg, M.D.
Clinical Associate Professor of Psychiatry, Albert Einstein College
of Medicine, New York, New York

Mark D. Sullivan, M.D., Ph.D.
Associate Professor of Psychiatry and Behavioral Sciences, University of Washington School of Medicine, Seattle, Washington

Julie R. Van der Feen, M.D.C.M.
Instructor in Psychiatry, Harvard Medical School; Attending
Child Psychiatrist, Richmond Psychiatry Service, Children's Hospital, Boston, Massachusetts

Stuart J. Youngner, M.D.
Professor of Medicine, Psychiatry and Biomedical Ethics, Case
Western Reserve University; Director of Clinical Ethics Program,
University Hospitals of Cleveland, Cleveland, Ohio

Acknowledgments

This book originated in the work of the American Psychiatric Association (APA) Subcommittee on the Psychiatric Aspects of Life-Sustaining Technology, chaired by Maurice D. Steinberg, M.D., from 1992 to 1996. The authors are grateful for the strong support given to the project by the respective chairpersons of the APA's Committee on Consultation-Liaison Psychiatry and Primary Care Education: Tom Wise, M.D.; Fawzy Fawzy, M.D.; Jimmie Holland, M.D.; and Mary Jane Massie, M.D. We would also like to thank Jim Shore, M.D., former Chairman of the Council on Medical Education and Career Development, and James Scully, M.D., former APA Deputy Medical Director, for their constant support and endorsement of the subcommittee's efforts.

M.D.S. and S.J.Y.

I would like to express my particular appreciation to Stephen Saravay, M.D., Chief of Consultation-Liaison Psychiatry at Long Island Jewish Medical Center (LIJ). For 25 years he has promoted the clinical and academic growth of his colleagues and staff through his selfless leadership, stimulating intellect, and wise counsel. I am grateful also to my colleagues in consultation-liaison psychiatry at LIJ, who have so graciously shared their wisdom and understanding with me. This book would not have been possible without the Herculean labors of Barbara Federlein and Marie Stercula in the preparation of the manuscript.

M.D.S.

I would like to extend my gratitude and thanks to Jan Casey-Liber for her assistance to me in the preparation of this volume.

S.J.Y.

Foreword

Paul S. Appelbaum, M.D.

As the debate over physician-assisted suicide and euthanasia swirls through our society, physicians are buffeted by conflicting interests and concerns. Arguments about the fairness of denying patients the assistance they may require to end their suffering vie with worries that physician involvement in ending life will alter the essence of what it means to be a doctor. The professions, the media, and, more recently, the courts all have struggled with these issues. If there is an easy answer, it has eluded everyone to date.

Sometimes lost in the welter of controversy is the simple reality that is portrayed so well in this volume. Regardless of the outcome of the policy debate over assisted suicide and euthanasia, physicians—especially psychiatrists—can be of enormous help to patients as they make decisions near the end of their lives. Indeed, however many patients might opt for affirmative steps to accelerate their demise, their numbers pale beside the legion who face seemingly less dramatic choices about potentially life-sustaining care. It is these commonplace events on medical and surgical wards, in outpatient clinics, and in hospices that offer important opportunities for psychiatrists to be of assistance to patients, families, and other caregivers.

How ought we to conceptualize psychiatrists' roles in these venues? I suggest we view a key goal as maximizing the clarity with which patients and their loved ones can make difficult decisions in the face of death. The obstacles are many. Some, like dementia, delirium, or psychosis, may be obvious. Psychiatrists are often asked to determine whether these syndromes so interfere with patients' decision making as to render the patients incompetent, necessitating allocation of the power to choose to patients' surrogates. Since many of these disorders are treatable, psychiatrists' roles also encompass identification of the etiology of these disorders and recommendations for treatment. The ultimate hope, not always achieved, is the restoration of patients' functioning sufficiently to allow them once again to make decisions on their own behalf.

Other impediments to meaningful decision making by patients may be more subtle. They do not undermine patients' competence in the usual sense of that term, but nonetheless alter the outcomes of decisions in ways that may not be consonant with patients' underlying values. Multiple factors may play a role here. Depressive affects, though not severe enough to be granted a diagnosis, can induce patients to give up hope sooner than they otherwise would, perhaps so soon as to lead reasonable people to question their judgment. Psychodynamic conflicts, ranging from fears of dependency to overwhelming anger, may undermine the process of weighing risks and benefits, resulting in impulsive, counterintuitive choices of questionable authenticity.

Since patients do not operate in interpersonal vacuums, their relationships with significant other people in their lives may also shape their decisions. Many patients fall victim to the quicksands of family dynamics. Unspoken familial rules may mandate that one member sacrifice his or her interests for the others. Medical decisions are sometimes seen as the opportunity to act on long-held grudges, retaliating for incidents that occurred decades before. And, since patients' relationships with caregivers can be just as complex as those with family members, infelicities in the doctor-patient relationship can be acted out in the rejection of proffered care or demands for additional interventions of dubious efficacy.

To all of these situations the psychiatrist brings two indispensable virtues: a knowledge of how people think and behave, and the ability to step back from the hurly-burly to offer some perspective on the unseen forces shaping each party's actions. Typically, the psychiatrist is called to the scene when an impasse has been reached between patient and physician, patient and family, or family and caregivers. The first steps can be the most important. Often merely by listening to what the participants have to say, the psychiatric consultant can uncover some critical piece of information, some unspoken need or assumption, that breaks the decisional logjam. When that is not enough, brief psychotherapeutic interventions may be of help. And sometimes simply helping everyone to understand the maelstrom that surrounds them makes it possible for the clinical team to continue to do its work and for patients and families to tolerate unavoidable pain and uncertainty.

As important as it may be to facilitate decision making by patients and families, this is not the outer bound of the psychiatrist's role. Few of us truly welcome death, ready to depart this world without any sadness or regrets. The more unexpected the announcement of the approaching end, the more difficult it is for most people to cope. Helping patients at a time like this is a low-tech enterprise. What is required is the willingness to listen and to empathize. Regretfully, the often frantic world of contemporary medicine has less and less time for such functions today. Psychiatrists, sometimes by default, find themselves called on to play this role with patients and families. It is an honorable and humane function, albeit a sad one.

The chapters that follow contain a wealth of practical wisdom about these very difficult situations. Together, they represent a striking endorsement of the critical place of psychiatry in decisions at the end of life. They remind us all that helping people cope with death can be a decidedly life-affirming act.

1

Introduction

Maurice D. Steinberg, M.D.
Stuart J. Youngner, M.D.

The process of dying has become complicated over the past three decades. Although the development of medical technology has not enabled us to ultimately defeat death, we can almost always postpone the moment of death for months, weeks, days, hours, or minutes. At the same time, our society has rejected an absolute vitalism—that is, an insistence on preserving life for as long as possible regardless of its quality and the degree of human suffering. We now have in our power both the ability to control the timing of death and the awesome responsibility to decide when to prolong or shorten life. Decisions to limit some treatment are now commonplace and may occur in as many as 90% of deaths (1).

Our society, through its legal system, has clearly endorsed patient autonomy—the right of competent patients to accept or reject medical treatment—as the gold standard for making end-of-life decisions. Although emphasis has shifted from physician to patient authority in decision making, many persons advocate *shared decision making,* in which patients, families, and physicians work in a collaborative, rather than adversarial, model (2).

Yet, the patient-autonomy and shared decision-making models present their own challenges. For example, these models put a premium on good communication, a skill and practice that too often falls short of the ideal, especially in the context of medical failure, death, and dying (3). Moreover, seriously ill and dying patients frequently suffer from medical or psychological problems such as delirium, depression, or deep ambivalence that cloud, and sometimes even preclude, their ability to make decisions. These issues raise questions about when someone other than the patient should step in as surrogate decision-maker and who that surrogate should be. Surrogate decision-makers may themselves be burdened by guilt or conflict of interest. Because the morally correct decision is so often a matter of judgment rather than fact, people of good will often find themselves in disagreement over the proper course of action. Conflict between and among family members, patients, and health professionals is common. Each person brings his or her own values, life experience, and coping style to the situation at hand. Matchings of key persons may be salutary or problematic independent of the specific decision-making context.

Certain characteristics of modern hospitals, especially tertiary-care centers, aggravate problems of communication and trust. Monthly rotations of house officers and attending physicians, the involvement of multiple subspecialist consultants, and the absence or lack of involvement of a primary care physician contribute to fragmentation and discontinuity of care. In these circumstances, psychological and interpersonal problems both blossom and go unrecognized (4).

The acceptance of decisions to limit interventions that prolong life has facilitated a renewed interest in more active forms of help in dying, such as physician-assisted suicide and active euthanasia. Twenty years ago, it was major news when a major medical journal published a report documenting a prominent hospital's practice of issuing do-not-resuscitate decisions (5). Today those same medical journals print articles reporting cases of physician-assisted suicide accompanied by editorials endorsing the practice, as well as surveys documenting the extent of its use (6–8). Now two-thirds of the public and the majority of physicians support physician-assisted suicide in some circumstances (9–11). The issue became the subject of a United States Supreme Court ruling in 1997 which held that there was no constitutional right to physician-assisted suicide but which left open the possibility of individual states legalizing it (12, 13). Oregon recently became the first state to do so after passage there of two separate referenda authorizing physician-assisted suicide (14). Major healthcare organizations continue to strongly oppose the legalization of physician-assisted suicide despite the strong public and professional support for it (15–17).

Things have moved quickly in the past 20 years. What was once controversial—that is, withholding and withdrawing life-sustaining treatment—is routine practice now. What could not be publicly discussed then is now a matter of open debate, a Supreme Court decision, and legislative process—i.e., physician assistance in dying. Although much of our society has intellectualized the acceptability of limiting life-sustaining treatment, many patients, families, and health professionals remain uncomfortable with some powerfully symbolic treatment limitations such as mechanical ventilation and tube feeding or practices such as the liberal use of analgesic medication in dying patients. Thus, what counts as acceptable behavior varies tremendously.

The Role of Emotional and Psychological Issues

Over the past two decades, the legal and ethical aspects of limiting treatment and physician-assisted death have been discussed extensively. More recently, the demographic dimensions have been considered. For example, studies have confirmed anecdotal clinical experience that age, religion, ethnicity, and socioeconomic status influence the treatment choices not only of patients and their families (18–23) but also of physicians (24–26). Young age, greater education, affluence, and white race are all predictors of patient preferences for less aggressive treatment and in favor of physician aid in dying (27, 28). Now there is increasing concern about the impact of finances on the families of critically ill patients (29). Many fear that an increased emphasis on cost saving in the setting of managed care will drive treatment decisions in the terminally ill that were previously made on a clinical basis (30). It is clear that end-of-life decision making is a complex process influenced by many factors, including religious, cultural, economic, legal, political, and psychosocial ones. This volume primarily addresses the psychosocial influences, a subject that has been too often neglected in both academic and public discussion.

There are several explanations for this neglect. Physicians' discomfort in dealing with their own feelings of sadness, fear of death, or guilt for failing too often leads them to avoid the emotional aspects of dying. In addition, the development of life-sustaining treatments has fostered in physicians what Gruman has called a "heroic positivist" attitude toward disease that emphasizes active interventions (31). Callahan has argued that scientific medicine has rejected the acceptance of death, seeing it instead as an enemy to be conquered at all costs (32). Such attitudes interfere with the physician's willingness to anticipate or attend to patients' many concerns and fears about the experience of dying in a high-technology hospital environment.

Another significant factor has been the extensive involvement of the legal system in the area of decisions about life-sustaining treatment. Legal tradition has focused primarily on a delineation of rights, rather than underlying psychological and emotional factors. Furthermore, many of the most persuasive voices in the debate have been nonclinical bioethicists, often analytic philosophers, who, while accepting the importance of social, cultural, or religious aspects of patients' decisions, have been somewhat mistrustful or ambivalent about psychiatric issues. Many have regarded psychiatric involvement as likely to medicalize or pathologize issues that, they believe, can only be resolved by application of universal, rationally derived moral principles. Finally, in its understandable zeal to promote patient autonomy in an era of unbridled medical paternalism, the patients' rights movement and its more controversial offspring—the popular groundswell in favor of physician-assisted suicide and active voluntary euthanasia—have largely ignored the complex emotional and interpersonal factors that influence decisions at the end of life.

More perplexing, however, has been the relative inattention of psychiatrists and other mental health professionals to the impact of life-sustaining technology on emotional aspects of dying. Relatively few have addressed the emotional or psychiatric aspects of withdrawal or withholding of treatment, or the complex motivation of patients seeking futile treatment (33–37). Psychiatrists have only recently entered the debate on physician-assisted suicide, drawing attention to the important psychosocial and psychodynamic issues (38–44).

This situation contrasts strikingly with the explosion of interest in the psychological aspects of death and dying that led to the development of the new field of thanatology in the 1960s. Extensive clinical and empirical research by sociologists (Glaser, Straus, Sudnow) (45–47), psychologists (Feifel, Shneidman, the LeShans) (48–50), psychiatrists (Eissler, Kubler-Ross, Weisman, Parkes, Cassem, and Pattison) (51–56), and other physicians (Saunders, Hinton) (57, 58) profoundly increased our awareness and understanding of the plight and needs of dying patients. The common fears of the terminally ill—abandonment, isolation, uncertainty, and pain—were described extensively, and dying was conceptualized as proceeding along predictable stages or phases. Emphasis was placed on the crucial importance of good communication, characterized by careful listening, openness, and honesty.

The impact of these writings in stimulating interest in dying patients was profound. Psychiatrists, who had been generally little involved in the care of the terminally ill until then, began to work much more with dying patients.

But attention to the broad emotional concerns of dying patients stimulated by the new discipline of thanatology was soon eclipsed by the intense interest in the ethical choices thrust on society by the new medical technology in the 1970s. The focus seemed to shift from helping patients come to terms with their impending death to helping them decide whether or not they wanted a chance at having their lives prolonged with ventilators, dialysis machines, and cardiopulmonary resuscitation. Clinical ethics consultation, carried out by ethics committees or individual ethics consultants, emerged as a response to the growing complexity of decision making at the end of life (59). Over time, the relevance of psychosocial issues in such decision making became more and more apparent as clinical ethics regularly confronted problems of competency assessment, communication, interpersonal conflict, and emotional distress. Psychiatrists and other mental health professionals, who were exposed to clinical ethics through their participation on institutional ethics committees, became interested again in the complex issues facing dying patients. In addition, the expansion of consultation-liaison psychiatry, with its specific work with oncology and AIDS patients, and the growth of geriatric psychiatry also stimulated the interest and involvement of psychiatrists and other mental health professionals in the experiences of dying patients and their families.

The increased attention to the terminally ill has made it clear that providing end-of-life care requires a broad biopsychosocial approach. Few aspects of clinical medicine in fact demand such simultaneous awareness of the biological, emotional, social, cultural, economic, and spiritual influences on patients as end-of-life treatment. Appropriate treatment of the dying by clinicians and institutions entails important roles for a broad spectrum of mental health and allied professionals, including psychiatrists, psychologists, nurses, social workers, and pastoral counselors. Although a significant portion of this book addresses issues from a psychiatric viewpoint, many of the considerations apply to the broad range of mental health professionals and other physicians concerned about optimal biopsychosocial care of the dying.

Factors Affecting Patient Decision Making

Because of societal emphasis on patient rights, physicians are far more likely than before to try to ascertain and honor patients' preferences for terminal care. In the process, they commonly accept at face value patients' decisions to hasten death by limiting care, viewing such choices as reasonable and appropriate to their dire circumstances. The underlying emotional factors affecting patient choices are often minimized or disregarded, even though such factors may compromise authenticity of those choices. For example, the debate about physicians' authority to unilaterally deny patient or family insistence on "futile" life-sustaining treatment has too often ignored the emotional factors such as guilt, mistrust, or denial of death that may underlie such "unreasonable" demands (60–62). Indeed, psychiatric consultation is rarely sought in end-of-life decisions except when severe psychopathology such as major depression or cognitive disorder appears to be impairing patient or family judgments. The importance of the role of major psychiatric disorders in affecting patient autonomy is addressed in several of this book's chapters—those by Youngner (Chapter 2), Sullivan (Chapter 3), Beckett (Chapter 7), and Block and Billings (Chapter 8).

However, major psychopathology that compromises capacity is less common than the wide range of other emotional or psychological factors associated with decision making that influence the autonomy of patients. The process of dying itself inevitably entails mental pain associated with ongoing and anticipated losses, mourning, or grief, that can be especially intense and difficult for some patients and families. The desire to hasten death may be an expression of patients' inability to deal with the anguish of dying. Anxious and fearful states are common in terminal illness, varying in severity and structure from well-defined Axis I anxiety and adjustment disorders to less organized, more transient conditions. Anxious and depressive symptoms are often influenced by the patient's physical status and vice versa. The wish to accelerate death, when it occurs in dying patients, is labile, probably because of the influence on mood of changes in physical distress (63).

Decisions to hasten death may arise out of patients' guilt or fear associated with the feelings of being a burden. Such concerns occur in a majority of older adults and affect end-of-life decisions (64) (in 90% of patients in one study [65]). Families in turn may exert subtle or overt pressure on patients to discontinue therapy because they are emotionally, physically, or financially stressed. Prior experience with terminal illness in family or friends may also profoundly influence treatment choices, especially when the experiences have been painful or traumatic. The impact of the family on patients' end-of-life decisions is explored extensively in Chapter 4 by Rothchild.

Sometimes, the need to gain control over the experience of dying may influence patients to hasten death. Feelings of helplessness and vulnerability are widespread in patients anticipating or experiencing dying in the hospital. An increasing number of cancer patients are electing hospice care, which moves the location of their dying to a more private setting in which they and their families can exert greater control over the dying process. Feelings of helplessness can be particularly difficult for patients with exaggerated needs for independence and control, who see the deterioration associated with terminal illness as frightening. Patients with controlling characterologic styles or overt character disorders dominated by such features are especially likely to execute advance directives that restrict treatment and be receptive to the idea of physician-assisted suicide. Personality disorders may impair coping, interpersonal relationships, or the ability to accept help in the terminally ill.

The psychological influence on patient decision making least well recognized by physicians is the impact of the patient-physician relationship itself. Physicians can unwittingly create feelings of abandonment by withdrawing from patients when they are no longer responding to or need active treatment. Such withdrawal can also prevent informing patients and families about important palliative options such as hospice care. Physicians' attitudes toward the use of aggressive treatment also can profoundly affect patients' choices. The many factors influencing patient-physician interaction and communication around end-of-life issues are explored in Chapter 5 by Morrison.

Disease-related factors such as specific diagnosis, prognosis, and quality of life may also greatly influence choices by patients, families, and health professionals. The level of pain and suffering (anticipated or experienced) is a major determinant of patient treatment choices at the end of life. Patients' willingness to endure persistent suffering is itself strongly affected by personality, psychodynamics, and psychiatric disorders such as anxiety, as well as cultural and religious beliefs. The relationship of pain to the wish to hasten death is probably complex, as indicated by those studies that have not found it to be a major influence on interest in physician-assisted suicide (66–68). The relative importance of disease-related variables and psychological factors in patients' desire to reject treatment or hasten death requires further study. Some studies have shown psychological factors expressing the desire for autonomy to be more influential than disease variables in determining patients' interest in physician-assisted suicide (69, 70). However, physicians who have assisted patients' dying appear to weight the latter more strongly in their decision to help patients die (71).

The process of decision making about treatment itself in the terminally ill is poorly understood. Whether, for example, the weighing of the benefits and burdens of their end-of-life care is a continuous activity or related to specific events in the patient's clinical course is not clear. The inner experience of dying patients in the age of life-sustaining technology has also received little attention. In fact, the question of how technology has affected the normal psychology of dying remains largely unanswered—for example, does the inescapable need to make (or avoid) decisions about life-prolonging treatment change the experience of dying? If so, how? Are there things dying patients fear more than death itself? How should physicians balance giving patients control against maintaining their hope or minimizing their distress? Greater understanding of such questions will contribute to our ability to care for dying patients and their loved ones.

Patient Choices to Hasten Death

Although close attention to the emotional issues underlying treatment decisions is critical, experience with dying patients makes clear that in some patients choices to refuse treatment or hasten death are not associated with overt mental disorder. While recognizing that emotional factors play a role in all treatment decisions, many psychiatrists have come to believe that choices to reject treatment or hasten death can be based primarily on a rational and authentic assessment of the benefits or burdens not only of further treatment but also of continuing life itself (72). In the face of deteriorating and irreversible disease, patients may reject treatment because of their unwillingness to bear further suffering. Such decisions are often consistent with patients' prior convictions and expressed values.

We believe that the dichotomous view that holds life treatment choices to be either rational *or* emotional should be abandoned. A growing body of research data and clinical experience also calls for a revision in the traditional psychiatric opinion that when patients see death as the least worst alternative, their view is always the product of psychopathology (73–75). Although depression was strongly associated with a desire for hastened death in one study of terminally ill patients, 40% of patients expressing such wishes did not show evidence of depression (76). In a study of ambulatory HIV (human immunodeficiency virus) patients, the authors reported many patients who were interested in physician-assisted suicide who did not show high

levels of depression, or suicidal ideation (77). Although specific epi-
demiological data are not available, there are numerous indications
that patients are more likely to reject treatment now than in prior years.
Decisions to limit treatment occur commonly in outpatient settings
(78), nursing homes (79), general hospitals, or specialty hospitals.
A majority of patients and families agree to physicians' recommendations against resuscitation attempts and accept do-not-resuscitate
status. Studies of hopelessly ill patients in an intensive care unit setting
indicate that more than 90% of families immediately accepted withdrawal of treatment suggested by physicians (80).

Patients' increasing willingness to limit treatment in specific end-of-
life circumstances suggests it may be an appropriate response to terminal illness for some people. "Raging against the dying light" may have
lost its appeal in an era when doing so can lead to a prolonged,
irreversible, and isolated dependence on machines. In fact, health
professionals increasingly view the unrestrained pursuit of aggressive
therapy in futile circumstances as a maladaptive response, except when
determined by strong religious or spiritual convictions. Such a view is
specific to the end stages of terminal illness; an active fight against the
progression of disease earlier in its course is still widely encouraged
and admired. Decisions to reject treatment early in the course of illness,
or in the absence of major suffering, should be carefully evaluated.

Does the view that limiting treatment can be an appropriate and
reasonable choice for some patients apply equally to the desire for
physician-assisted suicide? The motivation for both choices is similar
in some cases, and the choice for both can be made in the absence of
overt mental disorders. Yet the desire for physician-assisted suicide is
far less common than the limiting of treatment, especially in the context of adequate palliative care, where it rarely occurs. This suggests
that physician-assisted suicide is a far more complex and difficult
choice emotionally for patients and family. Physician-assisted suicide
also raises particularly difficult ethical, legal, social, clinical, and emotional issues for many physicians and other health workers. Our goal in
this book is to examine physician-assisted suicide primarily from the
psychosocial perspective and to set it in the larger context of end-of-life
treatment decisions. We believe that the intensive focus on physician-
assisted suicide in recent years has taken place without sufficient

attention to the experiences gained and the lessons learned from more than 20 years of patients' forgoing life-sustaining treatment. Because of the close relationship between the clinical, legal, and ethical aspects of physician-assisted suicide, we have included a discussion of the legal issues by Meisel in Chapter 9, and two different perspectives on the ethical issues, in Chapters 10 and 11 by Mayo and Callahan, respectively.

Psychiatric Evaluation of End-of-Life Decisions

Psychiatrists are more commonly involved in evaluating requests by patients to withhold or withdraw treatment than in evaluating the infrequent requests by patients for physician-assisted suicide. Yet, psychiatrists see only a very small number of the many patients who choose to limit treatment, since the decision to do so often generates little opposition among family members or the treating physician. Psychiatric consultation for decisions to limit treatment is generally sought only when such choices result in conflict between the patient, family, physician, and/or institution. Should physician-assisted suicide become legally permissible, it is possible that the evaluation by a psychiatrist or other mental health professional would be a requirement. The psychological factors that underlie patient wishes to hasten death by limiting treatment or by seeking physician aid in dying are often similar, although no actual studies have compared them.

A central thesis of this book is that patients choosing to hasten death by limiting treatment, especially those seeking physician-assisted suicide, should have a careful evaluation of the biopsychosocial influences in their choice. This assessment is important in all decisions to limit treatment, but is especially so when patients make such choices early in the course of illness or in the absence of obvious suffering. The evaluation should have two major components. The first is to determine whether a mental disorder or specific psychosocial suffering is unduly affecting the patient's desire to accelerate dying. The second is to determine the reversibility or treatability of these factors. When the decision to reject treatment or hasten death is due to factors that are amenable to intervention, such as psychotherapy or medication, such treatment should be made available. In addition, the psychiatrists may contribute to the care of such patients through consultation to the patients' treatment team.

Much of this volume is directed toward helping the consultant to identify the potential psychiatric and psychosocial factors that can compromise patient autonomy. Although we do not believe that the psychiatrist is the only health professional capable of providing adequate assessment and intervention, we think the psychiatrist is most likely to have the full range of necessary skills to do so. However, this would apply primarily to psychiatrists who work extensively with the medically or terminally ill, in general or specialty hospitals, hospices, or nursing homes, or to consultation-liaison or geriatric psychiatrists. Psychiatric involvement in end-of-life care is time consuming and labor intensive. Frequently, especially outside of major hospitals or academic centers, appropriate intervention by psychiatrists or other mental health physicians is not available, and the issues must be dealt with by the treating physician or nursing staff—whose time is also limited. Financial remuneration for such services is often problematic. A recent proposal to establish an ICD-9 classification for end-of-life care would be a major step in ensuring the adequate provision of indicated services to the terminally ill population (81).

The issue of whether all patients seeking to accelerate their death should have a mandatory evaluation by a psychiatrist or mental health clinician is a complex one, particularly with respect to patients who are seeking physician-assisted suicide. A majority of psychiatrists favor mandatory evaluation and do so because of the importance they attach to the influence of psychiatric factors on decisions to seek physician-assisted suicide. In addition, they are concerned about the willingness or ability of nonpsychiatric physicians to address these issues with their patients. In Holland, where mandatory psychiatric evaluation for physician-assisted suicide is not required, only 3% of patients seeking physician-assisted suicide receive a psychiatric consultation (82). Although Dutch psychiatrists have generally supported a policy that does not automatically involve them in requests for physician-assisted suicide, more recently some have called for mandatory psychiatric evaluation (83). American mental health professionals generally have been more active in the ongoing debate over physician-assisted suicide in the United States than their Dutch colleagues have been in Holland and have sought a more central role in any such policy. However, although mental health professionals generally support mandatory evaluation, and many legislative proposals to legalize physician-assisted suicide would require such evaluation, some psychiatrists question the appropriateness of doing so, on clinical and ethical grounds (84). They argue that mandatory psychiatric determination of competence is unreasonable because psychiatrists may lack objectivity in evaluating the capacity of patients to choose physician-assisted suicide, and that their judgment is sometimes influenced more by personal values than by clinical expertise (85). In addition, requiring psychiatric approval for patients seeking physician-assisted suicide would undermine the value of such a right (86). Patients might see obligatory psychiatric evaluation as highly intrusive and demeaning and, therefore, avoid exercising an important right. It is likely that the passage of any physician-assisted suicide legislation in the United States will mandate evaluation by a mental health professional, as is the case, for example, in Oregon (87). It remains to be seen however, how strictly such a requirement will be observed, or if it persists as a requirement over time.

Conclusion

In the early 1960s Weisman and Hackett introduced the concept of "appropriate death" (88). An appropriate death is one in which the person 1) is pain free; 2) operates on as effective a level as possible; 3) recognizes and resolves residual conflicts; 4) satisfies realistically possible wishes; and 5) is able to yield control to trusted others. Psychiatrists and other mental health clinicians are in a unique position to bring an important perspective to the end-of-life treatment decisions and policy, to maximize the chances that patients will have appropriate deaths. By appreciating the complex emotional and psychological factors that accompany and influence all treatment decisions, psychiatrists offer an opportunity to both maximize patient autonomy and minimize suffering. Nonetheless, important human decisions have a personal, moral, cultural, and existential dimension that cannot be reduced to mere psychology. Each of these perspectives is essential to a robust understanding of a quintessentially humanistic question: How can we best manage both our new choices and our inescapable helplessness about how we die? The purpose of this book is to contribute a heretofore-neglected psychosocial perspective. Our hope is that through the integration of this perspective with others, the care of patients will be enhanced.

References

1. Fried TR, Glick MB: Medical decision making in the last six months of life: choices about limitation of care. J Am Geriatr Soc 42:303–307, 1994
2. President's Commission for the Study of Ethical Problems in Medicine and Biomedical and Behavioral Research: Deciding to Forgo Life-Sustaining Treatment. Washington, DC, U.S. Government Printing Office, 1983
3. The SUPPORT Principal Investigators: A controlled trial to improve care for seriously ill hospitalized patients. JAMA 274:1591–1598, 1995
4. Youngner SJ: Applying futility: saying no is not enough. J Am Geriatr Soc 42:887–889, 1994
5. Rabkin M, Gillerman G, Rice NR: Orders not to resuscitate. N Engl J Med 295:364–366, 1976
6. Quill TE. Death with dignity: a case of individualized decision making. N Engl J Med 324:691–694, 1991
7. Lee MA, Nelson HD, Tilden VP, et al: Legalizing assisted suicide: views of physicians in Oregon. N Engl J Med 334:310 315, 1996
8. Slome LR, Mitchell TF, Charlebois E, et al: Physician-assisted suicide and patients with human immunodeficiency disease. N Engl J Med 336:417–421, 1997
9. Blendon RJ, Szalay VS, Knox R: Should physicians aid their patients in dying? The public perspective. JAMA 267:2658–2662, 1992
10. Cohen JS, Finn SD, Boyko EJ, et al: Attitudes towards assisted suicide and euthanasia among physicians in Washington State. N Engl J Med 331:89–94, 1994
11. Bachman JG, Aleser KH, Doukas DJ, et al: Attitudes of Michigan physicians and public toward legalizing physician-assisted suicide and voluntary euthanasia. N Engl J Med 334:303–309, 1996
12. Vacco v Quill, 117 S Ct 2293 (1997)

13. Washington v Gluckshey, 117 S Ct 2258 (1997)
14. Alpers A, Lo B: Physician-assisted suicide in Oregon: a bold experiment. JAMA 274:483–487, 1995
15. American Nurses' Association: Position Statement on Assisted Suicide. Washington, DC, American Nurses' Association, 1994
16. American Geriatrics Society, Ethics Committee: Physician-assisted suicide and voluntary active euthanasia. J Am Geriatr Soc 43:579–580, 1995
17. American Medical Association, Council on Ethical and Judicial Affairs: Decisions near the end of life. JAMA 267:2229–2233, 1992
18. Blendon et al, Should physicians aid their patients in dying?
19. Harvard School of Public Health/Boston Globe Poll, National attitudes toward death and terminal illness. Needham, MA, KRC Communications Research, October 1991
20. Wood F: Editorial. New York Times, May 24, 1989
21. Sehgal A, Galbraith A, Chesney M, et al: How strictly do dialysis patients want their advance directives followed? JAMA 267:59–63, 1992
22. Danis M, Patrick DL, Southerland LI, et al: Patients' and family preferences for medical intensive care. JAMA 260:797–802, 1988
23. Cohen L, Germain M, Woods A, et al: Patient attitudes and psychological considerations in dialysis discontinuation. Psychosomatics 34:395–401, 1993
24. Wachter RM, Cooke M, Hopewell PC, et al: Attitudes of medical residents regarding intensive care for patients with the acquired immunodeficiency syndrome. Arch Intern Med 122:304–308, 1995
25. Wachter RM, Luce J, Hearst N, et al: Decisions about resuscitation: inequities among patients with different diseases but similar prognosis. Ann Intern Med 111:525–532, 1989
26. Curtis JR, Park DR, Krone MR, et el: Use of the medical futility rationale in do-not-attempt-resuscitation orders. JAMA 42:667–689, 1994
27. Garrett JM, Harris RRP, Norburn JK, et al: Life sustaining treatment during terminal illness. Who wants what? J Gen Intern Med 8:361–368, 1993
28. Caralis P: The influence of ethnicity and race on attitude toward advance directives, life prolonging treatment, and euthanasia. J Clin Ethics 4:155–162, 1993
29. Covinsky KE, Goldman L, Cook F, et al: The impact of serious illness on patients' families. JAMA 272:1839–1844, 1994
30. Sulmasy DP: Managed care and managed death. Arch Intern Med 155:133–136, 1995
31. Gruman GJ: Ethics of death and dying: historical perspective. Omega 9:203–237, 1978–1979

32. Callahan D: Ethics and the medical ambivalence toward death. Humane Medicine 10:177–183, 1994

33. Youngner, Applying futility

34. Cassem NH: Treatment decision in irreversible illness, in The Massachusetts General Hospital Handbook of General Psychiatry. Littleton, MA, PSG Publishing, 1987, pp 618–638

35. Gonda TA, Ruark JE: Dying Dignified: The Health Professional's Guide to Care. Reading, MA, Addison-Wesley, 1984

36. Sullivan MD, Youngner SJ: Depression and the right to refuse treatment. Am J Psychiatry 1151:971–978, 1994

37. Jackson DL, Youngner SJ: Patient autonomy and death with dignity: some clinical caveats. N Engl J Med 301:404–408, 1979

38. Baile WF, DiMaggio JR, Schapira DV, et al: The request for assistance in dying. Cancer 72:2786–2791, 1993

39. Block SD, Billings J: Patient requests to hasten death: evaluation and management in terminal care. Arch Intern Med 42:275–279, 1994

40. Conwell Y, Caine ED: Rational suicide and the right to die—reality and myth. N Engl J Med 325:1100–1103, 1991

41. Conwell Y: Physician-assisted suicide: a mental health perspective. Suicide Life Threat Behav 23:326–333, 1994

42. Hendin H, Klerman G: Physician-assisted suicide: the dangers of legalization. Am J Psychiatry 150:143–145, 1993

43. Zlauber TS, Sullivan MS: Psychiatry and physician-assisted suicide. Psychiatr Clin North Am 19:413–427, 1996

44. Muskin P: The request to die: the role for a psychodynamic perspective on physician-assisted suicide. JAMA 279:323–328, 1998

45. Glaser BG, Straus A: Awareness of Dying. Chicago, IL, Aldine, 1965

46. Glaser BG, Straus A: Time for Dying. Chicago, IL, Aldine, 1968

47. Sudnow D: Passing On. Englewood Cliffs, NJ, Prentice-Hall, 1967

48. Feifel H (ed): The Meaning of Death. New York, McGraw-Hill, 1959

49. Shneidman ES (ed): Essays in Self Destruction. New York, Science House, 1967

50. LeShan L, LeShan E: Psychotherapy and the patient with a limited life span. Psychiatry 24:318–323, 1961

51. Eissler K: The Psychiatrist and the Dying Patient. New York, International Universities Press, 1955

52. Kubler-Ross E: On Death and Dying. New York, Macmillan, 1969

53. Weisman AD: On Dying and Denying: A Psychiatric Study of Terminality. New York, Behavior Publications, 1972

54. Parkes CM: Bereavement. London, International Universities Press, 1973

55. Cassem N: Treating the person confronting death, in The Harvard Guide to Modern Psychiatry. Cambridge, MA, Belknap Press, 1978, pp 579–606

56. Pattison EM: The Experience of Dying. Englewood Cliffs, NJ, Prentice-Hall, 1976

57. Saunders C: The moment of truth: care of the dying person, in Death and Dying. Edited by Pearson L. Cleveland, OH, Case Western Reserve University Press, 1969

58. Hinton J: Dying. Baltimore, MD, Penguin Books, 1967

59. Kanote G, Youngner SJ: Clinical ethics consultation, in Encyclopedia of Bioethics. Edited by Reich W. New York, Macmillan, 1995, pp 404–409

60. Youngner, Applying futility

61. Youngner SJ: Futility in context. JAMA 264:1295–1296, 1990

62. Youngner SJ: Medical futility and the social contract. Seton Hall Law Review 225:1015–1026, 1995

63. Chochinov HM, Wilson KG, Enns M, et al: Desire for death in the terminally ill. Am J Psychiatry 152:1185–1191, 1995

64. Americans View Aging: Results of a National Survey Conducted for the Alliance for Aging Research. Washington, DC, Belten and Russonello Research Communications, November 1991

65. Zweibel NR, Cassel CK: Treatment choices at the end of life: a comparison of decisions by older patients and their physician-selected proxies. Gerontologist 29:615–621, 1989

66. Youngner, Medical futility and the social contract

67. Breitbart W, Rosenfeld BD, Passik SD: Interest in physician-assisted suicide among ambulatory HIV-infected patients. Am J Psychiatry 153:238–242, 1996

68. Back AL, Wallace JI, Sharks HE, et al: Physician assisted suicide and euthanasia in Washington State. JAMA 275:919–925, 1996

69. Breitbart et al, Interest in physician-assisted suicide

70. Back et al, Physician assisted suicide and euthanasia in Washington State

71. Back et al, Physician assisted suicide and euthanasia in Washington State

72. Sullivan and Youngner: Depression and the right to refuse treatment

73. Youngner, Futility in context

74. Sullivan and Youngner, Depression and the right to refuse treatment

75. Zlauber and Sullivan, Psychiatry and physician-assisted suicide

76. Chochinov et al, Desire for death in the terminally ill

77. Breitbart et al, Interest in physician-assisted suicide

78. Fried and Glick, Medical decision making in the last six months of life

79. Holtzman J, Pheley AM, Lurie N: Changes in orders limiting care and the use of less aggressive care in a nursing home population. J Am Geriatr Soc

42:275–279, 1994

80. Smeidira NG, Evans BH, Gross LS, et al: Withholding and withdrawal of life support from the critically ill. N Engl J Med 322:309–315, 1990
81. Cassel CK, Vladeck BC: ICD-9 code for palliative or terminal care. N Engl J Med 335:1232, 1996
82. Groenewoud JH, van der Maas PJ, van der Wal G, et al: Physician-assisted death in psychiatric practice in The Netherlands. N Engl J Med 336:1795–1801, 1997
83. Klijn I: Psychiatric consultation in euthanasia and physician-assisted suicide: the Dutch experience. Paper presented at the annual meeting of the Academy of Psychosomatic Medicine, November 1997
84. Zlauber and Sullivan, Psychiatry and physician-assisted suicide
85. Cassell and Vladeck, ICD-9 code for palliative or terminal care
86. Zlauber and Sullivan, Psychiatry and physician-assisted suicide
87. Ganzini L, Fenn D, Lee MA, et al: Attitudes of Oregon psychiatrists toward physician-assisted suicide. Am J Psychiatry 153:1469–1475, 1996
88. Weisman AD, Hackett TP: Predilection to death: death and dying as a psychiatric problem. Psychosom Med 23:232–256, 1961

2

Competence to Refuse Life-Sustaining Treatment

Stuart J. Youngner, M.D.

A 65-year-old man with end-stage cancer tugs at the endotracheal tube connecting him to the mechanical ventilator that keeps him alive. He writes a note, "I want the tube out." When asked if he wants to be allowed to die, he shakes his head "no."

An elderly woman is readmitted to the hospital's intensive care unit for the fourth time in as many months. Experiencing mild dementia and crippled by severe arthritis and severe congestive heart failure, she lives alone in an apartment, unable to adequately feed herself or take her numerous medications. Against the advice of her physicians and the entreaties of her family, she refuses nursing home placement. "I'd rather be dead than go to a 'home,'" she says. The family and house staff want her placed both for her own safety and to prevent the predictable "waste" of repeated hospitalizations if she is allowed to go home.

Three days following a bone marrow transplantation, a middle-age woman wants to sign out of the hospital against medical advice. When she is informed that such a move would be extremely dangerous, the patient replies, "I don't care. I just want to be home."

These cases present an inescapable aspect of modern, high-technology medicine: although we can still not defeat death, its timing and manner are often controlled by deliberate human decisions (1). These decisions and the inescapable need to confront them strain the clinical, emotional, and moral resources of patients, families, and health professionals alike. The increasing involvement of psychiatrists, then, is no surprise, and one of the psychiatrist's most important roles in such situations is the determination of patient competence. When life itself is at stake, the determination of competence takes on a special importance.

How are we to understand this critical notion of competence? In this chapter I explore the clinical/practical aspects of competency determination, grounding it in the unique moral and social context of the present-day United States. First, I locate competence within the more comprehensive notion of informed consent, which forms the moral and legal underpinnings for medical decision making. I argue that although a strict legal determination of competence is an all-or-nothing choice, psychiatrists are much more at home with the clinical concept of *decision-making capacity,* which represents a continuum of varying degrees of mental ability. Next, I review the major mental capacities or attributes necessary for making important medical decisions and some of the operational "tests" for determining the extent to which these attributes are present or absent. Finally, I address a number of problems for the psychiatrist in the assessment of competence—problems that arise from unavoidable discrepancies in power between patients and physicians and that are complicated by the value-laden nature of competence.

I will argue that a "scientific" or purely objective definition is unattainable because, ultimately, competence is a social construct, based to a considerable degree on subjective belief. It is used to resolve situations in which two extremely important social goals come into conflict: the promotion of self determination (autonomy) and the protection of innocent persons from harm (beneficence or nonmaleficence). Patients usually consult psychiatrists in order to enhance their autonomy, for example, by reducing symptoms of anxiety, unrealistic fear, and excessive guilt, and to help relieve the suffering that accompanies such symptoms. These goals comfortably fit the psychiatrist's traditional role as physician/healer. As we shall see, the determination of competence puts the psychiatrist in a quasi-legal role, as judge of matters not entirely clinical. Indeed, competence is not something we can objectively measure as we can the score on a psychological test, but is a more malleable entity that is inevitably molded to fit the particular interpersonal, emotional, clinical, and cultural context. The notion of harm, for example, is especially value-laden and is influenced by personal experience, religious belief, and cultural norms. This malleability of competence is a two-edged sword. On one hand, it allows competency to be used as a socially viable compromise between the conflicting values of autonomy and a wish to prevent harm. On the other hand, it can be used to manipulate psychiatrists to carry out hidden (or not so hidden) agendas of third parties, or used by psychiatrists to impose their own values on patients who do not share those values. Competency can be purposefully nurtured and enhanced, or it can be subtly undermined. Sometimes, the issue of competency boils down to who has the most power.

The greater the conflict a case generates between the values of autonomy and beneficence, the more controversial (and subjective) the competency determination will be. Thus, for example, when a seemingly "clear-headed" patient makes a choice others see as extremely harmful, the determination of competency will usually be problematic. Today, the greatest conflict of values comes in regard to physician-assisted suicide and active voluntary euthanasia, with much of our society (including the criminal law) viewing active intervention to end life as a harm that trumps autonomy. In such cases, competency will more frequently be called into question and its determination subjectively influenced by the evaluators' personal beliefs about whether suicide and killing are always great harms.

Competency and Informed Consent

Law, medical ethics, and our culture in general have increasingly emphasized the rights of patients to informed consent or refusal of medical care that is offered to them, including the right to refuse life-sustaining medical interventions (2). The doctrine of *informed consent* governs the complicated exchange of information about treatment options and the decisions that result from it. Informed consent is intended to promote the two important social goals discussed above: protecting patients from harm and respecting their right to self-determination (3).

Of course, when patients are no longer capable of participation, medical decisions must be made by surrogates—family members, physicians, legal guardians, or, in some instances, the courts. Without guidance from patients, surrogates must act to minimize harms and maximize benefits for the patient, who is relieved of both the right and the responsibility for making these judgments. Under such circumstances there is the risk that the patient's interests might be frustrated, mistakenly or otherwise. It is precisely because so much is at stake in decisions about life-sustaining treatment that informed consent remains the principle that must guide such decisions. It is the informed patient who is in the optimum position to know and protect his or her best interests.

Several elements of informed consent are required for an acceptance or refusal of medical treatment to be considered valid. Competency is one of those elements, and because of its interrelationship and dependence on the other elements, a closer examination of informed consent will be useful before we consider the specific capacities required for competence, the standards for making competency determinations, and practical issues in evaluating competency in the clinical setting.

Meisel, Roth, and Lidz identify five elements to a legally valid medical decision: voluntariness, provision of adequate information, understanding, competence, and making and expression of an actual decision (4). A decision is *voluntary* if the patient is "free from coercion and from unfair persuasion and inducements" (5). Many argue that health professionals have an affirmative obligation to nurture patients' sense of autonomy and to encourage them to exercise their right to choose between treatment options. Patients must be provided with *adequate information* upon which to base their treatment decisions, which includes information on 1) the recommended treatment, along with its anticipated benefits and risks; 2) alternative treatments, along with their benefits and risks; and 3) the expected consequences if there is no treatment at all. Merely giving patients information is not enough; patients must be given information in a form and manner that allows them to *understand* what they are told. As Meisel and his colleagues point out, "The act of informing someone does not assure that one will understand the information that his been imparted" (6). Information given in esoteric medical terminology or delivered in a language foreign to the patient does not fulfill the requirements of informed consent. Of course, for an informed consent or refusal to be complete, the patient must express an *actual decision.*

Voluntariness and the provision of information in a way the patient can understand it are largely in the control of health professionals. Competence refers to mental and decision-making capacities inherent in the patient. However, competence cannot be evaluated until adequate information has been provided in a form the patient is at least potentially capable of understanding in an atmosphere that not only allows but also encourages patient participation in decisions. And, although competence is "inherent" in the patient, circumstance and the attitudes and behavior of health professionals can have an influence.

A "moderately demented" man in his late seventies who had immigrated 7 years before from Eastern Europe was admitted to the hospital for increasing shortness of breath. Radiological studies revealed a mass in his left lung. His physicians wanted to perform bronchoscopy to obtain a tissue sample, but the patient repeatedly said, "No! No!" to their requests. Frustrated, they consulted Psychiatry to determine his competence. After sitting with the patient for several minutes, it became clear to the psychiatrist that the patient was hard of hearing and had only a rudimentary knowledge of English. With the use of a translator and the patient's hearing aid (which he had left at home), the patient showed no evidence of dementia and was able to understand his medical situation and the physicians' recommended course of action. He reported that the physicians were impatient with him. The psychiatrist found him competent, and the patient gave informed consent for the bronchoscopy.

Competence, Incompetence, and Decision-Making Capacity

Competence is, ultimately, a legal term and, as Buchanan and Brock point out, is a "threshold" concept—either you are competent and can make your own decision, or you are not and someone else has the legal right and responsibility to make it for you (7). From the law's perspective, there is no middle ground. Patients are considered incompetent when it is determined that they no longer have mental capacity *adequate* to make informed decisions. Both the law and social custom presume that all adults are competent until the opposite is demonstrated. The determination of competence is straightforward at the clinical extremes. A comatose patient, for example, is incapable of accepting or rejecting treatment. At the other end of the spectrum is the intelligent, calm, self-aware, and rational patient who is not only willing but also eager to participate in decision making.

These observations about competence must be contrasted with the clinical term *decision-making capacity,* which is used to describe varying degrees of mental ability, ranging, for example, from none to slight, moderate, or excellent. Psychiatrists and other clinicians recognize that most patients, especially those with significant morbidity, have some impairment of decision-making capacity. They also know that patients with significant mental impairment—for example, those with Alzheimer's disease—still retain some ability to make choices in their lives. In fact, the terms competence and decision-making capacity are often used interchangeably, an unfortunate occurrence because they signify two distinct concepts.

A competency determination is all or nothing. Therefore, in all but the most obvious cases, competency evaluations will put the psychiatrist in an unnatural position, sacrificing subtle analysis in favor of a reductionistic legal perspective that sees only the dichotomous choice of competent or incompetent. Thus, some patients with impaired decision-making capacity will be judged competent, while others who retain some capacity will be declared incompetent. When decision-making capacity is marginal and patients' choices appear to threaten their well-being, competence becomes a much more consequential, elusive, and controversial issue because it determines the primary locus of decision-making authority.

Competency to accept or refuse medical treatment is *decision specific* (8, 9). The relevant question is, does the patient have adequate mental capacity to give consent to or refuse a specific treatment? The concern is not about the patient's capacity to manage his or her finances, make a will, or even decide about other forms of medical treatment. Of course, a patient may be found incompetent to make all life decisions, but when the competence of a patient to accept or refuse life-sustaining treatment is questioned, the focus must remain on that decision and no others.

Finally, a refusal of treatment may alarm or dismay health professionals and family but is never in itself proof of incompetence.

Incompetence and Mental Illness

In many ways, the concept of incompetence is the mirror image of another social construct, insanity. Like incompetence, insanity is a legal/social rather than a medical term. Insanity is judged *retrospectively* and helps society determine if a person should be held responsible for an illegal act he or she has already committed. Incompetence is used *in the present* to determine if a person has the right and responsibility to make certain important life decisions. In both cases, mental illness or disruption is a necessary but not sufficient condition.

A patient cannot be found insane or incompetent without some evidence of mental illness. Irrationality, impulsiveness, selfishness, extreme anger, or even self-destructiveness alone, without an explanatory underlying mental illness, is not sufficient grounds. The courts have generally accepted severe and clearly recognizable mental illness such as schizophrenia, dementia, delirium, and severe affective illness as serious enough to excuse a person from responsibility, if such illness can be shown to affect judgment sufficiently. Neurosis, character disorder, and situational upset generally do not qualify as reasons to excuse persons from and deprive them of responsibility for their choices.

A patient can be mentally ill, even psychotic, and still be considered responsible for his or her actions. It must be shown that the mental illness has affected (insanity) or does affect (competency) the person's judgment in relation to the specific act or decision in question.

The law recognizes various types of competence: competence to make a will, competence to handle one's financial affairs, competence to stand trial, and, the subject of this chapter, competence to accept or refuse life-sustaining medical treatment as part of the informed-consent process.

Fundamental Attributes Required for Decision Making

Buchanan and Brock, in their thorough and thoughtful analysis of competence, suggest three types of mental attributes necessary for optimal decision making: 1) understanding and communication, 2) reasoning and deliberation, and 3) a stable set of values (10).

Understanding includes the abilities "to receive, process and make available for use the information relevant to particular decisions" (11). This is not an abstract concept. "Relevant" means that information which is necessary for making a specific decision—that is, recommended treatment, alternative treatments (including no treatment at all), and the benefits and burdens of each alternative. Appelbaum and Grisso note that "the capacities at issue here include a memory for words, phrases, ideas, and sequences of information" (12). It should be emphasized that understanding here refers to an *inherent ability* to understand. The understanding that is a separate element of informed consent concerns the provision of adequate information by health professionals in a manner in which it can be understood by the patient (e.g., in nontechnical terms). This latter sense of understanding is not a mental attribute of the patient, but rather a responsibility of the physician.

Patients must be able to *communicate* their questions, concerns, and decisions. Expressive aphasia is an example of a loss of capacity that might well render a patient incompetent. On the other hand, inability to speak (e.g., a patient who is intubated) may be circumvented by other means of communication such as writing or use of a letter board. Appelbaum and Grisso argue that communications must be stable "long enough for them to be implemented" (13).

The ability to *reason and deliberate* is also an essential attribute, requiring the patient to draw inferences about the consequences of making a certain choice and to compare alternative outcomes based on how they further one's good or promote one's ends. Some capacity to employ at least very rudimentary probabilistic reasoning about certain outcomes will commonly be necessary, as well as the capacity to give consideration to potential future outcomes in a present decision. (14)

Appelbaum and Grisso stress the importance of rationality in deliberating about treatment alternatives (15). Deciding what is rational is not an entirely objective process; a patient's choice may be viewed as irrational because the evaluator disagrees with it or considers it to be unusual. Moreover, few decisions in life are entirely rational: "Rational manipulation involves the ability to reach conclusions that are logically consistent with the starting premises. . . . Assessing the relevant capacities requires examining the patient's chain of reasoning" (16). What is important here, as Appelbaum and Grisso note, is that the patient has weighed the relevant information and has "recognizable reasons."

Finally, patients must have a set of values and a notion of well-being

that is at least minimally consistent, stable, and affirmed as his or her own. . . . Although values change over time and ambivalence is inevitable in the difficult choices faced by many persons of questionable competence concerning their medical care, sufficient value stability is needed to permit, at the very least, a decision that can be stated and adhered to over the course of its discussion, initiation, and implementation. (17)

Although each of the attributes (understanding and communicating, reasoning and deliberation, and possession of a stable set of values) is conceptually distinct, there is some degree of overlap. For example, in order to reason effectively, one must be able to understand the relevant information. Likewise, one can not deliberate effectively without values.

Although largely asymptomatic, a 45-year-old woman was diagnosed with metastatic cancer. She had a history of recurrent major depression. Her physicians recommended aggressive chemotherapy. The chance for cure was only about 10%, but the chance for 3 or 4 years of relatively comfortable life was much greater. Without treatment, she would likely die within months. The patient was usually an optimistic and socially outgoing person. She enjoyed her family and had looked forward to seeing her two daughters graduate from college and to traveling with her husband.

The patient refused chemotherapy but appeared profoundly depressed. She said that life held nothing for her. She brooded, disparaging herself about career opportunities she had never taken advantage of. She had difficulty remembering treatment options. The patient was diagnosed with major depression and treated with antidepressants. Two weeks later she brightened up and agreed to chemotherapy, focusing positively on the very real possibility of extended and meaningful life.

Depression had affected several aspects of this patient's decision-making capacity. Normally, her family and her life with them had always been of great joy to her. Depressed, the patient found that these values were of little importance. Moreover, she seemed to have an uncharacteristically harsh disregard for herself. Her ability to understand and process relevant clinical information was also impaired by depression.

There is no unique or consistent correspondence between various organic or psychological states and specific loss of fundamental attributes. For example, dementia might disrupt the ability to retain relevant information, but delirium or severe anxiety could also produce such a deficit.

One must also remember that each of the attributes necessary for decision making—the ability to understand and communicate, the ability to reason, and a stable set of values—is most often partially, rather than completely, compromised. In such cases, the person evaluating decision-making capacity must make a weighty decision as to whether the compromise is sufficient to declare that the patient is incompetent and no longer has the right or responsibility to make his or her own choices. There is no escaping clinical and moral judgment.

Tests for Evaluating Competency

Although competency evaluations always involve subjective judgments, and each case is unique and must be evaluated according to its own characteristics, there are some objective guidelines for making a judgment about whether the fundamental attributes necessary for sound decision making are so compromised that the patient has crossed the threshold of incompetence. Having explored the somewhat theoretical concept of fundamental attributes, let us turn, now, to the more operational matter of *tests* that can be used to determine competence in actual cases. Before doing so, however, some observations are in order.

Because competence is such a multidimensional concept, and because the tests for measuring it vary according to the circumstances of the case, there is no single, correct test. No specific psychometric or clinical tests exist to operationalize the determination of competence at the bedside. Tests like the Mini-Mental State Exam, which attempt to quantify cognitive ability, and more general tests like the comprehensive mental status examination do not, in themselves, provide the answer. A low score on a quantitative test or deficits detected on a clinical examination (e.g., loose associations, pressured speech, etc.) will certainly raise suspicions about competence. The key question remains, do these deficits impair the patient's capacity to make a specific medical decision *enough* that the authority for making that decision should be assigned to someone else? Answering this question requires a specific and focused exploration of the patient's abilities to understand and deliberate about the decision at hand. In fact, as we shall see, the specific test or standard is often chosen after, not independently from, a weighing of the consequences to patients of their choices.

Various tests for evaluating competency have been suggested in the literature (18–24). The discussion by Buchanan and Brock (25) is the most comprehensive and useful, and much of the discussion that follows is based on it.

Buchanan and Brock identify three tests of competence that are "more or less stringent" and "strike different balances between the values of patient well-being and self-determination" (26).

1. The first test is that the patient is merely able to *express a preference.* This is a minimal standard and leaves unexamined the patient's capacities for understanding, reasoning, and whether or not the decision conforms with the patient's own values.

2. A somewhat more stringent test relies on the *outcome of patients'*
   decisions—that is, patients are competent if their decisions seem
   reasonable to others. Although such a standard can often be expected to protect patient well-being, it does so in a manner that may
   not, in fact, reflect the values of the patient. It also makes inferences
   about patients' ability to understand and deliberate about their
   choices, inferences that may be mistaken. Therefore, this standard
   may fail to respect patient self-determination and, consequently,
   well-being.
3. The most stringent standard examines the *process of reasoning* that
   precedes and results in the specific decision in question. Of the
   three tests, the process test alone makes an attempt to evaluate
   decision-making attributes directly. Here, one examines the actual
   ability to understand, reason, and hold a stable set of values. And it
   is to evaluate the underlying process by which patients reach decisions that the psychiatrist is most often called upon.

Buchanan and Brock identify two broad kinds of process defect:
1) "'factual' misunderstanding about the nature and likelihood of an
outcome, for example from limitations in cognitive understanding
resulting from stroke . . ."; and 2) "failure of the patient's choice to be
based on his or her underlying and enduring aims and values, for
example because depression has temporarily distorted them so that the
patient 'no longer cares' about restoration of the function he or she had
valued before becoming depressed" (27). They suggest as the proper
focus of a process evaluation the following:

> Help me try to understand and make sense of your choice. Help me to
> see whether your choice is reasonable, not in the sense that it is what I or
> most people would choose, but that it is reasonable for you in light of
> your underlying and enduring aims and values. (28)

Let us consider two clinical cases that illustrate both the usefulness
and the limitations to Buchanan and Brock's suggestions.

> A psychiatrist was asked to evaluate an 80-year-old man who was refus-
> ing amputation of his left foot. Blind and with moderate dementia and
> diabetes mellitus, the patient had lived in a nursing home for 7 years. He

had no living family or friends. His left foot was gangrenous, and the surgeons said it must be removed to save his life. The specific request to the consultant was to "come and declare this patient incompetent."

The patient, who had been bedbound for years, was an extremely emaciated man. He was able to respond to questions but had severe cognitive impairment. He was not oriented to time or place. He knew his name and birthday but had poor recent and remote memory and was unable to do even the most simple calculations. He was able to tell the psychiatrist, "They want to take my foot off. I won't let them. I want to die with my foot on."

Despite the severe deficits, the psychiatric consultant refused to declare the patient incompetent, arguing that the patient, with control of little else, had clearly expressed a preference and grounded it in a value he held important—he wanted to die intact.

Although the patient did express a preference (passing Buchanan and Brock's simplest test), the surgeons clearly saw the outcome of his decision to refuse amputation as unreasonable (thus, he failed Buchanan and Brock's second test). Furthermore, although the psychiatrist thought the patient "passed" the test of making a decision that was consistent with his settled preferences and values, one could argue with this assessment. Without the benefit of a more complete history or corroboration from family, how could the psychiatrist know that the patient's wish to die intact was "enduring" or "settled" rather than whimsical or the product of his demented mind?

A man in his late sixties was evaluated for recurrent chest pain. Severe coronary artery disease was diagnosed, and bypass surgery was strongly recommended as having an excellent chance both to rid him of angina and to extend his life. The patient refused surgery, and a psychiatric evaluation was requested.

The patient had been a laborer and had grown up in the rural South. He was of average intelligence and showed no intellectual deficits, depression, or psychosis. He simply stated that the night before, his father, who had died in surgery, had come to him in a dream, warning him, "Son, don't go under the knife." The patient was frightened by the dream but clearly unwilling to consider anything but its manifest meaning. He did not want to die, he said, but would take his chances with conservative medical treatment.

Let us examine this case using Buchanan and Brock's theoretical framework. Two of the three fundamental attributes required for decision making were present. First, the patient was clearly able to understand the situation and the treatment options and to communicate his questions, concerns, and decisions. Second, the rural culture of the patient's childhood and the personal experience of his father's death during surgery certainly provided an enduring set of values, in the context of which his literal interpretation of the dream could not be simply dismissed as whimsical, impulsive, or inauthentic. But there is some doubt as to whether the patient was able to reason and deliberate. If one accepted the patient's interpretation that his dream was a warning, then one might conclude that the patient's reasoning was intact. But if one did not accept the patient's interpretation, the literal interpretation and the weight the patient gave it could be used as evidence that he could not reason effectively.

What about the tests we could apply to evaluate whether the patient's decision-making capacity was impaired enough to obviate his right to refuse surgery? He clearly passes the simplest test—he was able to express a preference—but fails the second—reasonableness of the patient's decision to others—at least from the perspective of the physicians who strongly recommended surgery. For them, the outcome of his decision to forgo surgery was definitely not reasonable. With the results of the first two tests in conflict, then, let us turn to the more stringent third test, an examination of the process by which the patient made his choice. Again we find conflicting answers. The patient had the ability to understand and reason, but he relied on an irrational process (i.e., a dream), rather than a rational one (i.e., the reasoning of the physicians) for reaching his conclusion. In this case, the psychiatrist said that the patient was competent. Although the patient's reasoning was not "scientific," it was in accordance with his own narrative history and values. It was genuine, not the product of psychological illness or disturbance.

Competency: Fixed or Decision-Relative?

Should the standard for determining competence be the same in all cases, or should it vary with each decision and clinical context? With a few exceptions (29), most commentators reject the notion of one standard, endorsing instead a sliding scale that demands a more stringent standard when patients' choices seem to threaten their well-being (30–33). According to Buchanan and Brock, "No single standard of competence . . . can be adequate for all decisions" (34). Roth, Meisel, and Lidz caution, "The search for a single test of competency is a search for the Holy Grail" (35). This issue is also addressed by Sullivan in this book (see Chapter 3).

The decision-relative approach is the one most often employed in the clinical setting and reflects health professionals' and society's effort to reach an acceptable compromise when patients' decisions threaten their well-being. For example, when patients agree to a recommendation for treatment that has an excellent chance of restoring health and without which they are likely to die, their competence is rarely called into question. That they have made a reasonable choice suffices. Competence is challenged, however, in similar clinical circumstances when patients refuse treatments that are likely to restore their health. So, for example, when a known schizophrenic patient is admitted to the hospital with acute appendicitis and agrees to the physician's recommendation for surgery, it is rare that the psychiatrist is called in to explore the patient's process of decision making. It is only when the patient refuses that we want to dig deeper, to see, for example, if psychotic thought processes have adversely affected the patient's ability to understand or reason.

When patients refuse treatments that are unlikely to benefit them and carry great risks (e.g., a highly invasive experimental therapy), their competence will not be challenged. Under these circumstances, it is likely that a decision to undergo a risky treatment will be subjected to greater scrutiny than a decision to reject it (36).

Practical Considerations in the Determination of Competency

Clinical Issues Influencing Competency

In a paper titled "Clinical Issues in the Assessment of Competency," Appelbaum and Roth address "clinical factors that are likely to affect the assessment of competency regardless of which substantive test [standard] is used" (37).

First, decisions are rarely made in an "affective vacuum":

> The idiosyncratic meaning for the patient of any suggested procedure is a function of each patient's unique matrix of previous experiences.
>
> If the treatment or procedure for which consent is being sought is sufficiently provocative of anxiety and fear, the patient may be forced to revert to more primitive, even psychotic, levels of defense for coping with it. Thus the recommendation for the procedure itself may force the patient into an apparently incompetent state and may preclude the obtaining of competent consent. (38)

Identification of psychodynamic factors allows them to be explored and offers the potential that psychiatric interventions may resolve the conflicts arising from these factors, enhancing patients' decision-making capacity and, perhaps, restoring their competence. The following case illustrates this point:

> A 45-year-old woman with polycystic kidney disease was told by her physicians that she would soon need to have hemodialysis and, eventually, renal transplantation. The patient said she would rather die than "be attached to one of those machines or have someone else's organ in my body." A psychiatric consultant learned that the patient's father had succumbed to the same illness when she was a child.
>
> The patient was able to share with the psychiatrist memories of her father's repeated hospitalizations and suffering. She recalled her feelings of anger and abandonment when her mother left her with neighbors to spend long hours with her father in the hospital. Her parents had never explained to her either the nature of his illness or the treatments he underwent. The psychiatrist was also able to enlist the help of the patient's nephrologist in explaining to the patient that her father had been treated in the early developmental phases of dialysis and transplantation, which had advanced a long way since then. The patient became less fearful about the treatment and was able to focus on the positive aspects of the life she would be able to enjoy as a result of it. One month later she agreed to begin dialysis and to be put on a waiting list for a kidney transplant.

Second, Appelbaum and Roth urge that the person evaluating competence "authenticate" the history provided by the patient by obtaining information from others. "As a rule of thumb," they say, "the competency assessment should be considered incomplete unless the patient's history has been authenticated by someone who is familiar with his or her behavior in his or her natural environment" (39). Doing so not only confirms the accuracy of actual data presented by the patient, but also may give important insight into an impaired patient's settled values and preferences.

Third, one must make sure that patients have been given adequate information in a form they understand—that is, that the third element of informed consent discussed earlier has been fulfilled. Staff may have presented incomplete or even conflicting information, or the patient may have forgotten information since it was presented. Appelbaum and Roth recommend the following: "The psychiatric consultant should insist that an explanation or reexplanation of the relevant material take place in his or her presence. . . . This not only aids in helping to explain a patient's distortion, lack of understanding, or confusion, but will also help to clarify for the consultant the precise nature of the issues involved, including their urgency" (40).

Fourth, competency "may fluctuate [over time] as a function of the natural course of . . . [a patient's] illness, response to treatment, psychodynamic factors . . ., metabolic status, intercurrent illnesses, or the effect of medications" (41). Therefore, when competence is marginal and the situation is not emergent, more than one evaluation should take place. For example, elderly patients with dementia may be confused in the late afternoon but quite clear in midmorning. Such information may often be easily discoverable by talking with nursing staff.

Finally, the social and interpersonal context may influence competence. Appelbaum and Roth note that "the setting in which the consent is sought and the nature of the person who is seeking it can have similar effects. That a patient is unwilling or unable to attend to a presentation of information from a physician he or she dislikes or in a hospital at which she or he is furious does not warrant the conclusion that the patient is necessarily unable or unwilling to hear the information from another person or in another place" (42). Differences in race or social class and incompatibility of personality styles are reasons to attempt the competency assessment with a more compatible physician presenting the choices to the patient or even conducting the competency evaluation (43).

From the identification of these important clinical issues, an important ethical inference must be drawn. The psychiatrist—and, indeed, all involved parties—has an affirmative duty to enhance the patient's decision-making capacity. At stake here is the right of the patient to make his or her own decisions. There are few critically ill or dying patients for whom some measure cannot be taken to maximize their sense of self-worth and their ability to reason.

Determination of the Threshold to Incompetence

As mentioned earlier, most patients lie somewhere in the spectrum between fully rational and unable to reason at all. For seriously ill patients, pain, lack of sleep, side effects of drugs, metabolic disruptions, and the infirmity of serious illness have direct "organic" as well as indirect "psychological" effects on the mental processes necessary for clinical decision making, such as self-esteem or the ability to reason, remember, concentrate, and postpone immediate gratification. Commonly encountered emotional reactions to serious illness, disability, and death include anxiety, fear, dysphoria, hopelessness, and anger. Coping strategies and intrapsychic defenses include, among others, avoidance, denial, withdrawal, passive-into-active (an effort to exert control), projection, and displacement. Sometimes, such defenses are part of a larger characterologic pattern. Finally, patients are frequently ambivalent because none of the options they face are particularly attractive (44, 45).

The task of assessing decision-making capacity and, ultimately, competence in the context of inevitable psychological disruption is both subtle and complex. The person evaluating competency must judge whether the emotional reaction or coping strategy is "normal" or "pathological." In the context of severe or terminal illness, these concepts are not only elusive but also subject to the personal values of the evaluator. Misapplication of the golden rule ("do unto others") is frequently a temptation (i.e., "If I were in that situation, I would or would not feel/act this way") (46, 47).

Another pitfall for the person evaluating competency is the confusion of the clinical categories "sick" and "healthy" with the moral categories "bad" and "good." This problem has plagued psychiatry since its inception as society either pressures it to use a medical model for handling behavior society finds morally or politically troublesome or excoriates it for doing so. (Witness the outcry against political abuse by psychiatry in Russia, or how American psychiatry has handled the problem of alcoholism, issues surrounding homosexuality, and a variety of women's issues such as the validity of the diagnostic categories "self-defeating personality" or "premenstrual syndrome.") The risk of confusing moral and clinical judgment becomes especially problematic (and unavoidable) when the patient is making a decision that the person evaluating competency finds morally unacceptable. The decision to end one's life—by treatment refusal, but especially by more active means such as suicide and euthanasia—is anathema to many psychiatrists. Some assert that suicide is always morally wrong, even if a person chooses it rationally. Others medicalize the issue entirely, arguing that anyone who wants to commit suicide is de facto "sick" and that suicide is always irrational and pathological. Although modern psychiatry has moved away from an extreme position of viewing suicide as always evil or pathological, the problem of confusing clinical with moral categories remains real. Psychiatrists who deal with these issues should be clear about their personal views and professional stance not only with their colleagues and patients but with themselves as well. The danger is that if one does not approve of a severely ill or dying patient's decision, one can almost always find some rationale for declaring the patient incompetent.

Practically speaking, determining whether an emotion or coping strategy is pathological or "natural" does not answer the question of competency. The essential question remains, does the emotion or coping strategy interfere with the patient's judgment to the degree that someone else should make decisions about life-sustaining treatment for him or her? If a patient is understandably depressed (e.g., "Who wouldn't be in this situation?"), or if a patient is pathologically depressed (e.g., the patient has a history of depressive illness and is not acting his or her "usual self"), our decision about incompetence will be based on two factors: 1) our assessment about how much the depression is interfering with the patient's ability to understand, reason, and make choices consistent with his or her settled values and preferences; and 2) our estimate of how poorly or well the patient is being served by the decision he or she is making. Similarly, if a patient is in an anxious, fearful, angry, or numb emotional state, or if the patient is using unpleasant or unproductive coping strategies such as avoidance, projection, denial, or displacement, we still must determine if these factors disturb the patient's decision-making capacity *enough* to take away the patient's right and responsibility to make what may be the most important decision in his or her life.

Of course, few of us make important decisions (such as those involving career, marriage, friends) on purely rational grounds. Most patients who seek the help of psychiatrists do so voluntarily as outpatients, many with the expressed intent of improving the way they make life choices. With such patients it is not dementia or psychosis that poses the problem, but subtle influences such as character, neurosis, or habit. Whichever of these problems is at work, the psychiatrist is striving to make the patient a better decision-maker, not to decide if the patient should even be the decision-maker.

In the hospital setting, however, the playing field is very different. The request for competency evaluation almost always comes from the physician, not the patient. Moreover, the question asked is not often the subtle one of "What factors might be hampering this patient's judgment?," but the one framed by the dichotomous choice, "Does this patient have the ability to exercise the right to make his or her own treatment decisions? Yes or no?" A clinical ambience that is heavily influenced by medical paternalism, legalistic thinking, and the rights language of analytic philosophy may exacerbate the tendency to see things in reductionistic terms. In some cases, the nuances that usually inform the work of psychiatrists must take a back seat to answering the pressing question of who gets to make the decision about whether the patient will live or die.

A Finding of Incompetence Used to Mask Paternalism

Not infrequently, the psychiatrist is called, not to evaluate patients, but to declare them incompetent—that is, to put the official seal of approval on a decision already made by the consultee. Often, such requests are uncomplicated; the patient clearly is incompetent. Sometimes, however, there is pressure to make the determination quickly, even when the psychiatrist needs more information (such as historical material from family) or wants to see the effect of a medication change on the patient's mental status. Usually, even when life-sustaining intervention is at question, there is some room for delay. The psychiatrist must not be stampeded into making a premature judgment.

At other times, the patient may not incompetent at all, but merely acting in a way that the consultee perceives (often correctly) as not in the patient's best interests. This commonly occurs in situations like that presented at the beginning of this chapter: an elderly patent living alone is repeatedly hospitalized because he or she is not able to take adequate care of himself or herself physically, even with the assistance of family or community resources. Falls, poor nutrition, and noncompliance with medication may all be consequences of physical infirmity. A pattern becomes established: the patient returns home, deteriorates, and is readmitted to the hospital for recouping of treatment gains.

Psychiatric examination reveals a patient who has, perhaps, some cognitive deficits but clearly understands the situation and chooses to go home, rather than give up his or her "independence" by going to a long-term nursing facility. Such patients often clearly articulate that they would rather take their chances at home, even if this means they are going to die. Health professionals and family may view this decision as self-destructive, burdensome to them, and "unfair" to the larger society that must "foot the bill" for repeated hospitalizations.

A similar situation arises when a patient impulsively insists on leaving the hospital when to do so risks death.

A woman in her midthirties underwent a bone-marrow transplant for breast cancer. In the period immediately after the transplant, she became anxious and insisted that she wanted to go home to be in familiar surroundings. Because the patient was severely immunocompromised, such a move would have been extremely dangerous. The psychiatrist was asked to declare her incompetent.

The patient was a somewhat immature, impulsive woman who had throughout her life had difficulty postponing gratification. Her husband

and children usually gave into her petty demands and manipulations. However, she showed no signs of delirium, psychosis, or depression. She denied wanting to die. She simply insisted that she had to go home.

Cases such as this one pose special problems for the psychiatrist. In the case of an elderly patient who refuses nursing-home placement, the "incompetence" is physical rather than mental. In the case of the woman wanting to go home after the bone marrow transplant, however, the problem is characterologic or neurotic, not of proportions usually necessary to declare incompetence. In such cases, the right thing to do is not immediately obvious. Whose interests does the psychiatrist place first when the wishes of an apparently competent patient are patently harmful to himself or herself or to others? The patient's? The family's? Other health professionals'? Society's? Or is the patient's right to self-determination (as opposed to their best interests) the most important value at stake?

Before answering this question, we should consider several practical points. First, in a life-threatening emergency, any physician can declare a patient incompetent. A psychiatrist is not essential. Following emergency treatment, a patient can always go to court to object to both the treatment and the finding of incompetence. Although this is a possibility, it rarely happens. Either the patient dies or the patient is "saved" and, in retrospect, accepts the decision made by others. Second, if the situation is not emergent, the consultee has time to get another psychiatric opinion. In fact, physicians often ask for second opinions when the first one is not in accord with their own views. In nonemergent situations, there is always the possibility of going to the courts for authorization to treat against the patient's will. Of course, the fact that a psychiatrist has found the patient competent may influence a probate judge's opinion.

In part, the solution to the problem of "manipulation" will depend on the personal values and philosophy of the psychiatrist himself or herself. Some will not mind bending the meaning of competence to allow an officially sanctioned treatment of patients against their expressed will as long as the outcome is clearly beneficial for the patient and others. I have difficulty with this position because it sanctions paternalistic behavior without acknowledging it. Because the patient has been declared "incompetent," according to this view, we do not violate her right of autonomous decision making. After all, she is incapable of it. I find this line of reasoning to be disingenuous.

Why not call a spade a spade? Physicians have the option of exerting "old-fashioned paternalism"—that is, of acting against a competent patient's expressed (but foolish) wishes. In the case of the immature woman who wanted to leave the hospital following bone marrow transplantation, her physician could simply have told her that he would not let her leave. Judiciously chosen, this strategy avoids the deception of a bogus incompetence finding and allows the treating physician both to exert and to accept responsibility for what he considers to be an ethical decision. Although patients can always make a legal issue out of it, they rarely do.

Although the concept of competence is a social construct used to resolve conflicts between patient autonomy and society's wish to protect patients from harm, it can and should not be used to resolve all such conflicts.

Competency and Power

Howard Brody has written eloquently about the unrecognized importance of power in physician-patient relationships and decision making (48). His observations are quite relevant to competency determinations. In addition to the sliding scale that demands a more stringent standard for competence when patients' choices seem to threaten their well-being, there is a second sliding scale—one that reflects the power relationship between health professionals and family, on the one hand, and patients, on the other.

Physical Power

When patients are extremely weak (physically and emotionally), bed-bound, and unable to resist intervention, it is much easier to act on determinations of incompetence. In an outpatient setting, or in an inpatient setting when a patient is strong and mobile, forcing a treatment is more difficult, not only physically but from a psychological and social perspective as well. The physical strength and determination of the patient are most influential when the patient refuses an elaborate intervention (e.g., surgery) or insists that a simple one (e.g., feeding tube) be discontinued. Of course, if the patient is clearly incompetent and his or her decision to refuse life-sustaining treatment is clearly harmful to himself or herself, there is little or no problem in deciding what to do. But if decision-making capacity is only partially impaired, the physical struggle encountered by those imposing the treatment will act as a brake not only on their willingness to force treatment on the patient but also on their propensity to find the patient incompetent in the first place. In the case presented earlier of the man who refused bypass surgery because his father had come to him in a dream, a finding of competence had the added benefit of avoiding a distasteful, protracted, medically dangerous, and, perhaps, unsuccessful physical struggle.

Similarly, when a patient is clearly competent but helpless, the power of the healthcare professionals can easily trump the patient's autonomy. I once talked with a brilliant and highly successful lawyer in his seventies who spent several months in an intensive care unit, completely paralyzed from Guillain-Barré syndrome, from which he recovered fully. Throughout his experience he remained as level-headed and sharp as anyone I have ever seen under similar circumstances. He participated fully in all major decisions regarding his care. At one point he and his physicians seriously considered the possibility of discontinuing his ventilator and allowing him to die. "You know who violated my autonomy multiple times every day?" he asked me. "It was the nurses. 'Can we turn you? Can we weigh you? Can we give you a bath?' They asked, but they did what they wanted no matter what I said."

Bureaucratic Power

In a system that accords psychiatrists great authority in the determination of incompetence (technically, the patient can challenge such a determination, and a judge must make the final legal decision), psychiatrists will wield a certain amount of power (49). I have already discussed the danger of misapplying the golden rule or confusing illness with sin and thereby imposing one's own values on a patient who does not share them. Misuse of this power is unlikely in cases of treatment refusal, which has been widely recognized by our society as a basic human right.

The issue of physician-assisted suicide, however, remains highly controversial and is, therefore, much more likely to challenge the objectivity of the psychiatrist who is asked to evaluate competence. In addition, the right to refuse treatment is a *negative* right—the right to be left alone. The right to assisted suicide, if such a right exists, would be a *positive* one—the right to have another do something for or to the patient (as opposed to doing nothing). In both law and moral theory, positive rights are weaker than negative rights. For example, if a competent patient wishes to refuse a life-sustaining treatment, the physician must comply no matter what his or her personal beliefs. Participation in the more affirmative act of physician-assisted suicide will undoubtedly be a matter of moral choice for the physician (as is participation in abortion). It is also likely that the competency hurdle will be set higher for physician-assisted suicide by most physicians, who will be more likely to ask for psychiatric opinions. Thus psychiatrists are likely to wield more power in a world that allows physician-assisted suicide. This power would be magnified if the psychiatric evaluation for competency were mandated by law or custom. In such circumstances, the potential both for helping and for abuse would be heightened.

The Power to See What Is Not Obvious

One of the most important contributions psychiatrists make to the evaluation of competency is the ability to look below the surface, to recognize that patients' manifest demands may hide latent or unconscious wishes. One of the pitfalls of this perspective, however, is that the psychiatrist can pass off his or her own perspective as a glimpse into the unconscious of others. The following case illustrates both the promise and the pitfalls of the ability to "read the unconscious."

> A 50-year-old man with multiple sclerosis was admitted to the intensive care unit with an overdose of diazepam. The patient had been found unconscious by his wife and two sons when they returned home from a weekend out of town. When the patient awoke, he told a house officer in the intensive care unit that he wanted to be allowed to die with dignity. A psychiatric consultation was requested.
> The patient had lived with multiple sclerosis for 15 years. Despite significant handicaps, he had continued working as an extremely successful

management consultant until 2 years before his admission. His worsening physical condition had made him increasingly dependent on his wife and children, who were extremely devoted to him. This dependency had engendered considerable anger on his part, but when his wife left him alone for a weekend for the first time in their marriage in order to visit her own dying mother, the patient had become enraged and despondent. He was able to recognize that his overdose was not so much a wish to die, as an expression of anger at his wife. Suicidal ideation faded into the background as he focused on positive aspects of his life and family relationships.

The consultant psychiatrist continued to see the patient in psychotherapy for the next 3 years, during which time the patient became increasingly disabled. After 2 years, he could no longer dress, feed, bathe, shave, or take care of his bodily functions. His wife did everything for him. He was still able to watch television, however, and especially enjoyed sporting events. When his vision deteriorated, even this pleasure was unavailable. He began talking again of wanting to die.

The psychiatrist explored this issue with the patient at length. The patient's intellectual functioning was excellent. He had absolutely no signs or symptoms of depression except that he found his situation hopeless and felt helpless to change it. He had no physical pain or evidence of anxiety. He was not a complainer but, consistent with his premorbid character, was laconic about his feelings and matter-of-fact with his opinions. He did not talk with his wife about his wish to die because, devoted to his care, she would have none of it. He was now too weak and incapacitated to kill himself and asked the psychiatrist for assistance. The discussions went on for over a year, during which the patient never changed his position. Life had become intolerable for him. He wanted out. He was certain that, after an initial period of shock and grief, his family would adjust and move on with their lives.

The psychiatrist saw no displaced anger or other psychodynamic factors to explain away the patient's stated preference. When he suggested to the patient that, perhaps, there was something else going on, the patient sighed and said, "Doc, I know that's your business, to find things like that, but this is for real. You know me well enough to know that." When the psychiatrist presented the case to colleagues, those who viewed suicide as a moral abomination found various hidden messages and wishes in the patient's request for assistance in dying. "He wants you to argue against it so that he can argue for it. If you ever changed your stance, he would be devastated," one of them told me. Another was convinced that the patient had a "hidden" depression and that I should treat him with antidepressants. Others, less horrified by the notion of suicide in this context, thought the patient was entirely competent.

The psychiatrist did not help the patient die. In the last year of his life, the patient shriveled into a contracted ball, weighing less than 90 pounds. Despite the excellent care by his wife, he developed severe decubiti. His ability to speak was affected, and the sessions with the psychiatrist became difficult for both men. Often he uttered, "This is just bullshit." For the last 3 months of his life, his wife fed him liquefied food with an eyedropper.

In retrospect, the psychiatrist was convinced that whereas the initial suicide attempt did not represent a genuine wish to die, the later suicidal wish was emotionally and intellectually sincere. He did not agree with the comments by his peers about the patient's hidden agenda, expressed indirectly through his relationship with the psychiatrist, who "represented the side of life." Nonetheless, the possible existence of such dynamics troubled him, despite their dismissal by the patient. Moreover, he wondered about the family dynamics. Should he have made a greater effort to have the patient confront his wife about his wish to die? Would this have provided an opportunity for the patient to express and resolve unconscious rage, thereby allowing him to shed his wish to die? At other times he remembered the patient's last words to him, "This is bullshit." What right would he have had to push this man and his family into conversations and confrontations totally out of character for them? When was the patient's expressed wish enough?

A psychiatrist colleague once told me how, when he was a resident, he had presented a patient to a supervisor. The supervisor told him the patient was schizophrenic. "I didn't see any clinical evidence of schizophrenia," my colleague said, "but my supervisor told me that if I just listened long enough, the patient would reveal it. I listened, but the patient never did." Clinical hunches are a critical tool of a seasoned clinician. Hunches must, however, be backed by clinical evidence. Experience tells us all that seasoned clinicians often have different clinical hunches and that some clinicians' hunches are consistently influenced by a particular theoretical or personal outlook. How long can we hold patients hostage while we try to uncover the clinical evidence to support our hunches?

Judgments about the unconscious motives of patients who choose death as the least worst alternative are risky. Of course, psychiatrists working in this area, as in any other, must be aware of how their own personal values and experience influence their judgments. When it comes to the issue of physician-assisted suicide and euthanasia, however, I am not sanguine about how objective the current generation of psychiatrists can be. Perhaps, psychiatrists' role should be limited to what they do best: listen to patients, help clarify what they need and want most, and relieve their suffering. Of course, some persons would argue that active killing (either by patient or by physician) is sometimes the best or only way to relieve suffering. But that is exactly the issue that remains so clinically, emotionally, politically, and morally uncertain at the present time. For these reasons I would argue against psychiatrists being ultimate gatekeepers for or active participants in physician-assisted death.

When Patients Refuse Competency Evaluation

Psychiatrists are put in a difficult situation when patients who have refused life-sustaining treatment refuse to talk with them. Such refusals are often the result of failure of early communications and planning in the outpatient setting (50) or are expressions of patient protest against or mistrust of "an impersonal, alienating, and inhumane medical regimen" (51). Wenger and Halpern suggest several helpful approaches to this problem (52). First, if the psychiatrist "employs warmth, empathy, and persistence, the patient may accede to the consultation" (53). If this strategy is not successful, the psychiatrist should encourage the primary physician and healthcare team to temporize if possible, while keeping channels of communication open. Involvement of family members may be useful, and, finally, the psychiatrist can work "second-hand," coaching the primary physician or other trusted health professionals to do the competency evaluation (54). Wenger and Halpern maintain that when these strategies fail and the patient persists in refusing competency evaluation, the patient should not be permitted to refuse consultation. Stone tilts more toward patient autonomy, arguing that "no adult should be deprived of any liberty interest, right, or privilege unless he or she has a severe mental disorder" (55).

In practice, if the patient is obviously incompetent and the psychiatrist is really being asked to confirm or support this conclusion, or if the patient's refusal of treatment is viewed as reasonable, the direct involvement of the psychiatrist becomes less critical. A patient's competency refusal will be most problematic when 1) there is a serious question about the patient's decision-making capacity, and 2) healthcare professionals perceive that the patient's decision is clearly not in his or her best interest (causes more harm than benefit). Under these circumstances, it should be made clear to patients that the evaluation is intended to maximize their decision-making authority. A continued refusal to cooperate will be viewed as evidence of a wish for others to make the decision. Whereas some persons might view this strategy as coercive, I believe it provides a reasonable balance between respect for autonomy and the responsibility to protect patients from harm.

Tough Cases: The Ambivalent Patient

In some cases, competency evaluation seems almost impossible. Patients who otherwise have excellent decision-making capacity sometimes simply cannot make up their minds or vacillate between a decision to accept or reject life-sustaining treatment.

A 70-year-old man with end-stage chronic obstructive lung disease was admitted to the intensive care unit, intubated, and put on a mechanical ventilator. After 2 months it was clear he would never be weaned. Sometimes, he would tell the staff that he wanted the ventilator turned off and that he be allowed to die. At other times, he said he wanted to live as long as he could. His family urged him "not to give up" and his wish to live seemed related, at least in part, to their visits. When he asked to be allowed to die, the staff asked him to repeat the request in front of his family. He agreed but then did not follow through.

Faced with two unattractive alternatives (in the case above, certain death or prolonged life on a ventilator), it is not surprising that some patients cannot make up their minds. In evaluating and trying to resolve ambivalence, psychiatrists should look for psychiatric disorders that may underlie it—for example, Axis I disorders like depression or Axis II disorders like obsessive-compulsive personality disorder. Family and other interpersonal dynamics may also explain difficulty making a firm decision. Absent an Axis I or II disorder, however, I do not think we can call such patients incompetent and let others decide for them. I suggest instead that such patients be told, "We understand how hard it is for you to make up your mind. Until you do we will err on the side of life. We will continue to talk with you about this difficult decision. If and when you firmly and consistently choose a course of action, we will respect your wishes."

A variant of ambivalence occurs when patients make choices that are contradictory. An example is the first case presented at the beginning of the chapter, in which a patient asked to be extubated and disconnected from the ventilator but made the contradictory statement that he did not want to be allowed to die. Overcome by the discomfort and fear engendered by his intubation, he was unable to reconcile his contradictory wishes. Was he incompetent? Should someone else have made the decision? If so, what decision? Since the patient could not come to a workable decision, others had to, but in such cases the decision should always be to maintain life, with the patient kept informed and as involved as possible until either he or she can resolve his or her contradictory wishes or the clinical situation resolves the inner conflict for him (i.e., either he dies on the ventilator or he no longer needs it).

Who Should Evaluate Competence?

Must psychiatrists be called in to evaluate every case in which competency is called into question? Some persons have argued that the primary physician can adequately evaluate competence in most cases and that it would be cumbersome and even insulting to patients to "make" them see a psychiatrist every time a question of competency arises (56). To explore the issue of who can best determine competence, it is helpful first to identify the relevant skills. Sometimes, of course, the answer is so obvious that it is not necessary to call in an expert—for example, if the patient is comatose or the patient's decision-making capacity is clearly excellent.

Because competency is part of the informed-consent process, the person evaluating competence should be familiar with the elements of informed consent. Such knowledge is essential, because it allows one to determine (rather than to assume) that the other necessary elements of informed consent have been fulfilled—for example, that the patient has been given adequate information, in a form he or she is capable of understanding, and without undue pressure. Familiarity with diagnostic, prognostic, and therapeutic realities or the ability to ascertain them is useful in evaluating what the patient has been told. The person evaluating competence must feel comfortable questioning and even challenging, when appropriate, clinical assumptions that seem inaccurate or biased.

Before the specific clinical picture can be interpreted, the person evaluating competency should have some understanding of the moral implications of a competency determination—that is, the potential conflict between the values of patient self-determination and protecting patients from harm. Familiarity with both the theoretical concept of capacity for competence (e.g., understanding, deliberation, a stable set of values) and the more operational notion of standards of competency (e.g., processes underlying competent decisions) is essential.

The ability to recognize psychological and organic mental disturbances, and clinical acumen in using and interpreting the mental status and other clinical examinations, are also necessary for evaluating competency. In addition to the determination of competence itself, such knowledge may offer the opportunity to recognize reversible conditions and provide suggestions for treatment. For example, the patient may be confused secondary to an unrecognized delirium caused by benzodiazepine withdrawal. Or, a patient might be more confused at night or when family members are absent. Persons evaluating competency should also be familiar with the common psychodynamic issues and patterns of coping at the end of life—for example, denial, avoidance, guilt, and anger that has been turned inward and is expressed as self-loathing.

Familiarity with and comfort inquiring about the interpersonal, social, and even political aspects of the clinical setting is also important. What are the personal or professional agendas of the involved parties? Is the situation truly emergent, or is there time to do a more careful assessment? Has the patient been getting consistent information? Is there dissension within the treating team or between consultants about what constitutes a "reasonable" option? Sometimes, questions like these get to the heart of a competency dispute.

Finally, it is useful for the person evaluating competency to have some familiarity with the local laws, regulations, and administrative rules dealing with competency and guardianship issues.

It is no surprise that psychiatrists in general, and consultation-liaison psychiatrists in particular, are called in for consultation when competency becomes a question. However, psychiatrists are not the only persons capable of doing competency evaluations. Other physicians with adequate training and experience can and do evaluate competency adequately. Increasingly, physicians and nonphysicians are being trained as clinical ethicists, whose role includes the evaluation of competency (57, 58). Although some nonpsychiatrist physicians may have considerable experience and skill in carrying out these tasks, many do not. The failure by nonpsychiatrists to recognize significant psychopathology has been best documented with depression (59).

Being a psychiatrist does not, per se, make one the most qualified to do competency evaluations in medical, surgical, or critical care settings. A psychiatrist who is not familiar with the hospital setting, the interaction between psychiatric and medical illness, and both the theoretical and practical aspects of competency evaluation will be ill-suited to tease apart the subtle and elusive issues raised by a complex competency problem. With the proper experience and interest, however, the psychiatrist is the ideal expert. Psychiatrists are trained to recognize both psychological and organic factors that might compromise decision-making capacity. They have the ability to appreciate both interpersonal and family dynamics. They are in the best position to recognize and treat clinical depression in the medically ill, an issue that complicates many refusals of life-sustaining treatment.

Conclusion

Strictly speaking, a finding of incompetence is a legal matter; in practice, however, most determinations of incompetence (and competency) are made at the bedside. Moreover, consultees need not accept
the opinions of consulting psychiatrists. In practice, however, the psychiatrist's opinion usually determines the outcome. Consultees usually
accept the psychiatrist's pronouncement, and few cases are ever taken
to court. Even when the courts become involved, "the psychiatrist's
assessment often serves as the major source of data for the judge's
decision" (60).

As life-sustaining technologies multiply, and physician-assisted
death is increasingly debated and, perhaps, practiced, the determination of competence will gain increasing importance as the way society
assigns decision-making authority when the timing of death is a matter
of choice. Because the notion of competence is inextricably intertwined
with cultural and personal values, the involvement of psychiatrists in
decisions to hasten death (passively or actively) is both inevitable and
desirable. Psychiatrists have an important role to play not only in
clinical evaluations of competency but also in the study of this inevitably challenging issue. But they should beware lest they are used by
others to answer questions best resolved by broader and more democratic
social institutions such as federal and state courts and legislatures.

References

1. President's Commission for the Study of Ethical Problems in Medicine and
   Biomedical and Behavioral Research: Deciding to Forgo Life-Sustaining
   Treatment. Washington, DC, U.S. Government Printing Office, 1983
2. President's Commission, Deciding to Forgo Life-Sustaining Treatment
3. Faden RR, Beauchamp T: A History and Theory of Informed Consent. New
   York, Oxford University Press, 1986
4. Meisel A, Roth LH, Lidz CW: Toward a model of the legal doctrine of
   informed consent. Am J Psychiatry 134:285–289, 1977
5. Meisel et al, Toward a model of the legal doctrine of informed consent,
   p 286

6. Meisel et al, Toward a model of the legal doctrine of informed consent, p 287
7. Buchanan AE, Brock DW: Deciding for Others: The Ethics of Surrogate Decision Making. Cambridge, UK, Cambridge University Press, 1989, pp 26–29
8. Buchanan and Brock, Deciding for Others, pp 18–20
9. Roth LH, Meisel A, Lidz CW: Tests of competency to consent to treatment. Am J Psychiatry 134:279–284, 1977
10. Buchanan and Brock, Deciding for Others, pp 23–25
11. Buchanan and Brock, Deciding for Others, p 24
12. Appelbaum PS, Grisso T: Assessing patients' capacities to consent to treatment. N Engl J Med 319:1635–1638, 1988; see p 1636
13. Appelbaum and Grisso, Assessing patients' capacities to consent to treatment, p 1635
14. Buchanan and Brock, Deciding for Others, p 25
15. Appelbaum and Grisso, Assessing patients' capacities to consent to treatment, p 1636
16. Appelbaum and Grisso, Assessing patients' capacities to consent to treatment, p 1636
17. Buchanan and Brock, Deciding for Others, p 25
18. Buchanan and Brock, Deciding for Others
19. Roth et al, Tests of competency to consent to treatment
20. Appelbaum and Grisso, Assessing patients' capacities to consent to treatment
21. Drane JF: The many faces of competency. Hastings Cent Rep 15:17–21, 1985
22. President's Commission for the Study of Ethical Problems in Medicine and Biomedical and Behavioral Research: Making Health Care Decisions, Vol 1: The Ethical and Legal Implications of Informed Consent in the Patient-Practitioner Relationship. Washington, DC, U.S. Government Printing Office, 1982
23. Culver CM, Gert B: The inadequacy of incompetence. Milbank Q 68:619–643, 1990
24. Appelbaum PS, Roth LH: Clinical issues in the assessment of competency. Am J Psychiatry 138:1462–1467, 1981
25. Buchanan and Brock, Deciding for Others
26. Buchanan and Brock, Deciding for Others, pp 48–51
27. Buchanan and Brock, Deciding for Others, p 56
28. Buchanan and Brock, Deciding for Others, p 56
29. Culver and Gert, The inadequacy of incompetence

30. Buchanan and Brock, Deciding for Others
31. Roth et al, Tests of competency to consent to treatment
32. Drane, The many faces of competency
33. President's Commission, Making Health Care Decisions, Vol 1
34. Buchanan and Brock, Deciding for Others, p 51
35. Roth et al, Tests of competency to consent to treatment, p 283
36. Roth et al, Tests of competency to consent to treatment
37. Appelbaum and Roth, Clinical issues in the assessment of competency, p 1463
38. Appelbaum and Roth, Clinical issues in the assessment of competency, p 1463
39. Appelbaum and Roth, Clinical issues in the assessment of competency, p 1464
40. Appelbaum and Roth, Clinical issues in the assessment of competency, p 1465
41. Appelbaum and Roth, Clinical issues in the assessment of competency, p 1465
42. Appelbaum and Roth, Clinical issues in the assessment of competency, p 1465
43. Appelbaum and Roth, Clinical issues in the assessment of competency
44. Jackson DL, Youngner SJ: Patient autonomy and death with dignity: some clinical caveats. N Engl J Med 301:404–408, 1979
45. Youngner SJ: Informed consent, competency, and the reality of critical care. Crit Care Clin 2:178–188, 1986
46. Jackson and Youngner, Patient autonomy and death with dignity
47. Sullivan MD, Youngner SJ: Depression, competence, and the right to refuse life-sustaining treatment. Am J Psychiatry 151:971–978, 1994
48. Brody H: The Healer's Power. New Haven, CT, Yale University Press, 1992
49. Appelbaum and Roth, Clinical issues in the assessment of competency
50. Wenger NS, Halpern J: Can a patient refuse a psychiatric consultation to evaluate decision-making capacity? J Clin Ethics 5:230–234, 1994
51. Stone AA: Iatrogenic ethical problems: commentary on "Can a patient refuse a psychiatric consultation to evaluate decision-making capacity?" J Clin Ethics 5:234–237, 1994; see p 235
52. Wenger and Halpern: Can a patient refuse a psychiatric consultation to evaluate decision-making capacity?
53. Wenger and Halpern, Can a patient refuse a psychiatric consultation to evaluate decision-making capacity?, p 232
54. Wenger and Halpern, Can a patient refuse a psychiatric consultation?
55. Stone, Iatrogenic ethical problems, p 236

56. Schneiderman LJ: Is it morally justifiable not to sedate this patient before ventilator withdrawal? J Clin Ethics 2:129–130, 1991
57. Fletcher J: Goals and process of ethics consultation in health care. Biolaw 2:37–47, 1986
58. LaPuma J, Schiedermayer DL: Ethic consultation: skills, roles, and training. Ann Intern Med 115:155–159, 1991
59. Sullivan and Youngner, Depression, competence, and the right to refuse life-sustaining treatment
60. Appelbaum and Roth, Clinical issues in the assessment of competency, p 1462

3

Depression and the Refusal of Life-Saving Medical Treatment

Mark D. Sullivan, M.D., Ph.D.

Long-standing traditions in medicine and tort law oppose treatment refusal when this refusal will result in the death of the patient. However, over the past two decades, courts and legislatures across the country have articulated a "right to die" for seriously ill medical patients. This has been done through both court cases and natural death acts. Although no absolute right has been recognized, no court has rejected the right-to-die in a wholesale fashion (1).

The recognition of the right to die has taken place in the wake of advances in medical technology that make it possible to prolong life

---

This chapter is a revised version of a paper published in the *American Journal of Psychiatry* (Sullivan MD, Youngner SJ: "Depression, Competence, and the Right to Refuse Life-Sustaining Treatment." 151:971–978, 1994). Used with permission.

even when there is no prospect of return to a healthy and functional existence. The case of Karen Quinlan was critical in this regard. As legal scholar Alan Meisel has stated:

> Prior to the *Quinlan* case, there was a great reluctance in case law to permit patients to refuse treatment when that refusal would probably lead to their death. *Quinlan* changed that by making clear to the courts what had long been apparent in the health professions, namely that there is an increasing range of situations in which treatment will keep patients alive but not restore them to health. (2)

Though the Quinlan case opened the issue of a right to die, the precedent regarding the right to end one's own life was limited by the extremity of Karen Ann Quinlan's condition. She was permanently comatose and therefore unable to express her wishes, but there was no indication of suicidal intent by her. The intention of her parents was solely to minimize her suffering.

The courts took an important further step toward the recognition of a right to die in the case of Elizabeth Bouvia, a woman with severe cerebral palsy and pain who sought the right to refuse feeding with a nasogastric tube while on the psychiatric unit of a general hospital. The attending psychiatrist, Dr. Fisher, provided the most vehement opposition to this refusal on the part of a patient who had been admitted because she was suicidal. Meisel explains the appellate court decision that upheld her refusal:

> Although hoping that the forgoing of artificial nutrition and hydration, and indeed spoon-feeding, would not constitute suicide because the patient "merely resigned herself to accept an earlier death, if necessary, rather than live by feedings forced upon her," the court also stated that "a desire to terminate one's own life is probably the ultimate exercise of one's right to privacy." (3)

Here, the court moved toward the view that the intent to die did not disqualify one's right to refuse medical treatment: "If a right exists, it matters not what 'motivates' its exercise. We find nothing in the law to suggest that the right to refuse medical treatment may be exercised only if the patient's *motives* meet someone else's approval" (4). It is also clear from the Bouvia case that the right to refuse lifesaving treatment is not dependent on the presence of a terminal illness. Ms. Bouvia was severely disabled from cerebral palsy but not at risk of dying from the illness in the near future.

Alan Stone has pointed out an important qualification to the right to die left standing by this case: "The lesson of Bouvia is that hospitals and doctors need not passively abet the suicide of a patient who is not terminally ill" (5). The court thus distinguished between what Ms. Bouvia had a right to do and what she had a right to ask the hospital to help her to do. Recent legal precedent with medical patients has therefore supported both the right of competent patients to refuse lifesaving treatment for whatever reason and the right of healthcare professionals not to be complicit in this hastening of death. As yet, our society does not recognize a right to a medically assisted or medically witnessed suicide. However, the evolving ethical and legal consensus is that medically ill patients are presumed to be competent to refuse even lifesaving medical treatment. The burden of proof concerning competence is on those who wish to override these refusals.

There has not been a corresponding development of the right to refuse lifesaving treatment among those with mental illness. Important developments concerning the right of mental patients to refuse treatment have occurred in other areas. Most notably, the right to refuse antipsychotic medication has been upheld in many states (6).

Traditionally, legal competence has been considered a global property of persons. Lack of competence in mental patients has implied an inability to decide about both the need for hospitalization and the need for antipsychotic medication. Among the factors that have changed law concerning treatment refusal is the trend toward a more specific, rather than global, understanding of competence. Meisel comments:

> The general incompetence approach has long been the dominant one used by the courts. However, it has fallen into disfavor in recent decades, spurred both by legislative changes and by litigation aimed at enhancing the rights of the institutionalized mentally ill and mentally retarded. (7)

There is now the requirement for separate independent review (judicial in some states, administrative in others) of competence to refuse antipsychotic medication even after recognized procedures have permitted involuntary psychiatric hospitalization.

This trend toward a more specific understanding of competence has not significantly changed the care of suicidal patients. For those patients who report suicidal plans, the desire to die is considered prima facie evidence of mental disorder and impaired capacity to make decisions concerning the need for psychiatric treatment. No distinction is made between competence to refuse hospitalization and competence to refuse antidepressant treatment. The ethical and legal literature concerning the rights of patients with concurrent mental and medical illnesses is sparse. It is not apparent that a distinction has been made between competence to refuse psychiatric treatment and competence to refuse medical treatment for a concurrent serious medical illness. Indeed, some persons have specifically urged that living wills *not* be honored following suicide attempts (8).

There are substantial data to support these policies limiting the rights to treatment refusal for suicidal patients. Postmortem psychological investigations consistently reveal a high rate of mental illness among those who complete suicide (9). Rates of treatable mental illness are high enough in suicidal patients that at least a temporary presumption of incompetence to decide about the need for psychiatric care is justified. Though occasional suicidal thoughts are encountered among the terminally ill, multiple authors have described how exceptional it is for these patients to have persistent suicidal thoughts, plans, or intent (10).

Unlike medical illness, mental illness leading to the desire to die is assumed simultaneously to put a patient's life at risk *and* to compromise his or her capacity to make a competent refusal of treatment. Refusal of lifesaving treatment by the suicidal psychiatric patient is seen as a symptom of an illness that mental health professionals treat rather than the choice of an autonomous patient.

Our legal tradition has relied on reference to causation as well as to intention in sorting out suicide from forgoing lifesaving treatment. The intention criterion (i.e., intention to die makes a treatment refusal equivalent to suicide) appears to have been undercut by the Bouvia decision—at least insofar as it applies to patient intentions. (Analysis in terms of physician intention persists in the doctrine of "double-effect," whereby actions intended to relieve suffering that do cause death are excused.) The causation criterion identifies suicide in terms of its proximate cause. As Meisel notes, "Under the causation rationale, the patient's death does not constitute suicide because it is caused not by the forgoing of treatment, but rather by patient's medical condition for which treatment has been forgone" (11). Since the pathophysiological process present will cause death unless interrupted, the omission of treatment is not thought to be the cause of death. Both withholding *and* withdrawing lifesaving treatment, which might be requested in an advance directive such as a living will, are justified under this analysis. The Washington (Natural Death) Act, like most others, states in part "that acts in accordance with a directive are not deemed suicide . . . and the cause of death shall be that which placed the patient in a terminal condition" (12). A recent Dutch study found that a decision to withhold or withdraw treatment was made in 39% of all nonsudden deaths (13).

Some feel that it is dishonest to ascribe death to the underlying disease process when withdrawing treatment is extended to include food and fluids. Kenneth Schaffner has expressed doubts that analysis of cases involving the suspension of artificial nutrition and hydration in terms of the causes of a patient's death can distinguish between killing and letting die, between suicide and refusing lifesaving treatment (14). He argues that such withdrawal is "morally equivalent to suicide" (15). He further challenges us "to acknowledge that granting such patients (as Bouvia) the right to forgo life-sustaining food and water is the first step toward recognizing a right to medically assisted, rational suicide, and that the implications and ramifications of such a policy need extensive further debate and analysis" (16).

In reviewing the psychological, legal, and ethical approaches to the refusal of lifesaving treatment and suicide, it appears that the crucial question in determining whether treatment refusals should be respected is, who bears the burden of proof concerning competence to refuse treatment? Should we assume patients are competent to make decisions about their own medical care unless proven otherwise, as is the evolving tradition in the medically ill? Or should we assume that patients desiring to die are suicidal and incompetent to make life-and-death choices until proven otherwise, as is the tradition in the mentally ill? The increasingly common phenomenon of patients being treated for serious concurrent medical and mental illnesses brings this conflict between ethical traditions into clinical practice (17).

Depression and Competence to Refuse Medical Treatment

Consider the following case.

> A 55-year-old widowed white female with advanced multiple sclerosis is admitted to an orthopedic service for open-reduction and internal-fixation of a humeral head fracture sustained during a fall. Her orthopedic resident found her sobbing in her bed on the second postoperative day. The orthopedic attending sought and obtained a transfer to a medical-psychiatric unit at the same hospital. She has a living will and an agreement with her primary care doctor that she not have any resuscitation attempted if she should experience cardiac or pulmonary arrest. On admission to the psychiatric unit, the attending notes that the patient has passive suicidal ideation—that is, she wishes her disease would kill her soon. He wishes to override the DNAR (do not attempt resuscitation) order in the chart because he wishes to start a tricyclic antidepressant in this patient with a left-bundle branch block and because he sees the desire not to be resuscitated to be arising from her depression.

In the Report of the President's Commission for the Study of Ethical Problems in Medicine and Biomedical and Behavioral Research, Appelbaum and Roth make special mention of depression as a cause for treatment refusal that is particularly difficult to evaluate:

> Of all the psychopathologic processes associated with refusal, depression is the most difficult to recognize, because it masquerades as, "Just the way I would think if it happened to me." It is also the most difficult to think causally about the refusal, because, unlike the grossly delusional patient . . ., the depressed patient is frequently able to offer "rational" explanations for the choices that are made. (18)

Mental health tradition and clinical intuition hold that severe depression compromises patient autonomy. Cautions based on case reports have been issued about accepting do-not-resuscitate (DNR) orders from depressed psychiatric inpatients (19), some including the recommendation that a trial of electroconvulsive therapy (ECT) be employed prior to accepting a DNR order for patients in whom the role of affective disorder is unclear (20). At least one study supports the traditional view that suicidal ideas, even among the terminally ill, are usually linked to a mental disorder (21). Clearly, *some* patients desiring death are not acting autonomously. However, mental health professionals may be inappropriately extending their views concerning suicide in the medically well to the refusal of treatment among the seriously medically ill. Beck and associates have demonstrated that hopelessness is a good predictor of suicide (22). But it is very difficult to discern pathological hopelessness among the terminally ill. Mental health professionals tend to minimize the difficulty of this discernment—sometimes to the point of denying that there can be an autonomous wish to hasten death—even among the terminally ill. Determining whether someone with a serious, or especially terminal, medical illness is competently assessing his or her quality of life can be exceedingly difficult. Alan Stone has accused some psychiatrists of resurrecting the myth of the "omniscient psychiatrist" to combat the myth of the autonomous patient (23).

Clinical tradition may be overestimating the impact that mild to moderate depression has on preferences for life-sustaining treatment. In one study, mildly to moderately depressed elderly did choose less aggressive treatment in hypothetical scenarios with good medical prognosis than nondepressed elderly. However, depression accounted for only 5% of the variance in responses, and its effect was limited to the good-prognosis scenarios (24). More important than depression in shaping treatment decisions was patients' assessment of their overall quality of life. In a follow-up study on this same population, recovery from mild to moderate depression was *not* associated with changes in preferences concerning life-sustaining treatment (25). These results are congruent with findings from other studies that have shown depression to be a poor predictor of preferences concerning life-sustaining therapy in the medically ill elderly (26–28). On the other hand, treatment of severely depressed elderly who are initially very hopeless does appear to increase their interest in life-sustaining medical treatment

(29). One study found that treatment of 10 patients with advanced Alzheimer's disease and depressed affect with sertraline improved affect in 8 and diminished food refusal in 6 of these patients (30).

It would be a mistake to assume that depression—especially when severe—could not have a significant effect on capacity to decide about medical treatment. But it also appears inappropriate to assume that depression, when present in the mild to moderate form common among medical patients, is distorting patients' judgments about lifesaving treatment. Discriminating those cases in which depression impairs the capacity to make medical decisions from those cases in which it does not is best accomplished through a systematic approach to competence assessment.

The clinical assessment of competence or capacity to consent to medical treatment has traditionally focused on cognitive capacities. Appelbaum and Grisso outlined four categories into which legal standards of competence fall (31). In order of increasing a priori rigor, these are 1) communicating a choice, 2) understanding relevant information, 3) appreciating the current situation and its consequences, and 4) manipulating information rationally. We will not go into detail here about the implementation of these tests. It is interesting to note, however, that a recent empirical study by these same authors applying these standards failed to confirm a hierarchy of rigor (32). When tested on schizophrenic patients, depressed patients, and coronary disease patients and community members, each standard identified a similar percentage of subjects as impaired. However, each standard identified a slightly different group of subjects. When standards were combined, an increased proportion of patients were identified as impaired. This study reminds us that we do not yet clearly understand the structure of competence as it appears in our patient populations.

These standards for decision-making capacity are intended to assess the thought *process* behind a *product* of thought, namely, the treatment decision in question. If the thought process is intact, then a treatment refusal should be honored, even if the medical team disagrees with it. In practice, the assessment of process and product are not as independent as implied by the theory. Many authors have suggested that more stringent tests of competence are appropriate when the consequences of respecting a refusal are serious. Grisso and Appelbaum propose "in life-threatening circumstances to lower the threshold at which a determination of probable incompetence will be made" (33). Drane has argued for a "sliding-scale" of competence tests (34). Buchanan and Brock have also proposed flexibility in their "process-standard" of competence (35).

Such flexibility appears to be a reasonable way to protect patients' liberty *and* well-being. However, it can erode the independence of the competence determination from the specific medical treatment decision in question. Buchanan and Brock issue this cautionary note:

> Treatment refusal does reasonably serve to *trigger* a competence evaluation. On the other hand, a disagreement with the physician's recommendation or a refusal of a treatment recommendation is *no basis or evidence whatsoever* for a finding of incompetence. (36)

Alan Meisel similarly condemns a finding of incompetence on the basis of a refusal as "paternalism in the extreme" (37).

Charles Culver and Bernard Gert claim that the concept of competence cannot withstand the flexibility required to make it responsive to the clinical consequences of treatment refusal. If the harms incurred by such a refusal far outweigh the benefits, then, they argue, the refusal is properly overruled regardless of an otherwise intact thought process. They contend that this irrationality of the treatment refusal itself must be taken into account in determining whether the refusal should be honored (38).

It is specifically refusals of lifesaving treatment by depressed persons that prompt these debates about the concept of competence. Medical instinct rails against honoring refusals that will result in death or permanent impairment. Yet finding a procedure that accords with clinical intuition concerning patient welfare *and* protects patients' right to refuse treatment has been perplexing.

Evaluating the competence of the depressed patient has raised questions not only about the independence of the assessments of the process and product of thought, but also about the focus on cognitive aspects of competence. Bursztajn and colleagues have succinctly stated that "patients with major affective disorders can retain the cognitive capacity to *understand* the risks and benefits of a medication, yet fail to *appreciate* its benefits" (39). Understanding medical facts in the abstract is different from understanding how they apply to your own life. It is this transition that is so often impaired in the seriously depressed patient.

Utilizing a competence standard that moves beyond the assessment of understanding (i.e., asking the patient to paraphrase the clinician's statement of a treatment's benefits and risks) to an assessment of appreciation (i.e., asking the patient to describe how these facts count as pros and cons in his or her own life) is a reasonable response to the clinical challenge presented by the depressed patient who is refusing treatment. Using such a standard holds a risk, however, of invalidating the patient's values if they are different from those of the treating physician. Physician and patient may differ, for example, in the importance accorded to individual versus family well-being, sanctity versus dignity of life, or value versus futility of suffering. The doctrine of informed consent is intended to protect the right of patients to hold and exercise values different from those of physicians. James Childress has phrased the problem as follows: "While false beliefs about a medical condition may be a reason for viewing a patient as an incompetent, false beliefs about goods are not" (40). We want to make sure that patients have their facts right about a life-and-death decision, but should we be making sure that they have their values right?

Role of Psychological Assessment and Treatment in Refusal of Life-Saving Treatment

There appears to be substantial difference of opinion in the medical community concerning the role of mental health professionals in evaluating patients who are refusing treatment. In their study of medical treatment refusal, Appelbaum and Roth noted, in their review of more than 700 treatment refusals, that

> [p]sychiatric consultants were called upon to examine patients who had refused in two circumstances: first, when the patient had a known psychiatric history, and second, when the patient appeared to be suffering from an obvious psychiatric disorder and the refusal was potentially serious. (41)

This study suggests that treatment refusal should prompt more frequent psychiatric consultation. However, some psychiatrists have argued against more extensive involvement of psychiatrists with patients when there are problems obtaining informed consent. Gutheil and Duckworth have warned against utilizing psychiatrists as "informed consent technicians" (42). They see a danger in the psychiatrist's being consulted solely to facilitate the process of "getting the consent" or having the patient declared incompetent. This abrogates the appropriate role of the treating physician in establishing a consent dialogue with the patient and trivializes the expertise of the psychiatric consultant. Greater attention by mental health professionals to the depressed patient refusing treatment need not fall prey to this criticism, however.

Depression is especially common among the medically ill. While 2% to 4% of persons in the community suffer from major depressive disorder at any one time, 5% to 9% of ambulatory primary care patients are affected. When medical inpatients are assessed by self-rating scales, 22% to 33% are found to have an affective disorder. In a study utilizing a structured psychiatric interview, 15% of medical inpatients were found to have an affective disorder (43). The Medical Outcomes Study recently compared persons in the community with and without one of eight chronic medical conditions (44). Those with one or more of these conditions had a 41% increase in the relative risk of having any recent psychiatric disorder. Studies have also revealed that the most frequent precipitant for depression in the elderly is physical illness (45). Furthermore, the rate of depression has been shown to be higher in those elderly persons who are more severely ill (46). Actual rates of depression vary by illness and population studied as well as by diagnostic method. Among cancer inpatients, for example, a recent review documented studies demonstrating between 1% and 38% prevalence of major depression. Rates of major depression appear to vary considerably by type of cancer, from 50% of those with pancreatic cancer to 1% of those with acute leukemia (47).

This kind of data would seem to indicate that these depressions were "reactive" in the sense that they are a "reasonable response" to such illness. Seeing serious depression in the face of severe medical illness as reasonable is one of the most common forms of "pseudo-empathy" against which physicians must be warned. Such interpretations of these depressions as purely reactive minimize the value that biopsychosocial assessment and treatment might have in these cases. This risk may be particularly marked in cases of dysthymia, in which depression has become so chronic that the family sees it as "just who he is." The risk may also be high in the minor depression typical of the medically ill elderly.

Healthcare workers opt to withdraw treatment in the same circumstances in which a depressed patient might refuse treatment. A recent survey of Canadian healthcare workers using hypothetical scenarios revealed liklihood of short- and long-term survival, premorbid cognitive function, and age of the patient as the most important factors in the decision to withdraw life support from the critically ill (48).

The potential for successful treatment of major depression in the presence of serious medical illness is well documented. Antidepressants have been shown to be superior to placebo in double-blind trials for the treatment of depression in patients with medical illness (49), stroke (50), heart disease (51), cancer (52), chronic obstructive pulmonary disease (COPD) (53), Parkinson's disease (54), and tinnitus (55). Psychostimulants such as methylphenidate and dextroamphetamine have been demonstrated to be effective for depression in the medically ill in retrospective studies (56). ECT also has demonstrated effectiveness for depression treatment in those who are medically ill (57). The efficacy of cognitive-behavioral therapy and interpersonal psychotherapy for depression has been demonstrated in randomized controlled trials (58). Efficacy of psychotherapy specifically in the depressed, medically ill patient has not been tested in randomized trials.

Making the diagnosis of major depression in the medically ill can be difficult. Determining which symptoms are due to depression and which are due to the medical illness poses a considerable clinical challenge. Cohen-Cole and colleagues have recently reviewed four strategies for diagnosis of depression in the medically ill (59). The "inclusive" strategy considers all the signs and symptoms of depression presented by the patient, disregarding the possible role played by the medical illness in their production. The "exclusive" strategy systematically omits depressive symptoms likely produced by the type of medical disorder present (e.g., anorexia in cancer patients). The "etiologic" strategy, in accord with DSM-IV, seeks to determine, on a case-by-case basis, whether a depressive symptom is due to the medical disorder. In this strategy, only those symptoms not demonstrably related to the medical disorder in that particular person count toward psychiatric diagnosis. The "substitutive" strategy, as proposed by Endicott (60), replaces some vegetative symptoms of depression with further cognitive symptoms. A recent study of 130 palliative care patients revealed large differences in rates of major and minor depression (total: 26% vs. 13%) when low vs. high threshold diagnostic criteria were used (61), but did not show differences between types of diagnostic criteria (e.g., Research Diagnostic Criteria vs. those in DSM-III-R). This was true both when Research Diagnostic Criteria (which include somatic symptoms) were used and when Endicott criteria (which substitute cognitive for somatic symptoms) were used. For research purposes, where diagnostic specificity is most important, the exclusive or substitutive approaches are likely the best choice. However, in clinical practice depression tends to be underdiagnosed in the medically ill (62). Therefore, when refusal of lifesaving treatment lies in the balance, it is important to maximize diagnostic sensitivity with the inclusive approach.

Personal and family histories of depression are also useful information. Biological markers of depression (e.g., dexamethasone suppression test) have not been shown to be clinically useful and may well be confounded by the concurrent medical illness. In cases of persistent diagnostic uncertainty, a treatment trial may be necessary to determine whether a treatable depressive disorder is present. Psychostimulants have an especially rapid onset of action and may be particularly useful in this regard.

Limitations of Psychiatric and Psychosocial Assessment and Treatment

Biopsychosocial assessment and treatment have much to offer those who are refusing lifesaving treatment or seeking to hasten their death by other means. However, there are important limitations in mental health expertise and therapeutic power that must be acknowledged. Although clinical severity of depression is generally well correlated with its impact on competence to make medical decisions, this is not always the case. The presence of a major depressive disorder may be neither necessary nor sufficient for the impairment of competence. Symptoms that are the most important for the diagnosis of depression may not be the same symptoms that are most critical in determining the effect of that depression on competence. There is a strong emphasis on vegetative symptoms in the DSM-IV approach to depression diagnosis. Although insomnia and anorexia may significantly decrease a patient's quality of life, they are less likely by themselves to impair competence to make medical decisions.

The depressive symptoms that are most likely to impair a patient's capacity to accurately appreciate his or her medical situation are those distorted assessments of self, world, and future that typify depressive thinking (63). Depressive helplessness produces an underestimation of one's possible effectiveness in the face of serious illness. Guilt and worthlessness may make one believe that suffering and death are deserved and should not be forestalled. Anhedonia may make it impossible to imagine that life will offer any pleasures for which it is worth enduring the discomforts and indignities of medical illness. Depressive hopelessness can make it impossible to imagine that life will ever offer a better balance of pleasure and pain than it does at present. If some of these cognitive symptoms are present, competence to make decisions concerning life-sustaining medical treatment may be impaired in the absence of a diagnosable major depressive disorder.

Even after clinical attention has been directed toward anhedonia, helplessness, hopelessness, and worthlessness, determining their status as symptoms of depression can be perplexing. In the traditional young and medically healthy psychiatric patient, it is less difficult to determine that these are mental distortions than in the intractably suffering terminally ill patient. In the latter case, activities providing pleasure may no longer be available. One may be unable to help oneself or others in any meaningful way. Intolerable symptoms may in fact persist for the short remainder of one's life. It is sometimes impossible to determine that hopelessness is pathological in the terminally ill. A recent survey of Oregon psychiatrists revealed that two-thirds thought that physician-assisted suicide should sometimes be permitted (64). However, only 6% felt very confident that they could adequately assess in a single session whether a psychiatric disorder was impairing the judgment of a patient requesting assisted suicide.

Consider the following case.

A 75-year-old married white male with prostate cancer had metastases to his vertebrae that were causing great pain. He was in the hospital, receiving oral and intrathecal hydromorphone. However, he was still in severe pain, crying nearly constantly and asking to die. A psychiatric consultant thought that he met the criteria for major depression and recommended ECT. After long talks with his wife, the patient reluctantly consented. After five treatments, he experienced a marked improvement in mood and pain level. Eight treatments total were given, and the patient was sent home with oral and intrathecal pain medications. The patient did well for 3 months. He was then readmitted with new metastases and compression fractures. His pain again was severe, and he was asking to die. He refused repeat ECT and requested extra pain medication. The extra pain medication lowered his respiratory rate to 6, and he died in 2 days.

It is essential for psychiatry to accept that the choice to die by a seriously ill person *may* be rational, especially in situations in which the medical prognosis is very poor. However, acceptance of the desire to die as rational in any particular case is fraught with peril. Not only are the consequences serious and irreversible, but the temptations of pseudo-empathy are great. Physicians have been shown to underestimate seriously ill patients' quality of life and their desires for life-sustaining treatment (65). Physicians also neglect to adequately explore patients' reasons for refusing treatment. Appelbaum, Lidz, and Meisel issue the following caution:

> Patients are sometimes initially reluctant to reveal their reasons for refusal, feeling embarrassed about having inconvenienced their physicians or fearful of some retaliation if their reasons are not good enough. Sometimes patients may even lack a conscious awareness of all the reasons. Physicians need to take the lead in identifying the bases for refusal. (66)

Reluctance to explore the reasons for refusal can be particularly dangerous when combined with a superficial adherence to the ideal of patient autonomy and respect for the "right" to refuse treatment.

Inadequate physician exploration of reasons for the desire to die can unnecessarily turn situations that are remediable into tragedies.

When hopelessness, helplessness, and worthlessness are not present or not clearly of pathological origin, the mental health professional can be put into the uncomfortable position of validating a patient's request to die. The doctrine of informed consent implies that medical decisions have inescapable personal as well as medical elements. In a pluralist secular society like our own, it must be assumed that adults are competent to evaluate their own quality of life as tolerable or intolerable. We must learn to identify those refusals of lifesaving treatment that should be respected. The burden of proof concerning competence is on the clinician who is seeking to override a refusal. The desire to die is by itself not adequate evidence of incompetence. As explained above, a finding of incompetence cannot rest solely on the refusal in question.

There are some refusals in which the presence of depressive symptoms means that the refusal should *not* be respected. The boundary between these refusals and those that should be respected will not be clear because of the wide variability in values concerning life and death present in our society. Christian values concerning the proper balance between the well-being of the individual and that of his or her family or community, between the sanctity of life and the dignity of life, between redemptive and futile suffering, tend to favor the prolongation of life. But this is not true of other legitimate religious and philosophical traditions. In the first century A.D., the Stoic philosopher and statesman Seneca stated, "The wise man will live as long as he ought, not as long as he can" (67).

When depression compromises competence, it is advisable not only to treat it but also to consult advance directives and designated surrogate decision-makers. A living will can be used to verify that a current refusal is consistent with values and preferences expressed when depression was not an issue. Similarly, a family member can verify that a refusal is consistent with values present throughout a lifetime. If the patient has a long-term relationship with their primary care physician, this person can be an invaluable source of information about the patient's baseline mental status, medical care preferences, and deeply held values. These strategies are imperfect, however. When competence is questionable, it may not be clear when to defer to the advance directive, especially when it conflicts with currently expressed wishes.

Advance directives often do not address the exact situation within which the refusal arises (68). It is difficult to determine which differences in the actual situation would have changed the person's wishes and which would not. Families may not understand what the patient would have wanted or what the medical issues are (69). It is important to seek evidence of previously expressed wishes in order to verify that the desire to die is an authentic wish arising from the person rather than the depression. But there will always be uncertainties that require the application of clinical judgment to the particular case.

As documented above, depression *can* be treated in those with serious medical illness. Prior to acceding to a wish to refuse lifesaving treatment, it is important to optimize both medical and psychiatric treatment. Access to palliative and hospice care should be assured. Diminished severity of the medical illness (70) or of the pain associated with it (71) can improve psychiatric status. Both psychological and pharmacological treatment of depression can improve quality of life.

There are times when psychiatric treatment is not appropriate. Clearly, instances in which treatment refusal is not associated with a treatable mental disorder or symptoms are among these. Mental health professionals may also need to accept some depressions in the terminally ill as absolutely treatment resistant. These will be difficult decisions. How many different antidepressants must be tried? Are we willing to administer ECT to a terminally ill patient against his or her will? Just as internists must at some point decide "enough is enough," so might psychiatrists at some point appropriately stop trying to intervene and let the dying process proceed. There may be a role for palliative care (e.g., with benzodiazepines) in those for whom more definitive treatments for depression have not provided relief. There is always something that can be done to relieve suffering even if the disease cannot be cured or the life saved.

References

1. Meisel A: The Right to Die. New York, Wiley, 1989, p 45
2. Meisel, The Right to Die, p 44
3. Meisel, The Right to Die, p 66
4. Bouvia v Superior Court, No B019134 (Cal App 2d Dist, April 16, 1986)

5. Stone A: A reply to "Depression, self-love, time, and the 'right' to suicide." Gen Hosp Psychiatry 8:95–98, 1986

6. Appelbaum PS: The right to refuse treatment with antipsychotic medications. Am J Psychiatry 145:413–419, 1988

7. Meisel, The Right to Die, p 188

8. Karlinsky H, Taerk G, Schwartz K, et al: Suicide attempts and resuscitation dilemmas. Gen Hosp Psychiatry 10:423–427, 1988; see p 426

9. Pokorny AD: Prediction of suicide in psychiatric patients. Arch Gen Psychiatry 40:249–257, 1983

10. Brown JH, Henteleff P, Barakat S, et al: Is it normal for terminally ill patients to desire death? Am J Psychiatry 143:208–210, 1986

11. Meisel, The Right to Die, p 67

12. Washington (Natural Death) Act, RCW 70.122.100. Quoted in Meisel A: The Right to Die, p 69

13. Pijnenborg L, van der Maas PJ, Kardaun JWPF, et al: Withdrawal or withholding of treatment at the end of life. Arch Intern Med 155:286–292, 1995

14. Schaffner KF: Philosophical, ethical, and legal aspects of resuscitation medicine, II: recognizing the tragic choice: food, water and the right to assisted suicide. Crit Care Med 16:1063–1068, 1988

15. Schaffner, Philosophical, ethical, and legal aspects of resuscitation medicine, II, p 1065

16. Schaffner, Philosophical, ethical, and legal aspects of resuscitation medicine, II, p 1065

17. Sullivan MD, Ward NG, Laxton A: The woman who wanted electroconvulsive therapy and do not resuscitate status: questions of competence on a medical-psychiatry unit. Gen Hosp Psychiatry 14:204–209, 1992

18. Appelbaum PS, Roth LH: Treatment refusal in medical hospitals, in President's Commission for the Study of Ethical Problems in Medicine and Biomedical and Behavioral Research: Making Health Care Decisions: The Ethical and Legal Implications of Informed Consent in the Patient-Practitioner Relationship, Vol 1. Washington, DC, U.S. Government Printing Office, 1982, pp 382–456; see p 434

19. Ganzini L, Lee MA, Heintz RT, et al: Do-not-resuscitate orders for depressed psychiatric inpatients. Hospital and Community Psychiatry 43:915–919, 1992

20. Swartz CM, Stewart C: Melancholia and orders to restrict resuscitation, Hospital and Community Psychiatry 42:189–190, 1991

21. Karlinsky et al, Suicide attempts and resuscitation dilemmas

22. Beck AT, Brown G, Berchick RJ, et al: Relationship between hopelessness and ultimate suicide: a replication with psychiatric outpatients. Am J Psy-

chiatry 147:190–195, 1990

23. Stone, A reply
24. Lee MA, Ganzini L: Depression in the elderly: effect on patient attitudes toward life-sustaining therapy. J Am Geriatr Soc 40:983–988, 1992
25. Lee MA, Ganzini L: The effect of recovery from depression on preferences for life-sustaining therapy in older patients. Journal of Gerontology 49:15–21, 1994
26. Cohen-Mansfield J, Rabinovich BA, Lipson S, et al: The decision to execute a durable power of attorney for health care and preferences regarding the utilization of life-sustaining treatments in nursing home residents. Arch Intern Med 151:289–294, 1991
27. Michelson C, Mulvihill M, Hsu MA, et al: Eliciting medical care preferences from nursing home residents. Gerontologist 31:358–363, 1991
28. Uhlmann RF, Pearlman RA: Perceived quality of life and preferences for life-sustaining treatment in older adults. Arch Intern Med 151:495–498, 1991
29. Ganzini L, Lee MA, Heintz RT, et al: The effect of depression treatment on elderly patients' preferences for life-sustaining medical therapy. Am J Psychiatry 151:1631–1636, 1994
30. Volicer L, Rheaume Y, Cyr D: Treatment of depression in advanced Alzheimer's disease using sertraline. J Geriatr Psychiatry Neurol 7:227–229, 1994
31. Appelbaum PS, Grisso T: Assessing patients' capacities to consent to treatment. N Engl J Med 319:1635–1638, 1988
32. Grisso T, Appelbaum PS: Comparison of standards for assessing patients' capacities to make treatment decisions. Am J Psychiatry 152:1033–1037, 1995
33. Grisso and Appelbaum, Comparison of standards, p 1638
34. Drane JF: The many faces of competency. Hastings Cent Rep 15:17–21, 1985
35. Buchanan AE, Brock DW: Deciding for Others: The Ethics of Surrogate Decision Making. Cambridge, UK, Cambridge University Press, 1989, p 58
36. Buchanan and Brock, Deciding for Others, p 58
37. Meisel, The Right to Die, p 198
38. Culver CM, Gert B: The inadequacy of incompetence. Milbank Q 68:619–643, 1990
39. Bursztajn HJ, Harding HP, Gutheil TG, et al: Beyond cognition: the role of disordered affective states in impairing competence to consent to treatment. Bull Am Acad Psychiatry Law 19:383–388, 1991
40. Childress JF: Who Should Decide? Paternalism in Health Care. Oxford, UK, Oxford University Press, 1982, p 170
41. Appelbaum and Roth, Treatment refusal in medical hospitals, p 448

42. Gutheil TG, Duckworth K: The psychiatrist as informed consent technician: a problem for the professions. Bull Menninger Clin 56:87–94, 1992

43. Katon W, Sullivan MD: Depression and chronic medical illness. J Clin Psychiatry 51 (No 6, Suppl):3–11, 1990

44. Wells KB, Golding JM, Burnham MA: Psychiatric disorder in a sample of the general population with and without chronic medical conditions. Am J Psychiatry 145:976–981, 1988

45. Murphy E: Social origins of depression in old age. Br J Psychiatry 141:135–142, 1982

46. Berkman LF, Berman CS, Kasl S, et al: Depressive symptoms in relation to physical health and functioning in the elderly. Am J Epidemiol 124:372–388, 1986

47. McDaniel JS, Musselman DL, Porter MR, et al: Depression in patients with cancer. Arch Gen Psychiatry 52:89–99, 1995

48. Cook DJ, Guyatt GH, Jaeschke R, et al: Determinants in Canadian health care workers of the decision to withdraw life support from the critically ill. JAMA 273:703–708, 1995

49. Rifkin A, Reardon G, Siris S: Trimipramine in physical illness with depression. J Clin Psychiatry 46:4–8, 1985

50. Lipsey JR, Robinson RG, Pearlson GD, et al: Nortriptyline treatment of post-stroke depression. Lancet 141:297–300, 1984

51. Veith RC, Raskind MR, Caldwell JH: Cardiovascular effects of tricyclic antidepressants in depressed patients with chronic heart disease. N Engl J Med 306:954–959, 1982

52. Costa D, Mogos I, Toma T: Efficacy and safety of mianserin in the treatment of depression in women with cancer. Acta Psychiatr Scand Suppl 72:85–92, 1985

53. Borson S, McDonald GJ, Gayle T, et al: Improvement in mood, physical symptoms, and function with nortriptyline for depression in patients with chronic obstructive pulmonary disease. Psychosomatics 33:190–201, 1992

54. Andersen J, Aabro E, Gulmann N: Antidepressant treatment in Parkinson's disease. Acta Neurol Scand 62:210–219, 1980

55. Sullivan MD, Dobie RA, Sakai CS: Treatment of depressed tinnitus patients with nortriptyline. Ann Otol Rhinol Laryngol 98:867–872, 1989

56. Masand P, Pickett P, Murray GB: Psychostimulant for secondary depression in medical illness. Psychosomatics 32:203–208, 1991

57. Dubovsky SL: Using electroconvulsive therapy for patients with neurological disease. Hospital and Community Psychiatry 37:819–825, 1986

58. Elkin I, Shea MT, Watkins JT, et al: National Institute of Mental Health Treatment of Depression Collaborative Research Program: general effectiveness of treatments. Arch Gen Psychiatry 46:971–982, 1989

59. Cohen-Cole SA, Brown FW, McDaniel JS: Diagnostic assessment of major depression in the medically ill, in Principles of Medical Psychiatry, 2nd Edition. Edited by Stoudemire A, Fogel B. New York, Oxford University Press, 1991, pp 53–70

60. Endicott J: Measurement of depression in patients with cancer. Cancer 53:2243–2248, 1984

61. Chochinov HM, Wilson KG, Enns M, et al: Prevalence of depression in the terminally ill: effects of diagnostic criteria and symptoms threshold judgments. Am J Psychiatry 151:537–540, 1994

62. Koenig HG, Meador KG, Cohen HS, et al: Detection and treatment of depression in older medically ill hospitalized patients. Int J Psychiatry Med 18:17–31, 1988

63. Beck AT: Thinking and depression, I: idiosyncratic content and cognitive distortions. Arch Gen Psychiatry 9:324–335, 1963

64. Ganzini L, Fenn DS, Lee MA, et al: Attitudes of Oregon psychiatrists toward physician-assisted suicide. Am J Psychiatry 153:1469–1475, 1996

65. Appelbaum and Grisso, Assessing patients' capacities to consent to treatment, 1988

66. Appelbaum PS, Lidz CW, Meisel A:, Informed Consent: Legal Theory and Clinical Practice. New York, Oxford University Press, 1987, p 196

67. Seneca: Epistle 70, in Epistula Morales, Vol II. Edited by Loeb L. London, Heinemann, 1925

68. Emanuel LJ: The health care directive: learning how to draft advance care documents. J Am Geriatr Soc 39:1221–1228, 1991

69. Appelbaum and Roth, Treatment refusal in medical hospitals, p 464

70. Kathol RG, Noyes R, Wald T: Criteria and symptom based depression in cancer patients. Paper presented at the 145th annual meeting of the American Psychiatric Association, Washington, DC, May 1992

71. Spiegel D, Sands S: Pain and depression in cancer patients. Paper presented at the 145th annual meeting of the American Psychiatric Association, Washington, DC, May 1992

4

Family Dynamics in Decisions to Withhold or Withdraw Treatment

Ellen Rothchild, M.D.

At Dr. Albert Schweitzer's famous clinic in French Africa, early in this century, families brought their sick to the clinic, along with their cooking utensils and bed rolls, and stayed, providing care for the patient and accepted as an integral part of the treatment team; decisions about life-sustaining technology were not an issue. By contrast, in today's high-tech, crisis-oriented intensive care unit, a busy treatment team may focus exclusively on the patient, viewing the family as an appendage to be relegated to a waiting room. Even in acute ward settings, families can be negatively perceived

An earlier version of this chapter appeared in *General Hospital Psychiatry* (16:251–258, 1994). The author wishes to thank Elsevier for permission to publish this expanded version. The author also wishes to thank Lynn Rustad, Ph.D., for certain case illustrations and Kathy Cole-Kelly, Ph.D., for her critique of the manuscript.

as persons who might demand prolonged, medically questionable treatment for their relative, and feared as potential litigants. Yet family members are usually supportive advocates or concerned proxies for the chronically or terminally ill patient. And when choices of withholding or withdrawing life-sustaining treatment arise, families are vital (if somewhat neglected) members of the team.

Why the ambivalence toward families? Has the technological promise of extended life and denial of its many costs conferred on patients and families a heightened sense of entitlement? Are physicians zealous guardians of scarce resources, too pressed for time to talk and listen? Has an uneasy balance of power permeated the physician-patient alliance in end-of-life decision making, threatening patient trust (1)?

Most often, patients, families, and healthcare providers are allies, in agreement about treatment. But when conflicts arise, medical caregivers are especially compelled to consider the psychological aspects of the situation.

This review will focus on family responses to and interactions with the patient and staff when life support is to be withheld or withdrawn. It will address issues about the process that must be discussed with families and interventions found helpful when conflicts over limiting treatment arise. First, the social context of decision making must be considered.

The Changing Milieu of Decision Making

Recent Legal and Ethical Decisions

While the remarkable life-support technologies of the late twentieth century enable prolongation of life even in the terminally ill, the quality of that extended time and the costs associated with bringing it about do not always justify aggressive treatment. The principle of *patient autonomy,* whereby the patient or his or her proxy may choose or reject aggressive treatment, is now generally recognized as a means of protecting people from automatic and unwanted life extension by machine; in practice, the application of this principle has many nuances.

For instance, patients are not always so autonomous as to be able to resist the pressure of family wishes contrary to their own; or they may be so disabled or incompetent that a surrogate (usually a family member) then must assume decision-making responsibility, sometimes with no knowledge of what the patient might have wished. Recognition that more guidelines were needed was highlighted by the cases of Karen Ann Quinlan in 1976 and, more recently, Nancy Cruzan, young women in coma who had never formally made known their wishes and whose families struggled in the courts to show that these women would not have wanted life-sustaining treatment in their current circumstances. Thus the concept of advance directives was promulgated, both to extend patient autonomy to a time when the patient might no longer be competent to choose and to ease family responsibility.

The Patient Self-Determination Act, passed in 1990, obliges Medicare- and Medicaid-funded hospitals and nursing homes to inform patients of their right to make decisions about medical care and to execute advance directives, including appointment of a healthcare proxy should the patient be unable to speak for himself or herself. The proxy, usually a family member, is expected to decide as the patient would if competent (the substituted judgment standard) or to choose according to the patient's best interests if the patient's wishes are unknown. Several forms of advance directives are recognized. *Informal advance directives* involve verbally communicating one's future treatment wishes to one's family and/or physician. *Formal advance directives* include a written living will describing one's future healthcare wishes, or a durable power of attorney for health care appointing a proxy to decide for one in the future.

Although the aim of the Patient Self-Determination Act was to support patient autonomy and empower surrogate decision-makers, it does have shortcomings. Families can still influence or feel influenced by patients, and they can still feel some burden of responsibility in decision making. Further, advance directives may be hard to interpret in a given clinical situation, leaving healthcare providers and families guessing and sometimes disagreeing over life-and-death decisions. Some also argue that the act disenfranchises the family; for instance, were a patient to want aggressive treatment, no matter what the cost or prognosis, other family members would be expected to subordinate their own health, educational, and other needs in order to support the sick member (2). And, paradoxically, despite recognition of patient autonomy, in practice families are sometimes granted too much authority, as when a physician, fearful of upsetting a perfectly competent patient with bad news, turns instead to the family for healthcare decisions (3–5). In fact, family decision making is considered optimal in some cultures, so that insistence on patient autonomy when this runs counter to patient and family beliefs could represent another form of medical paternalism (6)!

The Healthcare System

In the past, families formed long-term relationships with physicians that fostered patients' trust in medical care and enabled physician understanding of patient values. In today's climate of heightened family mobility and managed care, there is less time for patients and physicians to get to know each other. Moreover the hospital has replaced the home as the most common site for dying, and this has rendered aggressive treatment more accessible. In the hospital, care, communication, and accountability are often diffused among multiple specialists and workers on different shifts. Collaborative decision making may be further jeopardized by wide ethnic, age, and economic differences between healthcare providers and the family; thus, a physician who is unfamiliar with a family of limited resources may be unaware of the very difficult sacrifices he or she might request on the patient's behalf.

Because palliative care is now becoming more widely recognized as a humane alternative to aggressive treatment of the terminally ill, there is increasing movement of patients back to the home or hospice. Further, it seems likely that physicians are withdrawing and withholding intensive care much more often than they did at the start of this decade (7).

The American Family

During the latter half of the twentieth century, dramatic changes in family composition, mobility, and the role of women have ensued. In addition to the traditional family, the following possibilities exist: two-income couples, single parents, blended families (from previous divorces), multiracial and gay/lesbian families, and families that include children born as the result of new reproductive technologies, the legal status of whom with respect to parental decision making is sometimes in question. Although the law recognizes a simple hierarchy of next of kin (i.e., spouse, adult children, parent, adult siblings, in that order) when proxy healthcare decisions are to be made, the hierarchy does not include all the compositional variations described. Heightened geographic mobility for career purposes has diminished the availability of nearby extended family members to help out in crises. Working women lack the time that the traditional homemaker had to care for the ill at home. Less community support may be forthcoming if bias exists toward a multiracial or gay/lesbian family.

Common Family Responses to Decision Making

As a family member's life-threatening illness progresses, the emotional and material resources of other members are stressed in the effort to provide care, assume new roles and responsibilities, and prepare for possible loss. Resources may be anxiously guarded or, alternatively, lavished on the sick person, and this may jeopardize the quality of life of the well members. Dormant family conflicts may resurface, such as unsettled grievances or rivalries. Sometimes long-severed relationships are reestablished: a prodigal son returns for reconciliation; an ex-wife sits vigil with her former husband. Roles shift: younger family members may need to insist that an ailing family autocrat yield to others' decisions. The crisis can precipitate both conflict and problem-resolution; treatment decisions may be part of this process.

Families generally heed the competent patient's treatment wishes, if such are known. However, family members' own interests, fear, denial, and other emotions may intrude. Thus, families have been known to challenge a patient's decisions, either openly to the patient or privately with the treatment team, occasionally asking physicians not to share bad news with the patient. A family member who feels guilty or denies the hopelessness of the situation may pressure the patient to prolong treatment. One who is emotionally, physically, or financially burdened may pressure the patient to discontinue treatment. Gonda and Ruark observe,

Often patients become less able to stand up for their own wishes against the pressures of loved ones who may advocate choices which are contrary to the patients' desires. Many families react to their sense of guilt and hopelessness by pushing for maximal medical intervention until the bitter end. This often results in patients whose fires have burned too low to resist persuasion accepting treatments that they never would have chosen if left to themselves. Such a course may allow the family to postpone their loss for a short time, but at a high cost to the dying person. Further, the time thereby mortgaged is seldom of sufficient quality to justify its prolongation. (8)

Patients may also feel pressed to die quickly to relieve the family of care, cost, and emotional burden. Sometimes such a person expresses the wish to die as a way of testing the family, backing off if the family rallies around and demonstrates concern.

Sometimes it is the family that feels unduly pressured by the patient's treatment wishes. For example, Brody cites the case of a 13-year-old boy with leukemia who had already failed several courses of aggressive chemotherapy but insisted on trying another. The oncology team felt this would probably offer little and only worsen the quality of his remaining life. For a time the boy's parents and the team were torn between respecting the expressed wishes of this adolescent, who was old enough to understand the issues and exercise a degree of autonomy, or acknowledging his bravery, taking responsibility for limiting treatment and providing comfort care instead (9). Examples also abound in which families feel obliged to make great financial sacrifices for a sick member's requested heroic treatment, as in, for example, transplants with uncertain prognosis. Conversely, influenced by a patient's depression, a family might press for treatment limitation when in fact the patient has a good medical prognosis.

When the patient is unwilling or unable to make decisions, responsibility for doing so shifts to a surrogate, usually a family member. Although competent to decide, some patients (more often the elderly) avoid the issue, hope their physicians will decide for them, or trust that their families will advocate for them in an unpredictable medical environment. If the patient is not competent, a surrogate is sought. Advance directives and health powers of attorney can ease decision making, although a surrogate may still need to interpret the directive, weigh the unforeseen situation, and occasionally guess at what the patient might have chosen if able. Some surrogate family members decide without hesitation, sure of the patient's previously discussed wishes. Others find decision making an onerous responsibility with a potential legacy of uncertainty over having chosen right and of "executioner's guilt," as if equating treatment limitation with killing. Such feelings are often inversely proportional to the clarity of the patient's previously expressed wishes and may be manifested by avoidance of making decisions, stalling for time by seeking second and third opinions, or insisting on futile aggressive treatment.

Sometimes a surrogate bases decisions on what is best for himself or herself rather than the patient's wishes or best interests. Brody described an elderly man who requested resuscitation for his failing wife who had far advanced chronic obstructive pulmonary disease (COPD) because she had always taken care of him and he could not get along without her (10). Conflicts of interest arise from many sources including wishes to relieve the stress of caring for an elderly patient, eagerness for an inheritance, and wishes to continue receiving the patient's disability or pension checks by extending life.

Families usually respect both a patient's treatment wishes and a physician's treatment recommendations; conflicts can arise, however, over both limiting and pursuing care. As surrogates, families may request treatment withdrawal in situations in which physicians believe the patient should be treated because the patient has a reasonable chance for recovery or the physicians fear legal repercussions for withdrawing treatment. Alternatively, the family surrogate may insist on continued care that the medical staff regards as both futile and cruel.

Variables Affecting
Family Decision Making

Family responses and points of potential conflict such as those discussed above are shaped by a number of variables, both intrinsic and extrinsic to the family.

Patient's Role in the Family

The patient's family role (e.g., boss, scapegoat, or caregiver) influences family responses to anticipated loss. Families are apt to be more invested in keeping alive the parent of young children than an aging bachelor and to urge more aggressive lifesaving measures—whether or not the patient wants these interventions. Similarly, the family may derive hidden value in prolonging the life of a family scapegoat, as in the following example.

> The "black sheep" in a family of achievers, Max had never quite suc-
> ceeded despite earning a degree in psychology. He developed chronic
> alcoholism and had a prison record for passing bad checks, and the
> family no longer welcomed him when he came around for a meal or
> a loan. However, when they learned that Max would probably not sur-
> vive his most recent hospitalization for liver failure, they quickly ar-
> ranged for his transfer to a hospital closer to home and insisted that
> everything be done to maintain life. A sister observed that without Max
> the siblings would have to "jump higher."

Issues of control over treatment can arise when the patient has been accustomed to wielding authority in the family and now expects family members (and medical caregivers) to acquiesce with his or her wishes.

> Dr. Adams, a distinguished and now retired neurosurgeon, insisted on
> undergoing experimental treatment for his inoperable pancreatic carci-
> noma, although his physicians opined that his age and general condition
> placed him at substantial risk. Overruling the oncologists' recommenda-
> tions for more conservative care and his wife's pleas, he started the
> experimental protocol only to die prematurely and painfully from treatment
> complications. His wife, who was present at the time, suffered recurrent
> nightmares of the event and profound guilt that she had allowed him as
> always to dictate, and sought psychotherapy for depression.

Developmental Stage of the Patient and the Family

We tend to let go of the aged chronically ill more readily than the young person. Use of advance directives may differ with age. The elderly who have children are more likely to avoid advance directives with the expectation that family members would know their wishes and act responsibly—as if decision making diffused throughout the family might extend the older person's autonomy (11).

The impact of illness and death on a family may differ with the family's stage of development. There is a higher incidence of marital breakup in younger families faced with severe illness of a child than in older families (12). The older family often has had more experience coping with crisis and can usually sustain stress better than a couple early in their marriage.

> Donna and Chuck, in their early 20s, were married only 5 months when Donna's acute leukemia was discovered. Both were still in school and financially dependent on their parents. Donna's parents, who viewed the young couple as "children playing house," took over direction of her care, selected her physicians, and carefully monitored every decision. At first Donna felt uneasy about their intrusion, but, as Chuck sought support from his classmates, she encouraged her parents and siblings to spend more time with her. Chuck felt increasingly helpless and guilty, and when Donna died 4 months later, he was spending much time with Rosemary, Donna's best friend and "a good listener."

Degree of Family Cohesion

The degree of alliance with and responsibility felt by family members for each other influences the extent to which they will support and sacrifice for one another, though family size also affects responses. Families with broad networks of extended relatives and generations may withstand the stress of a member's protracted illness better than does a small but highly coordinated family, which can eventually weary under the strain of care and "extrude" the sick member (13).

> Ms. Lee, a single working parent, had reared her daughter and a retarded son with little help from her family or the children's father. Her daughter, Jan, was taught to be a big sister to Joey, walking him to special classes in school and baby sitting for him after school while mother worked. As the children entered adulthood, Jan continued to share in her brother's care, transporting him to and from the sheltered workshop,

and the family was proud of its "can do" attitude. When Joey developed kidney failure, the women agreed once again to oversee his special diet and to spell each other on trips to dialysis, rearranging their work schedules. In the ensuing months, Ms. Lee developed headaches and hypertension; Jan became depressed and complained that she had "no life of my own." For a brief time Joey was boarded with Ms. Lee's sister and aging mother, but his medical management was erratic, and within months he was placed in a nursing home.

If divorce has divided a family, the crisis of a member's critical or terminal illness can reignite old loyalty conflicts, as, for instance, when a patient's second wife (his next of kin) and children from a first marriage disagree. This can lead to polarization of views within the family and triangulation of the treatment team members who find themselves unwittingly taking sides. Treatment decisions for a terminally ill minor in custody of one or another parent can stir bitter parental conflicts.

Persons with distant, uninvolved, or no family are apt to feel they have less to live for, relatively lacking as they are in support, reciprocity, and commitment to and from others. The incentive to survive to provide for others or to see children or grandchildren grow up is attenuated. Such persons may have alienated themselves from family members secondary to abusive relationships or substance abuse, and depression may contribute to their rejecting aggressive treatment. However, those with no known relatives can also feel they have less to live for, without depression being evident. A variation on this theme is the individual who *claims* to have no living relatives (though in fact such exist) because he or she does not want relatives contacted; in this instance the patient may actually feel a strong tie to the family he or she is so vigorously avoiding. Of course, if such a person then becomes incompetent to make decisions, the treatment team's task is the greater.

Definition of the Family

Legal definitions of next of kin, as described earlier in this chapter, do not always correspond with actuality. For example, sometimes a patient's lesbian/gay partner is not consulted even though she or he may know the patient's wishes better than does the family of origin (14). And sometimes crises of health care foster shifts in family boundaries, as in the following example.

> Mary and Chris had been life partners for years. Mary's family had distanced themselves because they did not approve of the relationship, and the local gay community had provided the couple a broad substitute "family.". Mary developed an inoperable hepatoma, and Chris devotedly nursed her until Mary bled and became disoriented. The medical team, in this case recognizing the relationship, consulted Chris, who had known that Mary wanted no heroic measures. However, Chris believed that Mary's family should be given an opportunity for a final rapprochement. She managed to locate a distant nephew and a brother of Mary's, who flew in for a family meeting with the medical staff, and the three jointly agreed to stop all but comfort measures.

Granting a trusted person durable power of attorney circumvents the priority list of family members. Thus, the patient who deems her children to have views incompatible with her own could execute a durable power of attorney specifying a trusted friend.

Structural Characteristics of the Family

Role attributions and expectations, functionality, communication patterns within and outside the family, values, problem-solving styles, and mythology (e.g., "The Johnsons have always been fighters"; "No one on his father's side could make a decision") are all aspects of family structure.

In some families, authority to make decisions is determined by age or gender. Some families have rules about sharing information or feelings with those outside the family, with some distrusting outsiders or disparaging expression of emotion as weak. A "closed system" family may rebuff staff interest and share little, including information about their basis for decision making. Sometimes information is withheld to cover family secrets such as an incestuous relationship, or internal feuds over inheritance rights. A family member can become a self-appointed bastion for the patient against the world, as was the case with the patient's sister in the following case example.

Mr. Carr's surgeons had repeatedly asked his sister to consent to a do-not-resuscitate (DNR) order, and she had repeatedly refused. Mr. Carr was an elderly, African-American man with dementia, cardiovascular disease, and mesenteric ischemia who had twice suffered cardiac arrest and been resuscitated, and the team felt he was being subjected to pain and suffering that he probably could not understand. When the staff tried to explore Ms. Carr's stance, she shared little information other than vague statements that her brother needed her. An ethics consultation was requested, and Ms. Carr then shared her sense that the young, white surgeons, in their importuning, had not respected her just as her well-educated brother had never received appropriate recognition or jobs commensurate with his ability because of race. She felt it her duty to see that he was now accorded maximal treatment as a sign of respect. With this understanding, the consultant helped negotiate a rapprochement between Ms. Carr and the treatment team.

Members of enmeshed families may have exaggerated needs to protect and depend on one another; rather than focusing anxiety or anger on the patient, family members may divert these feelings to the treatment team. Thus, members might seek information from one staff person and another; eventually the information becomes contradictory, staff people feel misquoted and pitted against one another, and tempers flare.

When Mrs. Davis had a massive myocardial infarct, her three grown sons arrived in the cardiac ICU with imposing large yellow legal pads and made copious notes of every move by and conversation with the staff; they transcribed their mother's bedside flow charts and information on the overhead cardiac monitor. As the brothers made many requests and questioned minor inconsistencies in explanations and routine, the staff grew defensive and angry. Psychiatric consultation was requested. It was then learned that the voluminous legal pad notes were being taken to a friend who worked in the hospital cafeteria so that he—as a hospital representative—might interpret them. Recognizing that the brothers' monitoring of their mother's care was based on anxiety in a strange environment, the staff then designated the nursing coordinator as the central person who would answer all the family's questions. This allayed anxiety for a time until Mrs. Davis had a fatal stroke. At that point the brothers called the local newspaper to report what they perceived as bad hospital care.

Family myths and traditions may also influence decision making.

Sam's family was struck by tragedy twice in rapid succession. A year before, his brother's 3-year-old son had died in a house fire, probably caused by the child's playing with matches. At the time, the boy's mother was out shopping, having left her son in the care of her friend, who evidently had napped. Sam's family, devastated and unforgiving, labeled their daughter-in-law a "murderer." Soon after, Sam needed vascular bypass surgery; he developed a wound dehiscence that required care in the surgical ICU. As his mental status waxed and waned, his young wife would panic and bolt from the unit, fearful that she might have to become his surrogate and risk making a decision for which she too would be branded by his family as was her sister-in-law.

A family that has experienced great trauma may adapt to the lingering sense of vulnerability by mutual overprotection of family members across generations. Such persons become very anxious if medical caregivers seem indifferent to their perceived danger.

When her father was hospitalized for the workup of a slowly growing prostate tumor (the prognosis for which might be measured in years), Mrs. Miller, a social worker, sat vigil at his bedside as if death were imminent. Fearful of leaving her father alone even for a moment, she insisted that the attending physician meet her at the bedside to discuss treatment options. The busy urologist left a message that he would only be free to meet at a specified time at his office in another building. Upset, Mrs. Miller grew more insistent, a control struggle ensued, and she then tried to mount a campaign to have the physician removed from staff. After psychiatric consultation was requested, it was learned that Mrs. Miller was the daughter of concentration camp survivors, reared in an atmosphere of anxious overprotection; she had entered social work in part to rescue the oppressed. Special sensitivity was needed to reassure her.

Families with limited personal and financial resources are especially vulnerable to suspicion that caregiver institutions will withhold that to which they are entitled. This vulnerability may result from many factors, including general distrust of public institutions, anticipation of helplessness in potentially adversarial relations, and projected need to conserve limited resources.

Mr. Fields lived in squalid conditions with his wife and psychiatrically disabled son. A series of strokes had left him with dementia, bedbound, and unable to swallow without choking. The hygiene of the home was such that visiting nurses finally refused to visit, and he developed deep decubitus ulcers. He was then hospitalized for surgical repair of the ulcers, whereupon a series of treatment and ethical dilemmas ensued. After improving Mr. Fields's nutrition with tube feedings, the surgical staff planned to operate, and the patient would then be discharged to a nursing home. Mr. Fields's wife, as his proxy, supported the plan as well as a DNR decision. His son, on learning this, rejected the DNR as a signal that his father was not getting everything to which he was entitled; he exhorted his mother to reject the plan (thus effectively becoming the proxy himself) and take his father home, in effect to die. As Mr. Fields was not considered terminally ill, the surgeons were uncomfortable with such a plan and began tube feeding. Only then was it discovered that Mr. Fields had a large, probably inoperable, esophageal tumor. The staff now deemed it most humane for the family to take him home as they had wished. At this point the family members changed their minds and insisted on nursing home placement as a service to which they had a right.

The ambivalence felt by dysfunctional families toward an addicted, alcoholic, or abusive member can kindle ambivalence within a treatment team, resulting in indecision and vacillation over treatment decisions.

Mr. Grant, a 52-year-old man with chronic alcoholism and advanced cirrhosis, appeared to have "nine lives." He was admitted once again to the medical ICU, with bleeding from varices, sepsis, encephalopathy, and a coagulopathy. On each previous admission he had somehow pulled through and left the hospital. Now, the usual medical interventions failed; he was intubated and had received more than 100 units of blood products. His wife opposed a DNR decision, unsure that this was his final event; besides, what if he recovered and learned of her decision? Further, she loudly deplored not having hospitalized him at the most prestigious hospital in town. Her sons, who had witnessed much domestic violence in their father's drunken rages, were less inclined to oppose a DNR order. But given Mrs. Grant's insistence on "doing everything," a surgical bypass procedure was considered, although the surgical service deemed Mr. Grant too great an operative risk. The medical staff were divided: Should they tell the family that everything had already been tried and that it was time to stop? Should they pressure the surgical service to attempt the procedure? The two services met and negotiated criteria that the patient would have to meet before being considered a surgical candidate. Unexpectedly, the patient improved. The surgical service now delayed a final decision for 72 hours, at which time the patient again bled. An ethics consultation was obtained. The medical attending physician then declared further treatment futile, and the patient died. In retrospect, the medical staff wished that they had been more realistic with Mrs. Grant about the fact that all reasonable options had been exhausted despite everyone's best efforts toward recovery.

Individual Psychopathology

The treatment team may also become triangulated by psychopathology within family members.

> Mr. Harris, a person with chronic schizophrenia, was shot in an argument by his son, Jimmy, who also was schizophrenic. He was rendered paraplegic, and in the surgical ICU he developed failing kidneys and fistulous tracts. Jimmy went to jail; if his father died, Jimmy would be tried for murder. Mr. Harris refused most health care, only accepting dialysis on his better days. Despite his mental illness he was considered by his psychiatrist to be competent to make healthcare decisions. Sympathetic to both father and son, the staff were in conflict over how aggressively to treat Mr. Harris. Striving to resolve their conflict, they appealed to a second psychiatrist, who judged the patient incompetent. They were thus enabled—with family sanction—to force treatment. Despite treatment, Mr. Harris died and Jimmy went to trial.

Denial, Guilt, and Anger

That family members may press for cure rather than care—in effect, for prolonged dying—is not surprising if they are struggling with disbelief, helplessness, or guilt at the impending loss. The "Daughter from California Syndrome" is a classic example (15). In this scenario, a devoted, unmarried daughter cares for her mother, who is declining in health and has dementia, until nursing home placement becomes inevitable.

In the nursing home the mother becomes acutely ill, and after hospitalization, a DNR order is discussed with the daughter, who agrees, believing her mother would have wished this. A second daughter, from California, who has had no contact with her mother for years, arrives and accuses her sister of scheming to get the mother's estate, insisting that the DNR be withdrawn, and threatening to sue unless her mother is immediately transferred to the ICU. The first daughter withdraws, intimidated, while the hospital staff try to deal with the second daughter's denial and guilt. She returns to California, never to return for her mother's funeral. (In California, this is known as the "Daughter from New York Syndrome.")

Communication of Treatment Wishes to Proxies

Although patients assume that their families will make appropriate decisions for them by proxy (16), studies show that neither families nor physicians are good predictors of the patient's wishes without prior discussion (17–23) (Table 4–1). These studies generally involve presenting elderly patients with hypothetical illness scenarios and comparing their choices of more or less aggressive treatment with those that close family members and medical caregivers would make for them. Concordance with patient choice was no better than chance in many instances. Families tended to choose more treatment, and physicians less treatment, than the patient endorsed. In Hare's sample, patients and families each addressed what they considered to be issues for the other; deciding factors for patients were "burden on others" and "time left to live," whereas for families the deciding factor was the patient's degree of pain (24). However, family proxies for incompetent patients sometimes knowingly choose contrary to the patient's previously expressed wishes (25).

Even though these studies are only questionnaire-based and not comparable methodologically, they raise important questions. Why do families and physicians diverge from patients and from each other in their choice of treatment aggressiveness? One answer is that many people are unaware of the relatively low ICU survival rates among the aged and chronically ill; when older persons were given realistic information on ICU survival, their DNR choices tended to increase (26). Further, sick people tend to have more positive perceptions of their quality of life than do others (27, 28). Nor to be discounted is the role played by a proxy's anticipatory grief and guilt, which may foster requests to prolong life.

Whether families make good proxies is another question. Given their emotional involvement, the potential for conflicts of interest, the observation that they may choose contrary to their understanding of patient wishes, that they may be influenceable (as in the case of Mrs. Fields) and surrender decision making to others, and that they may even be incompetent (29), would it be wiser to regularly appoint persons *outside* the family as alternatives? Or would greater familiarity with advance directives help people to consider and communicate autonomous choices earlier, help minimize uncertainty and guilt among family members, and diminish the numbers of dubious proxies? These questions invite further study. However, the importance of communicating treatment preferences before proxy decisions are to be made is evident.

Sophistication

Unfortunately, not all families are medically sophisticated enough to be good decision-makers. For instance, some rural families, overwhelmed by high-technology monitors, tubes, and ventilators and the alien environment of an ICU, become withdrawn and seek to protect themselves and their loved one by insisting that "everything"—that is, cardiopulmonary resuscitation (CPR)—be done (L. Rustad, personal communication, 1993). Distrustful of the setting, and feeling the patient's vulnerability and their own, they may respond by feeling they must "do something" rather than give up. Better educated families are more likely to attend ethics committee meetings, confident in their ability to articulate their views, although they too may request "everything."

Ethnicity and Religion

Minority status can heighten a family's distrust of the treatment team. In a study of preferences of frail elderly for CPR or DNR orders, Torian

Table 4–1. Patient and proxy choice discordance

Authors	Subjects	Method	Outcome
Seckler et al. (17)	70 competent elderly clinic patients, their family members, and primary care physicians	Patient and "proxies" compared for choice of CPR under conditions for current health or progressive dementia	Patients assumed that both physicians and family members would choose as did patient; family members overselected resuscitation; physicians overwithheld care that patients wanted
Uhlmann et al. (18)	258 elderly outpatients, spouses, and primary care physicians	Patient and "proxies" compared for choice of resuscitation under conditions of present health, CVA, COPD	Agreement with patient no better than chance for physicians and only slightly better for spouses; spouses overselected, and physicians underselected, relative to patient choice
Ouslander et al. (19)	70 elderly residents of long-term care facility, close relatives, and medical staff person	Patients and "proxies" compared for choices of four high- and low-risk procedures	Overall rates of agreement were low; agreement with patient closer for relative than for physician
Danis et al. (20)	126 competent nursing home residents and 49 family members of incompetent residents	Competent nursing home residents and family members of incompetent residents compared for choices of CPR, hospitalization, ICU, ventilation, surgery, and tube-feeding if patient was critically/terminally ill or permanently unconscious	Family members chose less life-sustaining treatment when patient was incompetent than did competent patient for self

Study	Sample	Methods	Findings
Zweibel and Cassel (21)	55 elderly outpatients and 107 physician-designated proxy relatives	Outpatients and physician-designated proxy relatives compared for choices of CPR, ventilation, cancer chemotherapy, amputation, and tube-feeding in vignettes of incompetent patients	There was trend toward patients requesting CPR that proxies decline, and proxies requesting ventilation, amputation, and tube-feeding that patients decline
Cogen et al. (22)	102 family surrogates for nursing home patients with dementia	Surrogates asked intervention choices (CPR, hospitalization, ICU, ventilator, tube-feeding) in five hypothetical clinical situations	Surrogates favored aggressive hospital treatment, with their choice unrelated to previously stated wishes of resident
Hare et al. (23)	50 young outpatients and 50 patient-selected surrogates in a family practice	Patients and surrogates compared for intervention choices similar to those in study by Danis et al. (20); substituted judgment asked of surrogates	Agreement within pairs only 70% of time (no better than chance)

Note. CPR = cardiopulmonary resuscitation; CVA = cardiovascular accident; COPD = chronic obstructive pulmonary disease; ICU = intensive care unit.

and colleagues (30) observed in a New York hospital that some Hispanic patients and families feared that discussion about CPR was the
treatment team's indirect way of conveying a poor prognosis or that it
implied the team was reluctant to fully extend treatment. In a questionnaire study comparing African Americans, Hispanic Americans,
and non-Hispanic white American subjects' attitudes, Caralis and colleagues (31) found that African Americans and Hispanic Americans
wanted life-prolonging treatment more often than did non-Hispanic
white Americans regardless of illness states such as persistent vegetative state or terminal illness. Elderly Korean Americans and Mexican
Americans questioned in senior citizen centers were more likely to
hold a family-centered model of medical decision making than the
patient autonomy model favored by African American and European
American subjects (32).

Some cultures are more fatalistic and accepting of death than others.
Pious Muslims believe death is part of God's plan and that to struggle
against it is wrong, while Jews as a group prize survival and fight
against death (33). Mexican Americans appear to be more accepting of
death than are white Americans (34, 35). Catholics as a group may be
more ready to accept DNR orders (36). Fundamentalist Christians who
believe in divine intervention may incline toward doing everything to
maintain life ("God needs help healing the patient").

Economic Pressures

One day of ICU care now costs thousands of dollars. The cost of
prolonged health care can sway a family (or patient) to choose to
hasten death, particularly in countries without universal health care.

Rob had worked summers and weekends toward his college tuition, and
his parents had also helped with the fund. He was to enter college in the
fall. Meanwhile, his grandmother had been battling breast cancer for
2 years, undergoing chemotherapy and radiation treatments. As she
grew sicker, she moved in with her daughter and son-in-law. Rob gave
up his room, and the family vacation was postponed. When Grandmother developed bony pain, her physicians recommended bone marrow transplant as a next logical step. Because this procedure was not

covered by insurance, it would have to be financed from Rob's college fund. The family was faced with choosing between the futures of two of its members. Grandmother then declared that she had lived a good life and had had enough.

Illness Variables

Certain illnesses are more readily perceived than others to carry a poor prognosis. In Smedira's study of decision making in ICUs, families were more likely to agree with physicians' recommendations to limit care to patients with metastatic cancer and severe head injuries than to those with multiple organ failure or respiratory failure (37). An illness like AIDS, inviting fears of contagion and stigmatization of lifestyles, can reinforce family decisions to withhold and withdraw treatment.

Conversely, family members may feel especially identified with and want to rescue the patient who has a genetic or familial disorder, or with the critically ill transplant patient for whom a family member was a donor.

Anniversaries and Special Family Events

When the sick person is, say, 99 years old, the prospect of claiming a centenarian may blind family members to her suffering. Or the only unmarried daughter of the family may resist a DNR decision for her father, hoping he will survive to walk her down the aisle.

Talking With Patients and Families About Treatment Withdrawal

Miles describes just how hard it can be for physicians to talk realistically with chronically ill and dying patients about treatment planning and to gauge their quality of life because of the physician's dread of his or her own aging, disability, and death or belief that the patient is as demoralized by his or her condition as is the physician (38). Whether discussion involves DNR status, treatment options such as antibiotics or nutrition, or treatment futility, the time and effort spent in talk is critical.

Ideally, patient and family should be involved in decision making long before implementation is necessary. Youngner points out that a DNR decision may be an ideal vehicle to foster conversation about treatment goals, because it anticipates an event is yet to be and thus is not so immediately threatening (39). Of course, involvement of family members allows them to hear what the patient wishes and why (40–43). Even when a living will exists, it is important to explore specific treatment preferences—for example, resuscitation in the event of a persistent vegetative state, antibiotics, fluids, and nutrition.

When there is a medically preferred plan, such as stopping ventilation, the physician should recommend it rather than assume a neutral, "It's up to you to decide" position. Making a firm recommendation implies shared responsibility and helps to relieve a family's "executioner's guilt" (E. Cassem, personal communication, 1993).

Those who attend terminally ill patients attest to the importance of continued and frequent reports of progress (or lack thereof) with patients and family members in order to enhance mutual problem-solving and trust and to better understand a family's values and goals (44, 45). Thus, Lee and colleagues approach treatment withdrawal in the medical ICU by discussing projections of probable survival and functional outcomes with families and patients, also explicitly using a "therapeutic trial" of, say, ventilation, vasopressors, or dialysis; they emphasize that discussions are prolonged, decision making gradual, and the effort one of "patient-doctor accommodation" rather than acquiescence to a preconceived medical decision (46).

There is some debate over the discussion of futile interventions. Hackler and Hiller propose that in some cases in which CPR would be futile, physicians should be allowed to write DNR orders without family consent or discussion. They argue that "there is no point in making families agonize over the matter and worry that they are breaking faith with their loved ones. To do so may create unnecessary suffering, strife, or guilt and may produce deadlock with an unsophisticated, death-denying or guilt-ridden family" (47). Proponents for discussion of futile interventions (48–50) point out that, because of pervasive media coverage, most laypersons are well aware of the use of CPR and are likely to question why it was not invoked for their loved one; further, although families should not be offered the *choice* of futile interventions, they deserve the *courtesy* of being told why these should be withheld: ". . . once physicians have determined that CPR is futile and should not be performed, they should so inform patients and families. To do otherwise is to discourage communication and feedback at a time when they are essential" (51). Caralis and colleagues, in their study of ethnic and racial influences on end-of-life decisions, noted that the majority of their patients disagreed with doctors' making decisions unilaterally (52). In practice, however, physicians have indeed made unilateral decisions, both without any discussion or in opposition to family requests (53).

There are, of course, instances in which family wishes to maintain treatment in hopelessly ill patients are to be honored. For example, one might continue to ventilate a brain-dead patient another day or so to allow the family to cope with grief or to permit a distant family member to travel to the scene if scarce medical resources are not an issue (54).

Ruark and colleagues caution against rushing decision making with families. Setting time-limited goals based on clinical judgment is advised—for example, "If we see no signs that your father has improved over the next 72 hours, then we believe you should consider withdrawing life support." The time interval allows family members to express anger, grief, and mistrust and to let go emotionally. Ruark et al. give helpful examples of wording—for example, "It is my best judgment, and that of the other doctors and nurses, that your relative has essentially no chance of regaining a reasonable quality of life. We believe that life support should be withdrawn, which means that your relative will probably die" (55).

Disagreements Between the Family and the Treatment Team

When the patient is less able to speak for himself, life support decisions generally fall to the medical team and the family. However, as the data on proxy decisions without prior discussion suggest, families and physicians—each assuming the role of advocate for the patient—may disagree about the use of life support. Families can oppose medical recommendations both to treat and not to treat. In the historic Quinlan and Cruzan cases, families sought to stop life support when there seemed little chance for recovery, but they encountered hospital opposition in an era when judicial guidelines for treatment withdrawal in an incompetent patient had not yet been developed. In some instances, families have requested withdrawal of life support, but physicians have refused because they thought the patient still had a reasonable chance to recover and they believed the families might not be acting in the incompetent patient's best interests (56). Yet another area for disagreement lies in requests by families for treatment that the medical team deems futile.

How often do disagreements arise, and how are conflicts resolved? The few studies in this area indicate that disagreement is relatively uncommon. In Bedell's chart review of DNR orders among patients with end-stage illness, when families were surrogate decision-makers, disagreement was noted in only 6 of 335 cases. Factors thought to aid families in supporting DNR decisions included 1) awareness that the prognosis was virtually hopeless in the presence of coma or brain death, 2) support given by staff and their reassurances that the family was doing the right thing, 3) ongoing assurance that the staff would maintain medical care and comfort for the patient, and 4) the patient's and family's prior discussion about resuscitation (57). In Smedira and colleagues' questionnaire study of decision making in two ICUs, it was found that of 102 families with mostly incompetent relatives, all but 10 initially agreed with physician recommendations to limit care; of these 10, all but two agreed with medical recommendations to withhold treatment after having a few days to grieve and accept the severity of the illness (58).

Thus, prolonged conflict between the family and treatment team appears to be infrequent. But what about when family and physicians continue to disagree? And does physician bias play a role? Brennan reviewed 20 ethics committee cases in which physicians had written DNR orders for terminally ill, incompetent patients against family wishes, and compared them with 105 cases of patients for whom physicians and families agreed on DNR status. He found that in the 20 cases reviewed by the ethics committee the patients were much sicker and that the physicians' decisions were based on medical futility; these patients were no more poor, demented, alcoholic, disruptive, or older than the 105 patients in the control group (59). In discussing how the families of these 20 cases were approached, Brennan noted:

> The . . . [ethics committee] and the attending physician spoke with the family in each of these cases and stated that do-not-resuscitate status was appropriate because every effort had been made to save the patient, that now the patient's chances for survival were getting smaller, and that further care would not benefit the patient and could needlessly prolong his or her suffering. Families were told that the decisions about do-not-resuscitate status were based solely on the clinical status of the patient; socioeconomic and difficulty of care issues were not part of the decision. (60)

However, physician bias and deception of families can indeed occur (61, 62).

Interventions When Families Disagree

Family members may disagree both among themselves and with the treatment team. Family opposition to treatment team recommendations is likely to increase in proportion to the number of family members. Paradis notes that "family members who believe that termination of aggressive treatment is in the best interest of the patient, even if in the majority, will accede to the request of one individual to continue care" (63).

Discussing intrafamily conflict over decision making, as in the "Daughter from California Syndrome," Molloy and colleagues (64) offer a number of specific suggestions:

1. Convene a meeting with all family members wishing to be involved in decision making for the incompetent patient, and invite all members of the healthcare team.
2. Give the family a consistent, simple description of the patient's condition and prognosis.
3. Outline in simple terms the specific areas for decision making (i.e., resuscitation, antibiotics, routine laboratory tests, nutrition, and hydration).

4. Give over control to the family for reaching a consensus and then informing the treatment team of their decision.
5. Nominate one family member to communicate with a designated team member.
6. Set a deadline for the family to inform the treatment team of their decision; arrange follow-up meetings; and provide a mechanism for them to continue to ask questions and to receive updates on the patient's condition.

With respect to the dysfunctional family who splits the treatment team, Gonda and Ruark (65) devote an entire section of their excellent book to management. They advocate close attention to communication within the team and designating one team member as the person with whom the family should communicate.

When families and the medical team continue to disagree, second opinions, ethics committee consultations, and, on rare occasions, court interventions may be the next steps. We are now entering the era when local courts are recognizing the physician's right to withdraw treatment in medically futile situations (66).

Both an ethics committee and mental health professionals aid resolution of conflict by listening to all parties and helping them to clarify the issues. In addition, the psychiatrist can help resolve issues of patient competence, provide family assessment, offer counseling to the family around loss-related issues, help negotiate conflicts over control between family and staff, and facilitate resolution of disagreement among staff.

Conclusion

Families are clearly integral to the decision-making process. They can give one a sense of the patient's values and goals as well as their own. Though reluctance to discuss treatment wishes and planning sometimes occurs among patients, families, and/or medical caregivers, discussion is vital to understanding and communication of prognoses and helps mitigate conflicts. Though the present healthcare system allows little time to listen to and share information with families, this is especially critical for families in crisis.

Research issues that need to be addressed in the future include

1. *Effect of treatment decisions on family.* Although most families go along with physician and patient decisions, we know little about the actual incidence of unconflicted endorsement, ambivalence, or silent disagreement, or about the course of such responses over time or the outcome in terms of later behaviors. Nor, for that matter, do we know the outcome for those who openly disagree. What later happens to those experiencing regret over treatment decisions? Is the incidence of pathologic grieving greater among proxies who choose to restrict treatment than among those who do not? What later happens to the "daughter from California" and others with unresolved denial and guilt? What of the patient who regains the ability to speak for himself or herself and disagrees with family decisions? In such situations, what is the emotional fallout within the family?

2. *Identification of high-risk family members.* There is a need to identify high-risk family members. Demographic high-risk screening is now used in some hospitals to identify homeless, unemployed, and low-income patients; similarly, a family high-risk profile addressing questions of family values and previous experience with loss could be developed and tested for screening and follow-up.

3. *Development and testing of intervention strategies.* There is a need to develop and test intervention strategies. We now recognize the importance of heightening staff sensitivity to cultural diversity, educating consumers and caregivers about advance directives, and fostering communication among family and treatment team members. However, much of our information is anecdotal. Interventions such as the use of family support groups in hospitals might be tested with outcome parameters of, for example, incidence of near-term physical and psychological distress among participants and controls.

4. *Effects of changes in the healthcare system.* What will be the impact of looming changes in health care, such as managed health care, with its emphasis on cost containment and shortened lengths of stay? If HMOs further limit care, might families feel relieved of some responsibility for decision making?

These are just a few of the issues that have surfaced with the advent of new technology. As we approach the end of the twentieth century, we should anticipate growing experience in this problematic and emotion-laden area.

References

1. Brody H: The Healer's Power. New Haven, CT, Yale University Press, 1992, pp 183–184
2. Hardwig J: What about the family? Hastings Cent Rep 20(2):5–10, 1990
3. Evans EL, Brody BA: The do-not-resuscitate order in teaching hospitals. JAMA 253:2236–2239, 1985
4. Finucane TE, Denman SJ: Deciding about resuscitation in a nursing home: theory and practice. J Am Geriatr Soc 37:684–688, 1989
5. Caralis PV, Hammond JS: Attitudes of medical students, housestaff and faculty physicians toward euthanasia and termination of life-sustaining treatment. Crit Care Med 20:683–690, 1992
6. Blackhall LJ, Murphy ST, Frank G, et al: Ethnicity and attitudes toward patient autonomy. JAMA 274:820–825, 1995
7. Snider GL: Withholding and withdrawing life-sustaining therapy. Am J Respir Crit Care Med 151:279–281, 1995
8. Gonda TA, Ruark JE: Dying Dignified: The Health Professional's Guide to Care. Reading, MA, Addison-Wesley, 1984, p 138
9. Brody B: Life and Death Decision Making. New York, Oxford University Press, 1988, pp 221–225
10. Brody, Life and Death Decision Making, p 163
11. High DM: All in the family: extended autonomy and expectations in surrogate health care decision-making. Gerontologist 28:46–51, 1988
12. Lansky SB, Cairns NU, Hassanein R, et al: Childhood cancer: parental discord and divorce. Pediatrics 62:184–188, 1978
13. Reiss D, Gonzalez S, Kramer N: Family process, chronic illness, and death: on the weakness of strong bonds. Arch Gen Psychiatry 43:795–804, 1986
14. Steinbrook R, Lo B, Tirpack J, et al: Ethical dilemmas in caring for patients with the acquired immunodeficiency syndrome. Ann Intern Med 103:787–790, 1985
15. Molloy DW, Clarnette RM, Braun EA, et al: Decision making in the incompetent elderly: "The Daughter from California Syndrome." J Am Geriatr Soc 39:396–399, 1991

16. High, All in the family
17. Seckler AB, Meier DE, Mulvihill M, et al: Substituted judgment: how accurate are proxy predictions? Ann Intern Med 115:92–98, 1991
18. Uhlmann RF, Pearlman RA, Cain KC: Physicians' and spouses' predictions of elderly patients' resuscitation preferences. Journal of Gerontology 43:M115–M121, 1988
19. Ouslander J, Tymchuk A, Rahbar B: Health care decisions among elderly long-term residents and their potential proxies. Arch Intern Med 149:1367–1372, 1989
20. Danis M, Southerland LI, Garrett JM, et al: A prospective study of advance directives for life-sustaining care. N Engl J Med 324:882–888, 1991
21. Zweibel NR, Cassel CK: Treatment choices at the end of life: a comparison of decisions by older patients and their physician-selected proxies. Gerontologist 29:615–621, 1989
22. Cogen R, Patterson B, Chavin S, et al: Surrogate decision-maker preferences for medical care of severely demented nursing home patients. Arch Intern Med 152:1885–1888, 1992
23. Hare J, Pratt C, Nelson C: Agreement between patients and their self-selected surrogates on difficult medical decisions. Arch Intern Med 152:1049–1054, 1992
24. Hare et al, Agreement between patients and their self-selected surrogates
25. Cogen et al, Surrogate decision-maker preferences for medical care
26. Schonwetter RS, Walker RM, Kramer DR, et al: Resuscitation decision making in the elderly: the value of outcome data. J Gen Intern Med 8:295–300, 1993
27. Uhlmann et al, Physicians' and spouses' predictions
28. Schonwetter et al, Resuscitation decision making
29. McCrary SV, Allen WL, Young CL: Questionable competency of a surrogate decision maker under a durable power of attorney. J Clin Ethics 4:166–168, 1993
30. Torian LV, Davidson EJ, Fillit HM, et al: Decisions for and against resuscitation in an acute geriatric medicine unit serving the frail elderly. Arch Intern Med 152:561–565, 1992
31. Caralis PV, Davis B, Wright K, et al: The influence of ethnicity and race on attitudes toward advance directives, life-prolonging treatments and euthanasia. J Clin Ethics 4:155–165, 1993
32. Blackhall et al, Ethnicity and attitudes toward patient autonomy
33. Neuberger J: Cultural issues in palliative care, in Oxford Textbook of Palliative Care. Edited by Doyle D, Hanks GWC, MacDonald N. Oxford, UK, Oxford University Press, 1993, pp 505–513

34. Gonda and Ruark, Dying Dignified, pp 293–295
35. Kalish R, Reynolds D: Death and Ethnicity. Los Angeles, University of Southern California Press, 1976
36. Brennan TA: Incompetent patients with limited care in the absence of family consent. Ann Intern Med 109:819–825, 1988
37. Smedira NG, Evans BH, Grais LS, et al: Withholding and withdrawal of life support from the critically ill. N Engl J Med 322:309–315, 1990
38. Miles SH: Physicians and their patients' suicides. JAMA 271:1786–1788, 1994
39. Youngner SJ: Futility in context. JAMA 264:1295–1296, 1990
40. Snider GL: Withholding and withdrawing life-sustaining therapy. Am J Respir Crit Care Med 151:279–281, 1995
41. Bedell SE, Pelle D, Maher PL, et al: Do-not-resuscitate orders for critically ill patients in the hospital: how are they used and what is their impact? JAMA 256:233–237, 1986
42. Havlir D, Brown L, Rousseau GK: Do not resuscitate discussions in a hospital-based home care program. J Am Geriatr Soc 37:52–54, 1989
43. Ruark JE, Raffin TA, Stanford UMC Committee on Ethics: Initiating and withdrawing life support. N Engl J Med 318:25–30, 1988
44. Lee DKP, Swinburne AJ, Fedullo AJ, et al: Withdrawing care: experience in a medical intensive care unit. JAMA 271:1358–1361, 1994
45. Tomlinson T, Brody H: Futility and the ethics of resuscitation. JAMA 264:1276–1280, 1990
46. Lee et al, Withdrawing care
47. Hackler JC, Hiller FC: Family consent to orders not to resuscitate: reconsidering hospital policy. JAMA 264:1281–1283, 1990
48. Brody H: The Healer's Power. New Haven, CT, Yale University Press, 1992, pp 183–184
49. Youngner, Futility in context
50. Tomlinson and Brody, Futility and the ethics of resuscitation
51. Youngner, Futility in context, p 1296
52. Caralis et al, The influence of ethnicity and race
53. Schneiderman LJ, Spragg RG: Sounding Board: Ethical decisions in discontinuing mechanical ventilation. N Engl J Med 318:984–988, 1988
54. Schneiderman and Spragg, Sounding Board: Ethical decisions
55. Ruark et al: Initiating and withdrawing life support, p 29
56. Ashe DA, Hanson-Flaschen J, Lanken PN: Decisions to limit or continue life-sustaining treatment by critical care physicians in the United States: conflicts between physicians' practices and patients' wishes. Am J Respir Crit Care Med 151:288–292, 1995

57. Bedell et al, Do-not-resuscitate orders
58. Smedira et al, Withholding and withdrawal of life support
59. Brennan, Incompetent patients with limited care
60. Brennan, Incompetent patients with limited care, pp 823–824
61. Brennan, Incompetent patients with limited care
62. Edwards BS: Withdrawal of life support against family wishes: is it justified? A case study. J Clin Ethics 1:74–79, 1990
63. Paradis NA: Letter to the Editor. JAMA 265:354–355, 1991
64. Molloy et al, Decision making in the incompetent elderly
65. Gonda and Ruark, Dying Dignified
66. Court ruling limits rights of patients. New York Times, April 11, 1995

5

Obstacles to Doctor-Patient Communication at the End of Life

Mary F. Morrison, M.D.

In many ways, good communication is the key to good decision making at the end of life. As the dying process unfolds, however, patients become progressively less able to participate in discussions about their treatment options. Thus, there is a premium on early discussions—not only between patients and physicians but between patients and their families as well. Ideally, such discussions should take into account prognosis and how treatment decisions might best conform with the patient's goals and values. Most patients would like to discuss end-of-life decisions with their physicians in a timely manner, and most physicians believe that patients should have a role in these decisions (1, 2). Since neither patients nor physicians are likely to initiate them, however, early discussions are the exception, rather than the rule. Although the use of advance directives is now mandated by federal law, the situation has not substantially improved.

This chapter explores the obstacles to communication for both patients and health professionals. I argue that psychiatrists, who have traditionally been underinvolved, are strategically positioned to help investigate and resolve the barriers to communication among patients, families, and physicians. Finally, I offer some recommendations to facilitate patient-physician communication at the end of life.

The following case illustrates a typical situation involving end-of-life care:

> J.R. was an 85-year-old man who was transferred to a university hospital on an aortic balloon pump for an emergent coronary artery bypass. He had recently suffered his fifth myocardial infarction. On psychiatric evaluation, he was thought to be confused and to lack sufficient capacity to consent to surgery. No family members were involved with J.R. or were familiar with his wishes.
>
> By the next morning, the medical and surgical teams had decided that J.R.'s confusion and poor ejection fraction made him an inappropriate surgical candidate. After speaking to the resident, J.R. understood quite clearly that he was not a surgical candidate because his chance of mortality was too high. He was not able to comprehend, however, that he was on a balloon pump and that he would be weaned off; nor did he understand the consequences.

Even though J.R. had severe coronary artery disease, his end-of-life preferences had not been addressed. When it was important for physicians to know his preferences, J.R.'s mental capacity was too impaired for him to participate fully in decision making. There was no proxy for J.R. because family members were uninvolved and other support systems were not quickly identifiable. The healthcare personnel at the tertiary care institution did not know him and had had no opportunity to discuss his preferences. Although J.R. understood he was not a candidate for surgery, he had not been informed of the lifesaving importance of the balloon pump—or that his weaning from it would probably lead to his death. His lack of understanding may have been due to cognitive changes or to the difficulty his physician had discussing the withdrawal of treatment that would likely lead to his death.

Ideally, J.R.'s preferences regarding end-of-life care would have been addressed earlier by a physician with whom he had an ongoing relationship as an outpatient. At that time, his cognitive capacity most likely would have allowed him to participate in the discussion. The results of the discussion would have been recorded and accessible to health-care providers at the time of the crisis. Instead, the appropriate discussion was delayed until he was unable to participate; then, in the absence of informed family, a major decision had to be made.

J.R.'s experience reflects many of the problems in our present medical system, where end-of-life decisions are not addressed adequately with patients suffering from serious disease. Sometimes treating physicians are unaware of the wishes of patients who have addressed end-of-life decisions appropriately.

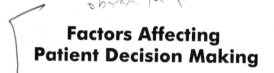

Factors Affecting
Patient Decision Making

Demographic Factors

Age, educational level, and gender are likely to be associated with different preferences for end-of-life discussion and decision making. Regardless of their ages, most respondents in a survey of outpatients in a family practice wanted the physician to bring up the issue of life-prolonging treatment (ages 18–40: 62%; ages 41–60: 73%; age 61 and older: 73%) (3). Only 11% did not want the physician to raise the issue.

In a 1982 survey that asked whether patients should make final choices, answers were influenced by age, income, health status, and education. Those patients in the poorest health (17%), the oldest (23%), the least educated (27%), and those with the lowest household incomes (32%) were far less likely to be in favor of patients making medical decisions in the face of serious illness than were their healthier (51%), younger (56%), better educated (52%), and wealthier (47%) counterparts (4).

In a more recent study of outpatient decision making that was not limited to end-of-life decisions, younger age was the strongest positive correlate of a patient's preference for making decisions (5). Other sociodemographic variables associated with stronger preferences for decision making were higher educational level; higher income; higher level of occupation; and divorced or separated marital status. Young, well-educated, and wealthy patients preferred making their own health-care decisions, whereas vulnerable patient populations appeared more likely to defer to physicians.

In the SUPPORT (Study to Understand Prognoses and Preferences for Outcomes and Risks of Treatment) study of seriously ill inpatients, a patient factor associated with not wanting to discuss cardiopulmonary resuscitation (CPR) was ethnicity and race other than black (6). In this study, being black and being younger were associated with wishing to discuss CPR preferences but not having done so. Similarly, Caralis found that in those who had not discussed preferences for life-sustaining treatment, more black (63%) and Hispanic (62%) persons desired such discussions than did non-Hispanic white persons (39%) (7).

Religious and Cultural Factors

Our social pluralism is reflected in the diversity of religious and cultural beliefs that inform individual moral decisions. Very little has been written about the role of these beliefs in end-of-life decisions, and they are not often discussed between doctors and patients. Moreover, the ways in which cultural and religious factors affect reactions to dying have not been well studied.

Religious denominations that have addressed end-of-life decisions all affirm the sanctity of life. However, there are different conceptions of the individual's obligation to accept treatment and the limits of that obligation (8), and physicians are not commonly aware of these teachings. The Vatican Declaration on Euthanasia specifies that a person does not have to accept "extraordinary" means to preserve his or her own life. "Extraordinary" means are all medicines, treatments, and operations that cannot be obtained or used without excessive expense, pain, or other inconvenience, or those that would not offer a reasonable hope of benefit. Many Protestant denominations also teach that a person may refuse life-sustaining measures that will "only prolong the dying process." Orthodox interpretation of Jewish law requires that one must accept all treatment that will preserve every possible moment of life until the patient is "very near" death.

Little is known about how the religious beliefs of the doctor and patient affect discussions and decisions about terminal care. If a physician is uncomfortable presenting all options to care because of religious beliefs, he or she is obliged to disclose that fact to the patient. It seems likely that a hospital with a religious affiliation may be biased in the presentation to the patient of end-of-life treatment alternatives; however, this phenomenon has not been studied.

To facilitate the interaction between religious beliefs about dying and secular medical institutions, some patients have opted for religious advance directives (9). Examples include the Catholic Health Association Affirmation of Life and the Jewish Health Care Proxy of Agudath Israel of America. Because the interpretation of these directives is subject to controversy, however, they can be more restrictive than the patient intended. Designating appropriate healthcare proxies and facilitating communication among patients, their agents, and healthcare providers are likely to better serve patient wishes.

Cultural factors also affect information seeking and reactions to death. The following case, described by Muller and Desmond (10), of a 49-year-old Cantonese-speaking woman from the People's Republic of China with metastatic lung cancer demonstrates some of the difficulties involved in relaying bad news, withholding treatment, and dealing with the family in a cross-cultural context.

Mrs. Lee (a pseudonym) was admitted to the hospital with a right-sided pneumonia secondary to metastatic squamous cell carcinoma. Neither Mrs. Lee nor her husband spoke English. Since their son Arnold spoke English, he became the spokesperson and assumed primary responsibility for decisions. Arnold did not wish to discuss his mother's diagnosis with her[,] and he did not want the physicians to speak to his mother through interpreters. The house staff caring for Mrs. Lee were concerned that the patient did not know her diagnosis and was unable to make her own decisions about the type and extent of treatment she should receive. Mrs. Lee's outpatient physician tried numerous times to discuss a do-not-resuscitate (DNR) order because of her poor prognosis. Arnold always accompanied his mother to her visits, however, and would not allow such a subject to be raised. Mrs. Lee developed and was treated for cord compression; two months later, she developed brain metastases. Two months after that she was admitted with a pneumonia and became unresponsive. The family adamantly refused to consider a DNR order and insisted that she receive all possible care. The house staff and attending felt that resuscitation would not only be medically futile, but would cause the patient great suffering and indignity. The attending physician wrote a DNR order in the patient's medical record and informed the patient's husband of the decision. The family reluctantly agreed to the order. As Mrs. Lee's condition worsened, her family became more visibly upset and vocal in their insistence on extensive and aggressive therapy. Arnold Lee insisted that his mother be intubated. When the attending physician denied his request, he became more distraught and accused the team of deliberately taking inadequate care of his mother because she was Chinese. The son's accusations of racial bias and threats of litigation continued until Mrs. Lee's death. (11)

Engaging in a discussion of prognosis or code status with a Chinese patient is viewed as casting a death curse, causing the person to despair and die even sooner (12). Chinese culture is a family-centered system. When a patient's illness is life-threatening, it is assumed that practitioners will talk with the family rather than the patient, who is to be protected (13, 14). The family in the case described by Muller and Desmond felt that the physicians' insistence on truth-telling was rude and dangerous to their mother. The differing values of the physicians and the family resulted in a breakdown of communication, mutual distrust, and frustration.

Mexican American patients also typically do not want to be informed that they have a terminal illness and are less likely to feel bound to communicate this information to a loved one (15).

If practitioners do not attempt to understand and bridge the gulf between their own values and those of their patients, they preclude meaningful and dignified deaths for their patients. Although some disagreements may not be able to be resolved, and not every patient may have wishes that mirror those of his or her culture, psychiatrists can be helpful in eliciting patient and family values. As objective physicians, psychiatrists can discuss the medical reality and its meaning to the patient and family. This process can then help the patient and family come to some understanding with the primary physician.

When the practitioner is dealing with terminal care issues with patients from cultures other than the practitioner's, it is critical to get as much information as possible about beliefs and values prior to the discussion. We, as American physicians, need to be sensitive to the fact that our culture as a whole is somewhat unique in its insistence on full disclosure.

Psychological Factors: Personal Preferences

The experience of most physicians suggests that patients do not bring up their preferences for end-of-life care. Several factors are involved in this omission. Dealing with end-of-life care is not an immediate priority when patients are healthy. Time is often at a premium during an outpatient visit, and end-of-life discussions can be particularly difficult and deserve not to be rushed. Denial of the possibility of becoming gravely ill and needing to address end-of-life decisions often plays a role. On the other hand, when patients do become ill, fear can make them reluctant to bring up end-of-life decisions. Patients may feel that if dying is not discussed, it will not be an issue. Some patients believe that it is the physician's job to initiate such discussions. A substantial proportion of patients appears confident that their physician will know their preferences for life-sustaining technology even though they have never been discussed (16). Finally, and unfortunately, patients may feel that their physician will not listen to or understand their concerns. Whether due to age, sex, cultural, or religious differences, these feelings of being unable to communicate become very important when an area as personal as dying is being discussed.

Personality Disorders

Personality disorders and poor coping styles can complicate discussions about end-of-life decisions and implementation of a plan for care. Although some degree of denial about one's illness may maintain hope and facilitate coping, severe denial or lack of insight about an illness and its consequences precludes meaningful discussion. A woman with widely metastatic breast cancer and a pathologic bone fracture who believes she has a routine arm fracture cannot participate in a meaningful discussion about her care. In fact, she may end up searching for another practitioner who agrees with her view.

The following case example illustrates how psychopathology can affect communication of end-of-life issues:

> A young man with borderline personality disorder developed leukemia. He would demand massive doses of benzodiazepines to cope with his chemotherapy and then, after having his request turned down, would abruptly leave the unit. This caused panic among the staff and anger toward the patient. The patient's level of sedation, his absences, and the resulting anger and frustration of the staff interfered with attempts to address his end-of-life preferences.

When psychopathology interferes with end-of-life discussion, psychiatrists can be helpful in identifying and ameliorating the problem.

Chronic Illness

A patient's disease and his or her prognosis affect end-of-life decision making and communication between the patient and physician. Despite the attention given to advance directives, and the fact that a majority of patients indicate a wish to discuss life-support therapy with their physicians before such therapy is required (17, 18), patients with chronic illnesses and limited life spans do not address end-of-life issues. Amyotrophic lateral sclerosis (ALS) is a motor neuron disease with a mean duration from diagnosis to death of 4 years. In one survey (19), the large majority of ALS patients (81%) said they wanted as much information as possible about their disease, with 70% saying that they would like to participate in decisions involving their own medical care. Although 81% said they thought their physician wanted to know their preferences about life-sustaining treatment, only 21% had actually discussed the issue. In the SUPPORT study of seriously ill, hospitalized patients, more medical comorbidity was associated with an increased likelihood of having discussed advanced directives (20). However, in this study the majority of seriously ill inpatients had not discussed and were not interested in discussing preferences for CPR (58%) or prolonged mechanical ventilation (80%). This important study suggests that there is a sizable population of hospitalized patients who do not want to discuss end-of-life issues.

Advance Directives

Advance directives were touted as a means of increasing physician-patient communication. A study of 115 cancer patients, however, suggests that advance directives do not significantly increase physician-patient communication about end-of-life decisions (21). Despite the fact that no study patient was estimated to have more than a 50% chance of surviving 5 years, only just more than half (55.7%) had executed some type of advance directive. It is also interesting to note that physicians usually do not know whether their patients have advance directives. When the physicians of the group of patients *with* advance directives were queried as to whether their patients had advance directives, 76% responded "no" or "I don't know." For the group of patients *without* advance directives, 90% of the physicians responded "no" or "I don't know." The study did indicate, however, that completion of an advance directive may increase the likelihood of the patient's having communicated his or her preferences to his or her physician ($P = 0.04$). Thirty-eight percent of patients with advance directives reported having a discussion of future treatment plans with their physicians, whereas only 20% of patients without advance directives described such discussions. In the SUPPORT study, having an advanced directive was associated with having discussed CPR preferences (odds ratio 2.4) (22).

Advance directives are often inconsistent with and poor predictors of specific procedural preferences. In an outpatient study of patients deemed to have life-threatening disease (defined as that associated with no greater than a 50% chance of surviving 5 years), Schneiderman and colleagues (23) found that "general instruction guidelines do not provide helpful guidance in specific clinical circumstances" (24). Individuals who chose explicit instructions for end-of-life care did not pick responses that correlate with one another. This suggests that these patients had a general sense that they might refuse life-sustaining treatment at some point but either do not know enough or are ambivalent about their choices. The inconsistency of patient choices found in this study reinforces the importance of a personal discussion with the physician.

The Nature of the Discussion of End-of-Life Issues

Surveys suggest three characteristics that are especially important for discussions of end-of-life issues: timeliness, direct communication with the physician, and honesty.

Timeliness

Patients would like to discuss end-of-life decisions with their doctors before immediate decisions need to be made. Patients who prefer to be the decision-makers want to be lucid when they communicate preferences with their doctor (25). Delaying end-of-life discussions often means that the patient loses the cognitive capacity to participate in decision making.

Direct Communication With the Physician

Ideally, end-of-life decision making would always be the result of direct consultation between the patient and his or her physician. Practical experience suggests that this does not always happen. Some decision making may be based on written documents drawn up with little or no consultation with healthcare providers.

Some patients will wish to discuss end-of-life issues alone with their physicians (26), and some will want to involve their families. The healthcare team should specify who should be involved, and preferences may change as a patient becomes more debilitated. Some patients defer to their physician's judgment before they have much experience with their illness and the medical system. Other patients take an active role in decision making when they are feeling well and cede control when they are feeling weak and fatigued.

Honesty

In an outpatient study of preferences for end-of-life discussion (27), a group of healthy patients put great emphasis on the desire for physician honesty. The patients had little concern about their ability to handle frank information, and they were not concerned when the physician could not make definitive statements about end-of-life care or about the variability of possibilities and outcomes.

Patient Reactions to Discussion of End-of-Life Issues

Discussion of end-of-life issues changes patient preferences for aggressive care. In a study of community-dwelling elderly, the response to positive or negative written descriptions of life-sustaining interventions was studied in different clinical scenarios (28). Acceptance of the interventions was significantly affected by the descriptions; subjects accepted the interventions 30% of the time when they were described positively, but only 12% of the time when they were described negatively. In another study, involving 371 patients age 60 and older, 41% opted for CPR (29). When educated about the low probability of survival after CPR, 22% opted for CPR; only 6% of patients age 86 and older opted for CPR. The physician's presentation of an option for life-sustaining technology has a strong influence on patient decision making.

When physicians and patients actually discuss end-of-life issues, patients' emotional reactions vary. In a randomized study of elderly outpatients, the intervention group felt that it was "a good idea" for doctors to talk to patients about these issues (30). The majority of patients in the intervention group denied having any particular reaction to the end-of-life discussion. Some patients wondered about their health when their physicians unexpectedly asked questions about end-of-life preferences. A few felt "puzzled," "uncomfortable," or "funny." On the positive side, a few felt "glad" and "safe." Levels of patient satisfaction were very high and similar to those in the control group. Most of the patients felt that end-of-life discussions were a good idea; they were not put off by the conversation and were highly satisfied with their encounters with their physicians.

Many ALS patients had positive reactions when their physicians brought up end-of-life issues (31). On the one hand, patients felt their physicians were concerned about them and were relieved that the topic had been broached. On the other hand, facing the issues of clinical deterioration and possible death understandably brought up feelings of sadness. Some patients acknowledged that they would rather avoid these feelings.

Another reaction to end-of-life discussions is that patients begin to actively imagine the process of dying and of being or not being on life support. Patients have difficulty discussing these issues because they have little experience with the clinical options at the end of life. Consequently, most patients can discuss only general feelings and not particular clinical scenarios. Patients do not know in advance how they will feel about their quality of life during a particular intervention.

Stability of Preferences Expressed in Advance Directives

Preferences expressed in advance directives and early discussions about end-of-life issues may not be stable over time, especially when death becomes more likely. Studies of people with serious illnesses found contradictory results about the stability of preferences for life-sustaining intervention over time. Thus, particular clinical scenarios need to be reevaluated periodically.

Among patients with ALS, "preferences for amount of information and locus of decision making were stable over six months" but preferences for CPR were not (32). In another study of patients with life-threatening diseases, preferences for interventions with life-sustaining technology were stable over 1 year (33).

Emanuel and colleagues conducted a study of end-of-life preferences in which 495 primary care patients with human immunodeficiency virus (HIV) infection and oncology patients were compared with 102 community subjects (34). Reassessments were conducted twice, with 6 to 12 months between each assessment. There was a 72% agreement between the first and second interview in the patient groups, indicating that end-of-life preferences were fairly stable. Interestingly, stability of preferences was similar for all patient groups. Moreover, severity of illness had little effect on stability of choices. Stability of preferences over time, however, was greater in patients with more education.

A study of community-dwelling Medicare recipients found that the preferences of 85% of people who desired less care at the end of life were stable at 2 years; those who desired more care had less stable preferences (35). Persons were more likely to want increased treatment if they had been hospitalized (23% vs. 18%), had an accident (29% vs. 18%), became more immobile (23% vs. 19%), became more depressed (25% vs. 15%), or had less social support (25% vs. 14%).

The stability of preferences is important because healthcare providers often must act on information provided at an earlier time. If preferences appear unstable, health providers may conclude that early conversations are useless and may neglect to bring up end-of-life preferences in a timely way.

Clinicians need to consider with caution a change in decision making by a patient facing imminent death. If decisions were previously stable, the change of heart may represent spurious, panicky, and ill-considered choices (36). Changes of preference may, however, reflect a genuine revision of understanding due to the unique experience of being near death (37). There is as yet no rule of thumb to guide the clinician.

Influence of Diagnosis on Physician Behavior

The likelihood that a physician will write a DNR order varies by diagnosis, even for illnesses with similar prognoses. DNR orders and written discussions were examined in one of four serious illnesses at three teaching hospitals (38). The illnesses—acquired immunodeficiency syndrome (AIDS), metastatic lung cancer, end-stage congestive heart failure, and advanced hepatic cirrhosis—are associated with similar short- and long-term mortality rates. Whereas approximately half of the patients with AIDS and cancer had DNR orders written, only 5–15% of the patients with cirrhosis and heart failure had DNR orders written. Patients with cirrhosis and congestive heart failure did not appear to be refusing DNR status at a higher rate. Therefore, the higher frequency of DNR orders for patients with AIDS and cancer was probably the result of more frequent discussions with patients about DNR.

Evidently, physicians feel more comfortable writing and discussing DNR orders for some diagnoses (e.g., AIDS and cancer) than for others with similar prognoses (e.g., end-stage congestive heart failure and advanced cirrhosis). Whether this difference reflects inaccurate perceptions of the mortalities associated with different diseases or some other psychological influence of the diagnosis is not known.

Diagnosis may also influence whether a patient is referred to hospice and whether insurers will be willing to pay for hospice treatment. Patients with terminal cancer and patients with AIDS are easily identified as potentially benefiting from hospice. A patient with end-stage restrictive lung disease may be less likely to be seen as benefiting from hospice treatment, even though his or her needs are similar.

Physician-Patient Communication in the Hospital Setting

Although lack of physician-patient communication is touted as the major problem in end-of-life discussions, attempts to facilitate this communication have failed to change established practices in the hospital setting. In a study of 4,301 patients with life-threatening diagnoses, only 47% of the physicians knew when their patients preferred to avoid CPR, and 46% of DNR orders were written within 2 days of death (39). Since there were substantial shortcomings in physician-patient communication, apparent from these findings, an impressive randomized clinical trial was designed to test the effectiveness of an intervention on patient care. The intervention sought to improve communication by providing timely and reliable prognostic information and information about patient and family preferences and fostering understanding about end-of-life treatment; a skilled nurse actively facilitated discussions, assembled relevant information, and arranged for meetings with participants. No difference was found in the proportion of patients discussing CPR (40% in the intervention group vs. 37% in the control group) or in the physicians' knowledge of patients' preferences for CPR. This study, which found that actively facilitating end-of-life discussions has no effect, demonstrates how difficult it will be for physicians to change their behavior. It is likely that there are other significant barriers to physician-patient communication that were not addressed by this study, although it is not obvious what those barriers are.

obstacles in phys.

Reasons Why Physicians Avoid End-of-Life Discussions

Lack of Knowledge of Advance Directives

A lack of understanding of the advance directive laws may cause physicians to avoid discussions of living wills. A survey of family physicians found that those who were more knowledgeable about living wills were more likely to discuss them with patients (40). Physicians may also be concerned about the best timing of end-of-life discussions. If the patient has already become sick, he or she may interpret such a discussion as meaning that the illness is terminal or that the physician is unwilling to provide necessary care (41). Although lack of knowledge about specific laws and concerns about appropriate timing may explain some part of physician reluctance to initiate end-of-life discussion, a major impediment is the natural emotional reaction to initiating a potentially painful discussion, as discussed below.

Fear of Causing Pain

Some of the discomfort with end-of-life discussions comes from our having normal human reactions to bad news. As physicians, we are afraid of causing pain. To consciously cause someone pain appears to upset the normal rules of the doctor-patient relationship; therefore, we try to avoid it. Physicians also experience discomfort in being with a person who has heard and is distressed by bad news (42).

Denial in the Physician Culture That Death Is Inevitable

In Western culture, death was once viewed as natural and expected but is now viewed as an enemy to be defeated (43). Because medicine in the United States emphasizes aggressive intervention, and new technologies that improve prognosis emerge quickly, death can be evaded successfully in many cases. When death appears unavoidable, physicians have a hard time imagining a role for themselves. Because of the fragmentation of medical care, the physicians caring for the dying often are not the physicians who cared for them when they were functioning independently; thus, there is no previous doctor-patient relationship (44). Often the majority of the care is directed by young physicians, many of whom are unfamiliar with the values of elderly persons and have little experience with dying and death. A "good death" is not thought of as a good outcome. Because they define a "good death" as a therapeutic failure, physicians feel incompetent and helpless, or blame themselves or others.

Fear of Being the Bearer of Bad News

Physicians do not like to give bad news. Almost universally, end-of-life discussions contain bad news. Doctors working with terminally ill patients experience several feelings—for example, helplessness, guilt, and anger about not being able to offer more. These feelings can affect physicians' behavior. Thus, although most physicians believe that patients should participate in end-of-life decisions and that physicians should initiate these discussions (45), few of them actually do so. At a university teaching hospital, more than 90% of private physicians and house officers believed that patients should at least sometimes participate in decisions about resuscitation (46). Of the physicians who believed in discussing resuscitation with patients, only 10% actually talked about this with these patients before their cardiopulmonary arrests; 21% discussed resuscitation with the family. When the probability of cardiac arrest was thought to be greater than 50%, the likelihood of discussion still did not increase. In a geriatric medical unit, only 18%

of the medical and nursing staff who had cared for 24 patients who died had discussed the diagnoses with the patients, and only 14% had discussed impending death (47).

Human beings are not good at dealing with bad news in the abstract. They therefore identify the news with the person bringing it and get angry at him or her. Physicians are taught throughout training that if a patient's health deteriorates, the physician may be blamed and possibly sued. The frequent advertisements for aggressive malpractice and injury lawyers in our litigious culture further reinforce these concerns.

Anticipated Disagreement With the Patient or Family Over Futile Treatment

Some physicians may not want to raise the issue of treatment options when there is ultimately no hope. Although many physicians think they know futility when they see it (48), defining it clearly has been a problem. Although many physicians consider it a matter of probability, there is no agreement on a level of statistical certainty as to when a treatment is futile (49). Providers are obligated to make every effort to understand why a patient desires treatment that a physician feels does not serve his or her interest, and to correct misunderstandings. Because inadequate or insensitive communication by providers probably accounts for a majority of unrealistic requests, such discussions may successfully resolve some conflicts. However, physicians struggle with their own ethics as to whether they have to provide treatment that they consider futile. The Council of Ethical and Judicial Affairs of the American Medical Association has concluded that physicians have no obligation to obtain consent for a DNR order when CPR is deemed futile (50).

Lack of Education

Doctors are not taught how to deliver bad news and often feel inept. Some healthcare providers do not feel it is appropriate to upset a patient under any circumstances and will blame the physician who does. Patients may ask questions that are appropriate but not answerable.

Not having concrete answers makes physicians feel even more incompetent and out of control. In terminal care situations, physicians may feel inept and helpless and abandon their patients, rationalizing that their jobs have been completed. Although it has not been addressed systematically in United States training programs, palliative care can be offered to patients at the end of life. Palliative care requires shifting goals from cure to maximizing comfort, independence, and quality of life. The American Board of Internal Medicine has recently incorporated the promotion of physician competency and training in the care of dying patients into internal medicine residency and subspecialty training (51, 52). Educational curricula, strategies for learning, and methods of assessing physician competence have been developed. These resources are an excellent model for training psychiatric residents and physicians in palliative care and should be used as guides by educators in psychiatry.

Physician Vulnerability and Fear of Death

Discussing end-of-life matters brings to the fore our own mortality and fears of death (53). Some people who go into medicine do so to conquer their own feelings of vulnerability to illness or in response to a personal traumatic loss. End-of-life discussions challenge feelings of being indomitable and can be an unpleasant reminder of our own mortality. A physician may feel a growing sense of separation when encountering someone who has no hope of survival (54). The physician's statement that the patient "can't take it" can be a projection of his or her own vulnerability; sometimes it is the doctor who "can't take it." Many physicians choose medicine because it is a profession that rewards empathy and is personally satisfying. Empathic healthcare professionals have more anxiety about talking with dying patients (55); as a result, they may reach out to their patients who are not dying and avoid their dying patients.

Patients who are dying often require the most active support and assistance of healthcare professionals in order to make informed and voluntary choices. Dying patients express a profound wish to be among the living and to be talked with and cared for (56). Yet, the limitations imposed on patients by severe illness (e.g., confusion, communication problems, personality changes secondary to pain, frustration, fear, dependency) may cause health professionals to withdraw from them, rather than to commit the additional time and energy that communication may require (57). In addition, professionals may feel that a dying patient represents a failure on their part and withdraw for that reason (58, 59). To stand by and watch a person slip away requires that we confront our feelings about death. Psychiatrists can be helpful to families and colleagues in this situation by enabling them to identify and cope with strong feelings and providing support and an environment in which to grieve.

Medical-Legal Concerns

Physicians' medical-legal concerns can influence end-of-life discussions and the type of treatment that is offered or withdrawn. This can be especially true when an adverse event has occurred or there is hostility among the patient, the patient's family, and the medical team. In this situation, the healthcare team may be inclined to offer futile treatment in order to reduce the likelihood of being sued.

Withholding Versus Withdrawing Treatment

Misunderstandings about the law influence discussions and decisions between doctors and patients at the end of life. Meisel noted that health professionals have many misconceptions about the law and life-sustaining treatment (60). For example, many health professionals erroneously believe there is a clear legal and ethical distinction between the *withdrawal* and the *withholding* of life-sustaining treatment, such as artificial respiration. This misconception about legal and ethical norms may inhibit treatment that may be beneficial to the patient. The belief that treatment cannot be withdrawn may make physicians less willing to initiate trials of potentially beneficial interventions— that is, they fear that the treatment will have to be continued even after it has proven harmful or futile.

In some cases, healthcare providers are aware that there is no *legal* distinction between withholding versus withdrawing treatment but feel an *emotional* distinction between the two. Some feel that with-drawal of a treatment is an active means of facilitating death, and they feel guilty when undertaking such a course of action.

Letting Die Versus Murder

Some healthcare professionals still confuse termination of life support with murder or suicide. To many physicians, it feels disingenuous to say "the illness killed the patient" when they have withdrawn extraor-dinary life support in accordance with the patient's wishes. For some, termination of life support feels like murder. Although there have been no successful criminal prosecutions for criminal liability for withhold-ing life-sustaining treatment (61), physicians' concerns about adverse publicity and stigma may influence their behavior. Uncertainty about common law and the applicability of preceding cases may also frustrate and frighten physicians who seek guarantees that they will not be liable for withholding treatment. Many physicians are cynical about the ability of the court to resolve ethical dilemmas in medicine.

Administrative Versus Physician Obligations

When physicians are concerned about legal risk, they often seek advice from hospital administrators, hospital attorneys, or risk managers. The primary obligation of these professionals is to the hospital, and they often want to minimize legal problems and bad publicity. Since the primary administrative concern is the overall good of the hospital, the legal advice given may not meet the more specific needs of physicians and patients.

The Role of the Psychiatrist

Psychiatrists have traditionally not been involved in end-of-life discus-sions with patients who have terminal conditions. In the past, some psychiatrists believed that no one, not even a patient with terminal illness, could have a rational wish to die. This view contributed to a schism between psychiatrists and their medical colleagues, who did not see psychiatry as helpful when they were working with dying patients. Recently, many psychiatrists have become more interested in the issues confronting medical patients. In addition, *medical-surgical psychiatry,* or *consultation-liaison psychiatry,* has come to be viewed as a distinct subspecialty within psychiatry. Even psychiatrists who work with medical patients, however, believe that the primary care physician or internist is the most appropriate person to raise end-of-life issues because he or she has the most information about prognosis and treatment alternatives. Many primary care physicians have long-standing relationships with patients, have known them through all phases of their illnesses, and have a sense of their values. When end-of-life discussions occur in the inpatient setting between physicians and patients who have no prior relationship, psychiatrists can be helpful in facilitating a complete and sensitive discussion of a painful subject and eliciting patients' fears and values.

Patients may feel more connected with their psychiatrist than with their primary care doctor, who may spend very little time getting to know them and their values. If the psychiatrist raises the issue, patients may sense that they have a caring advocate. Under managed care, psychosocial factors that contribute to increased medical utilization are likely to receive more attention, and psychiatrists may receive financial compensation for these important discussions. It is possible that psychiatrists may play a more visible role in the primary care setting and that, as clinicians and researchers in the psychosocial aspects of medical illness, they can contribute expertise. Indeed, their training as physicians can enable psychiatrists to help patients cope with the facts of their illnesses within the patients' own value systems and to improve communication between a terminal care patient and his or her primary medical doctor. Compared with psychologists, social workers, and other therapists, psychiatrists have a distinct advantage in the hospital setting. By integrating a knowledge of medical illness and treatment with expertise in understanding patient and family reactions to the stress of terminal illness, psychiatrists can assist patients in several possible roles.

Consultation-Liaison Psychiatrist

Psychiatrists can be quite helpful to the primary care physician by providing an objective opinion on the patient and family reactions and formulating a plan to enable effective communication. Although psychiatric input can be requested on a case-by-case basis, it is best for the psychiatrist to become a part of the healthcare team. Having close working relationships with nonpsychiatric colleagues facilitates the identification of problematic coping on the part of both patients and physicians and timely, supportive intervention. Psychiatrists can also address the withdrawal of the medical team that leaves dying patients feeling abandoned and facilitate implementation of palliative measures such as treatment of pain and depression.

There is increased emphasis on the role of psychiatry and the other mental health professions in primary care. A primary care outpatient clinic is another site for fruitful medical student and resident instruction in breaking bad news sensitively and addressing end-of-life issues. Such instruction may make the next generation of physicians more comfortable in dealing with death and, therefore, more likely to raise end-of-life issues. Both nonpsychiatric and psychiatric residents should receive this training. Nonpsychiatric residents will gain an understanding of what psychiatrists have to offer in facilitating end-of-life care. Psychiatric residents will gain experience in liaison work with patients and health professionals in the medical setting.

Ethics Committees

Psychiatric input is critical on hospital ethics committees, where the most problematic end-of-life situations are evaluated. Addressing treatable mental disorders is important in optimizing a patient's mental functioning and quality of life. Psychiatrists have special expertise in evaluating patients' decision-making capacities, which are often at issue at the end of life, and in helping to resolve conflict.

Cases before ethics committees often involve significant family and cultural issues. Psychiatrists have expertise in integrating the biopsychosocial model of patient care. Also, coping styles and values of patients and families can be accommodated more successfully with psychiatric input. (See Chapter 4 for a more detailed discussion of this topic.)

Recommendations for Facilitating End-of-Life Discussion

Mental health professionals working with seriously ill patients, either on an outpatient basis or in liaison work, may want to add a "patient review," similar to that devised by Delbanco (62), as a complement to the organ-specific review of systems conducted during patient encounters. The review includes discussion, as well as clarification and documentation, of end-of-life preferences/values. Seven dimensions of care are addressed:

1. Respect for patients' values, preferences, and expressed needs
2. Communication and education
3. Coordination and integration of care
4. Physical comfort
5. Emotional support and alleviation of fears and anxieties
6. Involvement of family and friends
7. Continuity and transition

Such an instrument could be used to focus on treatment goals and quality of life. Having an established instrument could give structure to a difficult discussion and help to "normalize" the process. Having the mental health team member broach the subject may help to decrease the patient's perceptions that the medical team is giving up—an unexpected consequence of having the regular physician bring up the issue. Preferences for amount of patient and family involvement in decision making can be elicited during the patient review.

Some mental health clinicians may interpret their role as helping primary care physicians in broaching end-of-life issues, rather than primarily addressing them. The following recommendations can be used in liaison work with primary care colleagues to address end-of-life issues sensitively and actively with patients in the outpatient setting.

1. *Develop a systematic approach so that end-of-life discussions become part of the clinical routine.* Build end-of-life discussions into the second or third visit, after rapport has developed, to increase patient and physician comfort.

2. *Organize the discussion with a written instrument appropriate for the patient population* (by age, culture, educational level) to provide a springboard for a discussion of patient values and desires for quality of life.
3. *Determine in advance who is to be included in end-of-life discussions.* Would the patient prefer to have this discussion with the physician alone, or should family or a friend be included?
4. *Ensure that the advance directive is available in all clinical sites.* An advance directive can be filled out by the patient and physician together. A plan should be developed to have the directive accessible should the patient be admitted.
5. *Develop a system of reevaluation of end-of-life preferences.* End-of-life decisions should be reevaluated periodically. The appropriate interval should reflect the acuity of the patient population.
6. *Organize a patient education group to discuss end-of-life care or incorporate this topic into existing patient groups.* Nonmedical leaders, such as religious leaders, may be helpful in organizing and participating in such a group.

Many end-of-life discussions occur in the inpatient setting. They are often precipitated by clinical deterioration and are, therefore, stressful and rushed. Care must be taken to assure the patient and family that treatment options have been adequately discussed. Psychiatrists can facilitate this process.

Some additional recommendations for end-of-life discussions in the inpatient setting are obvious but deserve mention.

1. *Ensure that the environment for discussion is private, quiet, and not chaotic.* Do not discuss end-of-life decisions in a hospital corridor (63).
2. *Keep language simple, and avoid medical jargon.* If it seems helpful, have another patient or family member speak to the patient about their experiences in a similar situation.
3. *Bring up end-of-life issues in a timely way.* End-of-life issues should be raised early in an admission to maximize the patient's cognitive capacity and ability to participate in decisions.

4. *Have the patient designate a decision-maker/spokesperson should he or she lose cognitive capacity.*
5. *Be as available as possible for questions.* Continue to meet routinely, even if only for a brief time.

These recommendations are based on common sense and very limited survey material. There are few opportunities for physicians to obtain formal training in how to conduct end-of-life discussions. Thus, physicians wishing to develop a rational, sensitive approach to this problem are obliged to formulate a plan and make themselves available to patients and physicians to help in this capacity.

Conclusion

begins

End-of-life discussions are highly personal and emotionally charged. They are influenced by one's personality, age, culture, ethnicity, religion, and personal values. Though both patients and physicians agree that such discussions are important, they rarely take place. In most clinical environments, the psychiatrist is the person most able to fill the gap. Indeed, it is likely that other physicians will expect psychiatrists to assume leadership in this important area. It is therefore incumbent on psychiatry as a specialty to contribute to the research that will optimize end-of-life communication and treatment planning.

References

1. Kinsella T, Stocking C: Failed communication about life-support therapy: silent physicians and mute patients. Am J Med 86:643–644, 1989
2. Finucane T, Shumway J, Powers R, et al: Planning with elderly outpatients for contingencies of severe illness: a survey and clinical trial. J Gen Intern Med 3:322–325, 1988
3. Edinger W, Smucker D: Outpatients' attitudes regarding advance directives. J Fam Pract 35:650–653, 1992
4. President's Commission for the Study of Ethical Problems in Medicine and Biomedical and Behavioral Research: Making Health Care Decisions. Washington, DC, U.S. Government Printing Office, 1982

5. Ende J, Kazis L, Ash A, et al: Measuring patients' desire for autonomy: decision-making and information-seeking preferences among medical patients. J Gen Intern Med 4:23–29, 1989

6. Hofmann JC, Wenger NS, Davis RB, et al: Patient preferences for communication with physicians about end-of-life decisions. SUPPORT investigators, Study to Understand Prognoses and Preferences for Outcomes and Risks of Treatment. Ann Intern Med 127:1–12, 1997

7. Caralis PV, Davis B, Wright K, et al: The influence of ethnicity and race on attitudes toward advance directives, life-prolonging treatments, and euthanasia. J Clin Ethics 4:155–165, 1993

8. Weir R: Abating Treatment With Critically Ill Patients. New York, Oxford University Press, 1989

9. Grodin M: Religious advance directives: the convergence of law, religion, medicine and public health. Am J Public Health 83(6):899–903, 1993

10. Muller J, Desmond B: Ethical dilemmas in a cross-cultural context: a Chinese example. West J Med 157:323–327, 1992; see pp 323–325 [Case reprinted with permission of the *Western Journal of Medicine*]

11. Muller and Desmond, Ethical dilemmas, pp 323–325

12. Muller and Desmond, Ethical dilemmas

13. Muller and Desmond, Ethical dilemmas

14. Li S, Chou JL: Communication with the cancer patient in China. Ann N Y Acad Sci 809:243–248, 1997

15. Gonda TA, Ruark JE: Dying Dignified: The Health Professional's Guide to Care. Reading, MA, Addison-Wesley, 1984

16. Virmani J, Schneiderman L, Kaplan R: Relationship of advance directives to physician-patient communication. Arch Intern Med 154:909–913, 1994

17. Kinsella and Stocking, Failed communication

18. Finucane et al, Planning with elderly outpatients

19. Silverstein M, Stocking C, Antel J, et al: Amyotrophic lateral sclerosis and life sustaining therapy: patients' desire for information, participation in decision making and life-sustaining therapy. Mayo Clin Proc 66:906–913, 1991

20. Hofmann et al, Patient preferences for communication with physicians

21. Virmani et al, Relationship of advance directives

22. Hofmann et al, Patient preferences for communication with physicians

23. Schneiderman L, Pearlman R, Kaplan R, et al: Relationship of general advance directive instructions to specific life-sustaining treatment preferences in patients with serious illness. Arch Intern Med 152:2114–2122, 1992

24. Schneiderman et al, Relationship of general advance directive instructions, p 2119

25. Pfeifer M, Sidorov J, Smith A, et al: The discussion of end-of-life medical care by primary care patients. J Gen Intern Med 9:82–88, 1994
26. Pfeifer et al, Discussion of end-of-life medical care
27. Pfeifer et al, Discussion of end-of-life medical care
28. Malloy T, Wigton R, Meeske J, et al: The influence of treatment descriptions on advance directive decisions. J Am Geriatr Soc 40:1255–1260, 1992
29. Murphy D, Burrows D, Santilli S, et al: The influence of the probability of survival on patients' preferences regarding cardiopulmonary resuscitation. N Engl J Med 330:545–549, 1994
30. Finucane et al, Planning with elderly outpatients
31. Silverstein et al, Amyotrophic lateral sclerosis
32. Silverstein et al, Amyotrophic lateral sclerosis, p 910
33. Schneiderman et al, Relationship of general advance directive instructions
34. Emanuel L, Emmanuel E, Stoeckle J, et al: Advance directives: stability of patients' choices. Arch Intern Med 154:209–217, 1994
35. Danis M, Garrett J, Harris R, et al: Stability of choices about life-sustaining treatments. Ann Intern Med 120:567–573, 1994
36. Emanuel et al, Advance directives
37. Emanuel et al, Advance directives
38. Wachter RM, Luce J, Hearst N, et al: Decisions about resuscitation: inequities among patients with different diseases but similar prognoses. Ann Intern Med 111:525–532, 1989
39. The SUPPORT Principal Investigators: A controlled trial to improve care for seriously ill hospitalized patients. JAMA 274:1591–1598, 1995
40. Edinger and Smucker, Outpatients' attitudes
41. Edinger and Smucker, Outpatients' attitudes
42. Buckman R: How to Break Bad News. Baltimore, MD, Johns Hopkins Press, 1992
43. McCue J: The naturalness of dying. JAMA 273:1039–1043, 1995
44. McCue J, The naturalness of dying
45. Edinger and Smucker, Outpatients' attitudes
46. Bedell S, Delbanco T: Choices about cardiopulmonary resuscitation in the hospital: when do physicians talk with patients? N Engl J Med 310:1089–1093, 1984
47. Graham H, Livesley B: Dying as a diagnosis: difficulties of communication and management in elderly patients. Lancet 2:670–672, 1983
48. Truog R, Brett A, Frader J: The problem with futility. N Engl J Med 326:1560–1564, 1992
49. Truog et al, Problem with futility

50. Truog et al, Problem with futility
51. Blank LL: Defining and evaluating physician competence in end-of-life patient care. West J Med 163:297–301, 1995
52. American Board of Internal Medicine, Committee on Evaluation of Clinical Competence: Caring for the Dying: Identification and Promotion of Physician Competency. Philadelphia, PA, American Board of Internal Medicine, 1996
53. Klocker JG, Klocker-Kaiser U, Schwaninger M: Truth in the relationship between cancer patient and physician. Ann N Y Acad Sci 809:56–65, 1997
54. Seravalli E: The dying patient, the physician, and the fear of death. N Engl J Med 319:1728–1730, 1988
55. Servaty HL: Relationships among death anxiety, communication apprehension with the dying, and empathy in those seeking occupations as nurses and physicians. Death Studies 20:149–161, 1996
56. Seravalli, Dying patient
57. Fox R: The Sociology of Medicine. Englewood Cliffs, NJ, Prentice-Hall, 1989
58. Seravalli, Dying patient
59. Feifel H: Death in contemporary America, in New Meanings of Death. Edited by Feifel H. New York, McGraw-Hill, 1977, pp 4–12
60. Meisel A: Legal myths about terminating life support. Arch Intern Med 152:1497–1502, 1991
61. Kapp M, Lo B: Legal perceptions and medical decision making. Milbank Q 64 (suppl 2):163–202, 1986
62. Delbanco T: Enriching the doctor-patient relationship by inviting the patient's perspective. Ann Intern Med 116:414–418, 1992
63. Clarke D, Goldstein M, Raffin T: Ethical dilemmas in the critically ill elderly. Clin Geriatr Med 10:91–101, 1994

6

Consultation to End-of-Life Treatment Decisions in Children

Julie R. Van der Feen, M.D.C.M.
Michael S. Jellinek, M.D.

Many factors contribute to making end-of-life decisions in children so difficult. Children are not supposed to die. In a culture that rarely, if ever, acknowledges that death is a part of life, the end of an unfolding life seems particularly unfair and out of our control. Children experience the world differently from adults. They relate differently to medical and mental health professionals, requiring distinct interventions and consultation approaches depending on their level of development. Concomitantly, their role in decision making evolves over time and always occurs within a family context. In addition to the expected cognitive, emotional, and physical changes, a chronically ill child and family evolve in a world characterized by stress, medical interventions, pain, and uncertainty, cycling through hope, fear, overattachment, distancing, overprotectiveness, and confusion. The end-of-life period ends this cycle as the child and family are forced to face separation and death.

Dying children elicit many emotions from their caretakers and family members, and this results in intense interactions that profoundly affect everyone (1). In an attempt to control the inexorable course toward death, we may withdraw, become overly involved, or seek refuge in our medical expertise or procedures. The clinician's challenge is to think of the child as a person, however tragic, rather than as organ systems, symptoms, or diagnoses. Thinking of a child as a "leukemia" or "adjustment disorder" may offer an escape from the tragedy but prevents us from being with the child and family as the end approaches.

Clinicians consulting to treatment dilemmas involving critically ill children often need to serve a variety of functions in order to best help the child and the family. The consultant's role often includes maintaining an emphasis on immediate and extended family and trying to support harmony and consensus with the pediatric team. The consultant needs a combination of interpersonal skills, forethought, empathy, and adequate training to deal with the complex issues raised by decisions involving dying children and their families. Interventions will vary, depending on the nature and predictability of the illness or trauma. Some deaths involve controversial decisions that elicit powerful emotions, including guilt, anger, denial, and distrust. A child's death, even without controversy, often requires work with individual families and treatment teams.

Consultation to Critically Ill Children

Consultations to children involve multiple medical and psychological factors. Individual psychological factors (such as a child's personality and developmental level), family factors (such as the current state of family functioning), and the role of the consultant all need to be carefully assessed before significant decisions about a child's care can be made. Medically, the consultant must be aware of the illness's natural course, unusual features with regard to the patient, the quality of the relationships between the physician(s) and the child and family, and any acute medical issues. Although the consultant cannot be a pediatric subspecialist, he or she should have a sense of a severely damaged neonate's prognosis or the consequences of intubating an adolescent with end-stage cystic fibrosis. Further, the consultant should try to develop a relationship with the pediatric team to appreciate their medical judgments and the quality of their relating to the child/family and to be aware of any conflict within the team regarding end-of-life decisions.

Optimally, a screening psychiatric consultation is scheduled soon after initial diagnosis so that the consultant can assess the family's and child's likely strengths and vulnerabilities as well as gather history concerning previous experience with life-threatening illness. Ideally, the screening psychiatrist is integrated into the specialty team and is an available, familiar physician as needed (pain management, compliance, parental problems, depression, decision making, etc.).

Ascertaining the child's level of cognitive development will help determine his or her understanding of the illness, especially as end-of-life decisions approach. The child's cognitive functioning may be altered or impaired by medical (e.g., concussion, leukemia) and affective (e.g., depression, anxiety) stressors. Many children regress secondary to physical injury and their emotional state; for example, a preteen child may suddenly change from increasingly autonomous to clingy, resisting his or her parents' effort to leave the bedside.

When major decisions about treatment arise, the consultant needs to evaluate the family's functioning, their life-cycle phase, their religious beliefs, their values, and their experience with and adjustment to previous losses or crises. For example, parents commonly feel guilty, believing they are responsible for protecting their child. The specifics of the child's illness may increase the guilt if the child's illness is genetic or the result of a possibly preventable accident (e.g., a near drowning, a fall from a building).

The child's illness must be placed in the context of his or her family's coping style and relationship to the healthcare team. Part of every consultation, especially at the end of life, is to assess the relationship between the child/family and the pediatric team. A sense of trust is critical between one member of the team, not necessarily the senior attending, and the child and family. Some pediatric teams (unconsciously) spread the emotional burden, often through "rotations," so that no physician has a full alliance. Occasionally, a senior psychiatric subspecialist will try to "do it all" and be overinvolved in psychiatric issues; the opposite may also occur if the subspecialist withdraws as the child's death (seen as a defect) approaches. Other pediatric teams may have ongoing, covert conflicts about "aggressive" treatment and facing end-of-life decisions. Forming a superficial alliance or giving confusing messages of hope and despair adds greatly to the family's and consultant's burden. A trusted alliance and overt cohesiveness within the pediatric team are highly supportive and allow both the family and the consultant to work on grief and essential resolution.

A number of approaches are available to adults to determine their care at the end of life directly, as with advance directives, or indirectly, through substituted judgments. These options are not as relevant to children. Specific to issues of consent at the end of life are the capacity of children and the family context. The child's capacity depends on cognition and development, emotional immaturity, and disease-related circumstances. Although generally age-related, cognitive and emotional maturity may vary widely and can be influenced by disease-related pain, handicap, or organic mental impairment. The family has a presumed right to speak in the best interests of the child. Preadolescents have a growing ability to contribute both to disease management and to decision making. Parents sensing the need and value of promoting autonomy share more information and authority with their child. Families, often in a quiet and subtle manner, reach an understanding of how to proceed at end of life. Open, sustained, or strident conflicts are uncommon, although when they occur, the ethical and dynamic issues are dramatic and consuming.

The progression to autonomy and control are on a continuum with increasing assent in school age and consent in early adolescence. As in other emotionally charged circumstances, consultants must be aware of their own beliefs as they attempt to discern the medical and psychological "best interests" of the child. Consultants are frequently called on to face end-of-life decisions during the most difficult times in a child's course of the disease or in the context of misunderstandings. The pressure from the pediatric team and from the family, and the large amount of data needed to assess the child, frequently lead the consultant to feel overwhelmed.

Developmental Considerations Affecting Decision Making by and for Children

An appreciation of important milestones in a child's development can help consultants understand the reactions of children to life-threatening diagnoses at different ages. How does the child understand the illness and prognosis, and death itself? How should the child be integrated into the treatment? How ready is the child to understand his or her downhill course, and how helpful is it to the child to include him or her in decision making?

Children pass through cognitive, affective, and physical stages that can be roughly divided into four groups, based on life periods. These age ranges are somewhat arbitrary, since each child matures at his or her own pace and in his or her own way. Usually a child's concept of death develops in an orderly sequence from ignorance to comprehension. However, children vary in their rate of development. Also, children are also influenced by their environment, which impinges on their cognitive, affective, social, moral, and physical growth. A life-threatening illness may result in depression, anger, or pain, causing a child to regress or to become mature beyond his or her years.

Infancy (Birth to 2 Years)

Infants experience the world through their senses and motor movements. They learn to adjust their behaviors based on feedback from the world around them (2). For example, infants require special efforts to have their parents present without interruption and to be in an environment that is consistent and contains familiar objects. Affectively, they begin to develop trust, based on the consistency of positive interactions with their caretakers. Because infants have little ability to differentiate animate from inanimate objects, they are far from an understanding of death (3). Much of their understanding comes from parental presence, from interactions with a primary nurse, and from being physically comforted and held.

Parental attachment to a baby begins at conception. Consequently, a relationship already exists between the infant and his or her parents at birth, and this attachment intensifies through the newborn period. If the child is born with or develops a life-threatening illness, the parents and the consultant face a serious dilemma: how to support the parents' attachment in the event of an uncertain future or tragic death. If the family has a history of positive attachment and a capacity for loss, it may be best to support the parents' attachment to provide meaningful memories for the future. However, if the parents have had past devastating losses or a history of incomplete grieving, or are affected by a mental illness or substance dependence that interferes with their ability to cope, the consultant may need to take a more cautious approach to encouraging attachment. These parents may have a particularly difficult time and need intensive support services while withdrawing from the infant if the prognosis is grim. This paradoxical situation can be difficult not only for the parents but also for the entire treatment team. One cannot underestimate the powerful attachment to a fetus or infant who dies.

During pregnancy, parents begin to construct their lives based on joyous expectations. If these hopes are shattered, parents can become disoriented: during the first few hours of learning their child has a life-threatening illness; during interactions with others, especially relatives; and even when asked to care for their child, who, because of physical deformities or limitations, may need attention in a way that a parent never imagined (4). It is often difficult for any healthcare professional to focus on the immediate practical concerns as well as longer-term follow-up. Involving both parents in decision making is important. They will face decisions involving situations such as seeing a less-than-perfect baby, being asked to provide care to a degree that seems overwhelming, altering their expectations for their child and family, and informing friends, family, and other parents of prognosis and decisions.

It is increasingly accepted to question whether life-prolonging treatments are in the best interest of a critically ill neonate. Many parents have their doubts when heroic measures are initiated and expect information and guidance from the doctors caring for their child (5). Parents are expected to make rational decisions that will alter their child's life course at a time when they are physically and emotionally bombarded by feelings of guilt, anger, fear, and sadness (6). The intensive care unit (ICU) can be a particularly bewildering and isolating experience for parents, since often they feel unable to do anything practical, such as holding or feeding their child (7). Communication is a major issue; the team must be sensitive to the use of jargon or inconsistent messages about treatment or prognosis. Parents may be unable to integrate communications from the treatment team because of depression, anxiety, or denial. At times, denial gives parents time to cope; however, sometimes rigid, prolonged denial interferes with a child's care and must be explored and gently confronted.

Late Infancy and Early Childhood (Ages 2 to 7 Years)

Young children during this age period tend to be egocentric and are learning to distinguish reality from fantasy (8). They attribute life and consciousness initially to inanimate objects (e.g., rocks and stuffed animals) and later to moving objects (e.g., clouds and cars). They believe that they can make objects obey by their actions and thought. Older children evolve superstitions such as avoiding stepping on cracks in the sidewalk. Consequently, children use an answer or reason to explain much that happens in their world and do not include the abstract concept of chance. School-age children actively incorporate their parents' values and guilt. For example, a 4-year-old hit by a car may believe the accident happened because he did not listen to his mother. A 6-year-old with leukemia may attribute fevers to being out in the sun too much or not using sunscreen lotion. Because of these limitations in their ability to understand and to reason, special skill is required to communicate and involve them appropriately in treatment. Nonetheless, incomplete comprehension of a disease process should not preclude children's participation in aspects of their care. Although they may not grasp the abstract concept of a "cancer," they will experience concrete symptoms such as hair loss or nausea. Explaining and helping a child to accommodate to necessary changes and symptoms should be an ongoing process.

At this stage, children may know the words "dead" or "dying," but they do not fully comprehend their meaning. Young children believe death is reversible. For example, they may believe that people who go to "heaven" can easily come back. Death is understood by using magical thinking or by parroting a notion they may have heard elsewhere. By the age of 4 years, most children are aware that other living things (e.g., insects, other animals) that die are no longer the same physically. Yet, they still do not relate this concept to themselves. Because they are egocentric (i.e., understand the world only as it relates to them), they may assign causality of illness to some aspect of their own behavior. They may believe their anger during an argument killed their parent. This can lead to feelings of self-blame, guilt, and fear of punishment or retaliation.

Older children in this age group will begin to grasp the notion that death is irreversible. At the very least, they will understand that death means leaving those they love behind. Practical implications of this progression in development are severalfold. End-of-life treatment decisions made for children at this stage may need to include time for the child to say goodbye to relatives and loved ones. Quality of life may play a larger role for some children than for others. For example, parents of a child actively involved as a player or fan of team sports may decide to cut short or eliminate a treatment regimen that may briefly prolong the child's life but leaves him or her unable to participate because of weakness or vulnerability to infection. Likewise, other meaningful events in a child's life (e.g., the graduation of a sibling, an upcoming season, a family trip or vacation) may influence a parental decision to complete a painful or difficult treatment regimen in order to give the child more time to reach this life event.

Children early in this stage are unable to understand cause-and-effect relationships between their health status and the need for painful and unpleasant treatments. Given the choice, they would naturally avoid treatments that involve even minimal pain, incapacitation, or separation from their families. They are often in pain, blame themselves, and are scared by the hospital's alien environment. With help, children will begin to appreciate these concepts. They may be distressed by changes in their body image, or focus on the possibility of bodily injury (9). Younger children have a poorly defined sense of their internal organs. They may even worry that their bodies cannot produce more blood, for example, or that their physical body does not exist beneath bandages. Older children may need repeated validation of their bodies via concrete pictures or dolls designed with removable internal organs. Most will be unable to appreciate the therapeutic intent of multiple, repeated procedures and may again feel that these are for punishment. They frequently feel that they can neither control nor influence their treatment. Consequently, they may become angry and irritable and regress behaviorally.

Children cope in different ways. One way to help them adjust is to allow them to have some control over a procedure (e.g., choosing from which arm to draw blood, ways to receive medication; scheduling treatments around special events) so that they feel involved in their own care. These simple choices can be extremely meaningful to children and may make the difference between a child who withdraws and one who remains actively curious and involved in his or her disease process. Child life specialists can help children rehearse different treatments or procedures with stuffed animals or dolls. Remaining sensitive to children with a poorly developed sense of time may involve telling them about procedures shortly beforehand to allow them to mobilize resources before elaborate fears develop. Permission to express anger and frustration is essential; aggressive play that is noninjurious can be helpful (10). Parents need to remain empathic and to validate their child's experience even if it is terribly painful or frightening. Often this may involve taking extra time to sit with the child and gently questioning her as she explains her understanding of the illness. Clarifying their child's stories can be invaluable in alleviating anxiety.

Parents and staff need to be consistent in their communications with the child to facilitate trust. Children will need constant reassurance that adults are not angry at them. Children's self-esteem can be boosted by listening carefully, offering encouragement, and recognizing a child's accomplishments (11). This confirmation of worth is critical in order for a child to cope and to realize that he or she will not be abandoned, rejected, or left alone.

Young children cannot fully participate in end-of-life decision making and will be highly reliant on their parents to balance any possible benefit to aggressive treatment when approaching death. The consultant's role is often to support parental agreement on the details of the child's final weeks—such as when to stop fully all curative efforts, and how to manage where the child will die—and to help the parents cope with issues or pressures as they arise from, for example, religious conflicts or as members of the extended family express their concerns. Keeping everyone involved—the subspecialist who has "failed," the housestaff who are "busy" with "new" patients, and both parents, who will soon have to go on without the child—is difficult and sometimes undervalued work.

Middle Childhood and Preadolescence (Ages 7 to 11–12 Years)

Older children begin to think more about themselves as individuals and their relationships to others. They gradually become more confident in their ability to master new tasks. However, they are keenly aware of differences from their peers and can easily feel inadequate or inferior (12).

The child slowly discovers that experiences are no longer explicable by magic and that death is something grave and permanent. If asked why death occurs, most children at this stage will give a concrete explanation, often based on physical causes. Thus, the child who has advanced in his or her cognitive development views death as a natural, universal, and irreversible event. Still, children are reluctant to personalize death and may regress, or become dependent as an expression of their feelings. These older children may develop separation worries not previously present.

These children's reactions to treatment may vary from feelings of anger to depression. They may become defiant, resistant to procedures, and hostile to staff as a way of battling their feelings of helplessness. Their behaviors may be ways of coping and solving problems but can be defensive and self-destructive. Parents and clinicians need to remember that anger is an appropriate feeling for the child that should be tolerated, not taken personally. Compliant children are often thought to be coping extremely well, whereas, at times, hopelessness and helplessness may be confused with compliance.

Caretakers may withdraw from these demanding, or alternatively complacent, children. The child's regression may alienate friends and staff who feel that the child should be "tough" or "act his age." Many of these reactions are to be expected, and children should be encouraged to verbalize their anger, frustration, and feelings. However, children may regress for other reasons: they may be in pain, feel lonely, feel a lack of control, or be depressed. As with younger children, finding opportunities to give children in this age group control is helpful. Interventions can be as simple as increasing visiting time or offering choices to help increase their participation. When possible, attending school or returning to school work with the help of a tutor can highlight the child's age-appropriate strengths, thus countering some of the regressive pull of the illness.

End-of-life treatment decisions for children in this age group may be particularly heart-wrenching. Children at this age lack the cognitive capacity and understanding of their illness to make informed decisions about their care. Their developmental maturity affects the meaning of information they receive. Many of these children may act pseudo-maturely, having spent long periods of time already undergoing treatments or multiple hospitalizations. Consequently, parents and staff may overestimate a child's decision-making capacity or ability to handle a treatment decision. They may be inclined to treat the child as a mini-adult, overinvolving the child in his or her care or asking the child to make decisions that would be overwhelming for him or her to consider.

Alternatively, parents and staff may be loathe to involve the child at all in the decision-making process, believing they are protecting the child from any difficult news or decisions and sparing the child emotional pain. In general, children tend to know and be aware of more than their parents acknowledge. Failure to involve them or giving them information they know is false will only confuse them and may jeopardize an already tenuous treatment alliance.

Psychological intervention may take the form of assessing the child's cognitive and affective level and advising parents and staff. A child who has not yet achieved abstract thinking and whose main goal in life is to master a certain talent will have to be involved differently than a mature 11-year-old who has begun to think abstractly and to form a discrete identity.

Late Childhood and Adolescence (Age 12 Years and Older)

During this phase of intellectual development, which continues into adulthood, the child achieves abstract thinking as well as a solid concept of reality. Children begin to generalize their thinking, formulate hypotheses beyond their experience, and reason deductively. Adolescents gradually begin to comprehend death, its irreversibility and universality. However, the thought of death as a personal event is overwhelming at this stage. Thus, they often use denial to cope with their anxiety and may engage in taking "dares" or trying out risk-taking behaviors. If they do experience the weight of impending death, they may feel angry and cheated.

The overall tasks of adolescence include identity consolidation, psychosexual differentiation, vocational planning, and separation from parents (13). Adolescents tend to be more concerned about the physical consequences of a disease and its treatment. They commonly feel a loss of control, frustration by their parents' overprotectiveness, and concern over peer relations and social isolation. A life-threatening illness may force them to become more dependent on their parents, less autonomous, and estranged from their peers.

Adolescents have the potential to cope differently than younger children. Some adolescents endorse clear religious positions at this stage and often develop a philosophical stance based on their belief system. Some cope by remaining physically active despite disabilities. For example, a teenage runner who has lost a leg may instead join the swim team. Often teens may try to maintain normalcy and their individual identities. Other adolescents may turn to substance use, sexual activity, or noncompliance in this struggle to affirm, or deny, their independence. These self-destructive behaviors may be a defense against the loss of invulnerability, attractiveness, or hope.

Clinicians need to accept the adolescent's struggle to be a normal teenager and his or her wish to maintain privacy. Flexible treatment schedules enable teens to feel more in control and to spend private time with friends. Establishing a positive atmosphere for communication enhances mutual trust. This will enable the adolescent child to verbalize his or her needs and work through his or her feelings. Noncompliance may respond to a clear explanation of the pros and cons of each procedure or treatment, appealing to the child's autonomy and ability to make decisions. Adolescent support groups can become a forum to share feelings and to feel less alone. Additionally, interactions with well peers who are informed and accepting can help the adolescent child feel less isolated and more understood.

The development of cognitive capacity for decision making occurs during adolescence. As a general guideline, most institutions require the assent of children age 13 or older (14). Brock has identified the required capacities for decision making as 1) understanding the medical information, 2) considering or reasoning about it, and 3) having or applying a set of values to choose various options (15). Leikin further defines having a set of values as a stable conception of one's good such that appropriate weight is assigned to future consequences of present decisions (16). Appreciation of a set of values allows the adolescent to evaluate treatment alternatives and weigh the burdens and benefits of various treatments, both in the present and in the future. The age for acquiring these capacities varies widely, from age 14 to adulthood. Older adolescents that refuse treatment need to be assessed for their understanding of the illness and its therapeutic outcome, and their competence for decision making. Also, the degree to which their values adequately reflect their future interests also needs to be considered. For example, an adolescent may refuse leg amputation for an osteosarcoma based on the decision that it will affect his or her appearance. However, if the treatment is lifesaving, the adolescent's ultimate well-being is not being served by refusing the intervention.

Case Example

Steven O. was a 16-year-old male who developed an osteogenic sarcoma of his lower extremity. After diagnosis and initial treatment, psychiatry and social service clinicians met with Steven and his father. During the meeting, Mr. O. stated that Steven's mother had died of breast cancer several years before, and he described her death as being prolonged and painful. He went on to say that if his son were to relapse, he would consider shooting Steven with a gun to prevent him from suffering the way his mother had. Steven did not know of this conversation. Because of this statement and other concerns, it was felt that it would be helpful for Mr. O. to meet with someone for support during the course of his son's treatment. He refused this offer but said he would ask for help when and if he needed it. Steven was offered psychiatric help while in the hospital, which he found helpful. After about a year of chemotherapy, Steven developed lung metastases, and it became quickly clear that he would not survive. Staff were concerned that Mr. O. would follow through on his possible plan to shoot his son when he was told about the relapse. A meeting was planned to tell the father and included the oncologist, psychiatrist, and social worker. During the meeting the father was asked about his statement to shoot his son. He was told that we were aware of his emotional pain but that he could not hurt his son. Mr. O. at first was angry but then began talking about his experience with his wife and his feelings that he was all alone with her while she died. He needed reassurance that he would not be alone, that every attempt would be made to minimize his son's pain, and that the staff would be accessible to him at all times. On hearing this the father relaxed and was able to talk about how his son would be told and how he would plan for the ongoing care of his son. Although he did not want to meet with someone face to face, he did use the telephone as a method of staying in contact with various caregivers after his son went home.

Case Example

Peter was a 15-year-old male who developed an osteogenic sarcoma in his hip. After initial surgery he was started on chemotherapy and seemed to do well. However, after about 18 months he had a recurrence of his tumor and developed metastases to his lungs. A new form of chemotherapy was used, without success, and Peter became sicker. He informed his nurses that he did not want any more chemotherapy, and he was urged to tell his parents. Peter could not tell his parents, who in fact wanted chemotherapy to continue. Peter felt he had to do what his parents wanted because he did not want to hurt them. Since the nursing staff knew of Peter's wishes, they became angry at the parents and angry at the oncologist for continuing to administer chemotherapy. Some, in fact, refused to follow the orders that were written for Peter's chemotherapy. Peter remained reluctant to tell his parents until it was suggested that a meeting could be held in which staff would be there and would support him while he spoke to his parents. Such a meeting was organized, and Peter hesitantly told his parents that he wanted to stop chemotherapy so that he could live the remaining period of his life feeling as healthy as he could and out of the hospital. After much discussion, which included the parents stating that they wanted to feel that they had done all that could be done and Peter assuring them that he felt that all had been done, his parents were able to accept Peter's decision. Everyone was now able to accept the inevitable, without conflict, and join together in their sadness.

Families

Each child should be viewed as constituting part of a homeostatic family system at a particular developmental stage in the life cycle (17). Each family member contributes to the system; consequently, anything that impinges on the life of one family member may disrupt or even overwhelm the balance of the system (18). A child's serious illness can provoke parental discord or isolation; open communication within the family has been found to help children cope more successfully (19).

Many factors affect the grieving process and a family's response to end-of-life decision making (20). It is important to identify the specific concerns of each member of the family. Living with a critically ill child has an impact on everyone. Each member will have his or her own way of expressing and tolerating feelings about the child's death. Assessing the role of the dying or deceased child, the emotional integration of the family, and the capacity for emotional expression is key (21, 22). Family resources, including physical, emotional, financial, social, and spiritual, should be estimated.

Given the crisis, the loss, and the values inherent in an end-of-life discussion, many family factors become evident. What was the quality of the marriage before the child's illness, and was the child planned, accepted, or conceived without mutuality? Strikingly long dormant tensions about one or another parent's never wanting the child or anger about behaviors like substance use during pregnancy or about one spouse's "bad genes" may burst forth in the rage that accompanies losing a child. How well do parents understand the disease? Have they overinvested in technical comanagement, or, for lack of sophistication, have they put their whole trust in the hands of a subspecialist who has now failed them? Do the parents share religious or cultural views of how the child should die? In particular, identification of previous losses in the family and coping patterns is essential (23). Did a sibling or parent die of a disease? What was the experience of the medical care, how did the family manage the end of life, and how did everyone cope thereafter? Are there unreserved angers or doubts? Frequently, former experiences with death will be highly relevant and predictive of how the individual parent will manage the current circumstances.

Distinct grieving patterns, whether related to gender or cultural or religious in origin, can dramatically affect decision making and coping with loss. Women's grief is generally more demonstrative than men's; in one study, women expressed more sadness, crying, difficulty sleeping, guilt, and irritability on a self-report questionnaire (24). This increased emotional expression may make some women appear indecisive and may unwittingly cause team members to exclude women (physically or emotionally) from meetings in which critical decisions are discussed. Men's response to grief often is expressed as an increased interest in work, a decrease in self-worth, guilt over their perceived lack of involvement, and an inability to ask for help (25). This seeming lack of emotion and controlled exterior may make men seem more decisive and may lead team members to assume prematurely some men are more informed or have conclusively decided the best interests of their children. Clinicians should be aware of these gender differences in coping because they may unwittingly encourage the stereotypes of highly expressed emotion or controlled passivity without giving each parent the time to verbalize her or his feelings in a safe place. Old angers, responses to death, and discord in the marriage traditionally require time to emerge; however, under the stress of end-of-life decision making, the historical and psychodynamic information is readily at hand. Empathically listening and offering straightforward explanations to clarify issues clears the air and allows parents to focus on the here and now, including coming together to get through the coming week. Potential guilt and grief are so overwhelming that it is best to avoid traditional "therapy" with couples and families, although it may be tempting to heal old wounds when they are so exposed.

The impact of culture and religion on a family's ability to make decisions and cope with loss also needs to be considered. Different societies have a variety of explanations for the phenomenon of death and its meaning. Rituals make up an important part of the grieving process for families and need to be respected in order to help individual members cope with loss. This may frequently involve altering or relaxing hospital policies around such routines as meals, visiting, passes, and so forth. Clinicians need not only to be sensitive to families' requests but also to actively ask in what ways they may be helpful or facilitate special religious or cultural arrangements. In addition, consultation with the hospital's Pastoral Services department can be invaluable.

It is not uncommon to overlook the involvement of siblings during the end-of-life period (26). Treatment decisions will profoundly affect siblings. Sometimes they are felt to be "too young" to be involved, and often the parents are so overwhelmed that they feel unable to assist them. In fact, siblings, too, are vulnerable to loss and may be at a greater risk for psychosocial problems than their ill siblings. Behavioral changes, mood changes, and/or a decline in school performance may indicate that a sibling is struggling. Siblings may suppress their grief secondary to unintentional messages that they be "strong and silent." Siblings fare better emotionally if they share the family's experience and remain active participants (27). Interviews with healthy, school-age siblings in a family with a child dying of cancer found that the siblings had three major concerns: 1) need for information, 2) need to feel important and not displaced, and 3) need to be a participant in the life of their dying sibling (28). Support groups are frequently helpful in alleviating common feelings and reactions that siblings of critically ill children experience (29). Parents need to be helped to understand that all members of a family will be grieving and that continued attention to their other children's emotional needs is necessary.

Many factors can impinge on our relationship with the patient, and each child should be approached uniquely. Clearly, a trauma that has occurred suddenly and involves a quick decision in terms of continuing or discontinuing treatment will affect the professional's relationship to the family differently than a chronic disease that has been treated over the course of many months or years and for which the consequences of that treatment have been long discussed and planned. Also, the opinions of the nursing staff, medical team, and other consultants will influence the consultant's decisions and consultations. Frequent, brief team meetings focusing on problem solving will help facilitate cohesiveness and a unified presence (30). Consultants may be involved supportively by assisting other team members, directly as leaders or collaboratively with other professionals.

Not uncommonly, mental health clinicians must care for families that are unable to work collaboratively with the team. All families will go through stages of shock, fear, anxiety, guilt, and shame. However, there are families who, because of their past experiences, will test the limits and patience of even the most cohesive treatment teams (31). These families should be identified early on, before their relationships with staff are irreparably damaged—a situation that could result in consequences to a child's care. Every family has its own unique way of responding to adversity and loss; there will inevitably be families whose coping styles and relationship to medical professionals are characterized by anger, alienation, and even obstructiveness. These maladjustive patterns of coping are best understood in their historical, religious, and ethnic roots. Forming an alliance with a family can be challenging under routine circumstances but is even more crucial with these so-called "difficult" families. Physicians and staff have been shown to use distancing tactics with these families; thus, team support is essential (32). Social service should be involved as soon as possible, as should the consulting mental health team. Team members can be of invaluable assistance in providing observations and impressions about these families. Frequent team meetings may be necessary to avoid divisiveness and to brainstorm on ways of working with these families to enhance their ability to cope.

Children and Decision Making to Limit or Withdraw Treatment

Communication with children, possibly even more than with adults, requires a sense of trust (33). Although in the past it was common not to tell dying children of their disease or prognosis, the question currently is how much to tell. The family's role is crucial. Assessing previous losses, coping, and hopes and expectations of the family will help the physician know the current capability of the family to deal with tragedy. Communication of the diagnosis in a thoughtful, empathic way is critical to parents' ability to cope with the disease and to come to terms with their child's impending death. The parents should be told in understandable language their child's diagnosis and the prognosis. Parents value private discussions with ample time for them to ask questions and absorb the information (34).

After the parents are informed, a decision needs to be made as to when and how much to tell the child. Every child is an integral part of a family system, with decisions made by and for a particular child dependent on understanding the child as an individual and as part of the system. A further complicating factor to consider is the child's developmental maturity. Two 11-year-olds with end-stage osteosarcoma may be at completely different cognitive, affective, and physical stages of development, necessitating completely different levels of involvement in their care. Obviously, careful consideration of a child's developmental stage, with the above information used as a guideline, is a good beginning.

Research has shown that children with a life-threatening illness develop an awareness of their prognosis and an awareness of death earlier than was believed in the past (35–38). Nonverbal cues such as excess anxiety or disguised verbal cues such as superficial questions may indicate that a child wishes to talk or ask further questions. Each child is different, and information should never be forced on a child, but should be revealed in accordance with the child's wishes. Delivery of a diagnosis, explained in terms appropriate to their developmental stage, can inspire a patient to become more fully involved in his or her own care (39).

Conversely, hiding a diagnosis from a child will almost always complicate the situation. Children are acutely aware of their parents' attitudes and levels of stress and rapidly sense changes that inevitably exist after parents are informed of their child's prognosis. If children are prevented from talking about their feelings, worries, or fears, they may be forced to deny them. This can lead to a retreat into lonely isolation complicated by depression, denial, or aggression. They may feel emotionally unsupported and abandoned by those they love, because an atmosphere of secrecy and "protection" has been unwittingly created by the family (40).

Slavin and colleagues (41) found, based on clinical interviews and standardized objective and projective tests, that patients' early knowledge of the diagnosis (i.e., informed early: told diagnosis by parent or physician within 1 year or diagnosed in infancy and told the diagnosis before age 6 years) was associated with better psychosocial adjustment. Learning the diagnosis later on (i.e., informed late: not told diagnosis within 1 year or diagnosed in infancy and not told diagnosis before age 6) was associated with more evident psychiatric symptoms and impairment of functioning. They associated an early telling of the diagnosis as a manifestation of family openness and willingness to help the child cope with his or her fears. The diagnosis should be communicated by the person who feels most comfortable conveying the information. This should be the parents if they are able, but often they find it helpful for the physician to be involved. The physician can be helpful by answering specific questions and helping to communicate in a thoughtful and frank manner.

How much input should children have into decisions about their care? Unfortunately, there are no easy answers. A determination of the child's understanding and integration of medical information is necessary. A child may not need to know all the details about a medical procedure to agree to it; nevertheless, he or she will need to know basic implications of diagnostic and treatment procedures. The child's ability to manage current and future circumstances also is a factor in deciding how much input children should have in treatment decisions.

What if parents or the child refuses treatment? Therapies that have little proven chance of even palliation can be refused. Justifications for withholding, withdrawing, or limiting therapy are 1) it can be shown that the therapy will not work, 2) the burdens of the treatment outweigh the benefits, and 3) the burdens of the disease outweigh the benefits of survival (42). The success rate of the refused therapy is crucial; if the therapy has been proven to be beneficial, physicians should not agree to requests to deny treatment (43). Parental refusal of a proven therapy can be overridden on ethical grounds if their choice results in deprivation of benefits such that harm or death to the child would occur (44). If the impasse cannot be solved through conventional interventions, ethics consultation should be requested (45, 46). Ethics consultation can assist patients in reaching decisions and help physicians guide patients and their families by developing a decision-making framework (47). An ethics committee brings together a variety of different professionals, such as a pediatrician, intensivist, layperson, religious representative, mental health clinician, and ethicist. It provides a forum for a multifocal case review from numerous perspectives. Such a committee allows for reconsideration of diagnostic questions, clarification of legal issues, explanation of physicians' judgments, and improvement of the decision-making process.

Refusal of treatment by adolescents is a more complex issue. If the patient is legally considered an emancipated minor (i.e., living separately from his or her parents, being self-sufficient economically and financially), then the patient is able to make an independent decision as his or her legal right. Recently, courts have accepted the claim that children with strong religious beliefs and "settled dispositions" might also fall into a similar category and thus be entitled to make healthcare decisions on their own behalf (48). Leikin (49) proposes that if a child has had an illness for some time, understands the benefits and burdens of treatment, can think and make decisions about the illness, and comprehends death and its implications for the family and for himself or herself, then that person, irrespective of age, is competent.

Most consultations should start with a medical evaluation to understand the child's current condition and to rule out organic factors affecting the child (e.g., medication side effects, anorexia due to nausea, or mood swings due to delirium). Depression, anxiety, confusion, and psychosis will all, obviously, have an impact on a child's ability to consent to or refuse treatment. Often, education of parents and medical staff unfamiliar with childhood psychiatric diagnoses is necessary. Not all children with terminal cancer become depressed, and not all children who have sustained a significant trauma develop anxiety. Children with preexisting psychiatric conditions are especially vulnerable to further decompensation under the stress of a terminal illness. Proper diagnosis and treatment of these psychiatric conditions is essential prior to any consideration of a child's decision-making capacity. Equally important to consider is the role of untreated fever, pain, suffering, and impaired cognition. These disease-related influences markedly affect a child's participation in his or her treatment and necessitate prompt and adequate treatment.

Ideally, children should be given as much control and decision-making power as possible in their own treatment to help alleviate feelings of helplessness. Allowing a child to choose the time and delivery route of a treatment, for example, will help him feel more involved in his care. Giving a child the chance to specify whom she wants to be present during a chemotherapy treatment, when she wants to see a mental health worker, and what time of day she can have a pass outside are also examples of how to make children feel more empowered. Consultants can intervene in many ways, by supporting parents' need to talk about their decisions with an informed adult and by providing a safe space for children to voice their feelings. Often the simple task of referring parents or siblings to a support group or counseling can go far and may be the best intervention we can offer when considering the best interests of the affected child.

Jellinek and colleagues (50) developed a set of questions for physicians and parents in the neonatal intensive care unit (NICU) setting. Modification of these questions for more general situations encountered in death and dying issues for children is a helpful way of beginning to address decision-making issues in children and adolescents (Table 6–1). When the physician or parent is asking these questions, it is best to refer to the baby/child/adolescent by name (we use "John" in Table 6–1) in order to emphasize the child as a person rather than a disease entity.

These discussions are among the most intense emotional experiences for both the parents and the physician; however, in the midst of tragedy, parents can still feel support and maintain a source of gratitude for the physician's effort, care, and companionship.

Discontinuation of Life-Sustaining Treatment

In adults, there is a general consensus that life-sustaining treatment may be ethically discontinued if the burdens of continued treatment outweigh the benefits of such treatment. In children, however, each case represents a composite of medical, developmental, psychosocial, and familial factors that renders such decisions uniquely complex. Life-sustaining treatment decisions are based on two major ethical values: the patient's well-being (best interest) and autonomy (capacity for self-determination) (51).

Current consensus is that there is an obligation to use only those therapies that offer a reasonable hope of benefit and are desired by the patient (or the patient's proxy) (52). Since children lack legal competence, and therefore autonomy as it is traditionally understood, the value of well-being becomes the standard for stopping life-sustaining treatment. Additionally, most experts feel that a distinction exists

---

Table 6–1. Questions for physicians and parents dealing with a critically ill child

---

1. How do you understand John's medical problems?

2. Has anything like this ever happened to you before?

3. What do you feel may have contributed to John's illness/accident?

4. Is there anything that we are doing or not doing to John that is worrying you?

5. Do both of you see John's medical problems and the decisions we are facing in the same way? Do either of you see anything differently?

6a. Have you been able even to consider that John, being this ill, is in danger of not getting better or actually dying?

6b. Just as we fear not being able to save every child, we also fear going too far, even worsening their suffering, when our efforts are futile. Do you think that this could happen to John?

6c. If we are sure that certain treatments will cause suffering for John without really helping him, then we won't be able to do those things. We always tell parents when we think this time is approaching. [Initially] For John things have not reached this point and we hope they do not. [Later] For John we could be there in a matter of days. [A brief period of silence will allow parents to respond.]

7. Do you feel we are helping or guiding you too much or too little?

8. How do your religious or cultural values influence your view of John's illness and any decision you may make about his care?

9. What was your main reason for deciding the way you did?

10. How do you feel about home or hospice care versus keeping John in the hospital?

11. How do you feel about staying with John during his last few hours and/or after the machines are removed? Are there ways in which we can make this time easier for you?

Source. Adapted from Jellinek et al. (50).

between legal competence and functional competence for pediatric patients. Functional competence in children (i.e., the criteria for decision-making capacity) has been described as the ability to reason, to understand, to choose voluntarily, to appreciate the nature of the decision, and to have an adequate conceptualization of death (53).

Freyer has taken the above approaches to life-sustaining treatment decision making in children and applied them to pediatric oncology (54); however, the concepts are easily applicable to life-sustaining treatment decisions in many cases (Table 6–2). Younger children, for example, lack legal and functional competence, such that decisions for them are made on their behalf (usually by a parent or guardian), and the decision carried out is described by Freyer as an "empathic choice." Adolescents can have functional competence, such that decisions can be made through a substitute decision-maker (in some states referred to as a *healthcare proxy*). Again, this decision-maker is often a parent or guardian. Explicit directives are communicated to this decision-maker, who legally executes the decision, enabling the patient's stated wishes to be enacted. In all such policy matters, consultation with the relevant hospital attorney should occur, because statutes regarding rights of minors vary from state to state.

Table 6–2.   Life-sustaining treatment (LST) decision making

Age group	Competence		LST by proxy	
	Legal	Functional	Standard	Type
Infancy–young school age	Absent	Absent	Best interest	Empathic choice
Older school age	Absent	Sometimes present	Best interest/autonomy	
Adolescence	Absent	Usually present	Autonomy	Increasing negotiation among parent, child, and physician

Source.   Adapted from Freyer (52).

The Consultant's Role

Are we, as consultants, being asked to be the diagnostician, healer, bearer of sad news, mediator, counselor, ethicist, or mourner? It is important to consider which roles we are being asked to provide and how we are expected to provide assistance. Sometimes we are involved in multiple roles. We may be asked to evaluate delirium in a critically ill child or to differentiate biological causes of symptoms from psychological ones. The consultant may be asked to help decide what is in the child's best interest; this is a task that is at best formidable and should never be an independent venture. We may be asked to help the treatment team cope with a difficult parent or family. Assessing a patient's, or parent's, competence to make a crucial decision about care may be necessary. The treatment team may request guidance in supporting a child or a specific family member at any point in the decision-making, bereavement, or treatment process. Our experience with pain and suffering may help a family member work through unresolved grief over past losses. We may be asked to play an indirect role via mediation or via supporting other team members and helping to bear their painful feelings.

Consultants are frequently asked to intervene when communication breaks down or is a barrier to decision making.

Case Example:
Child and Adolescent Psychiatrist,
Urgent Consult to NICU

Billy was born at 30 weeks' gestation, suffered a severe grade 4 intracerebral hemorrhage, and was now in the fifth week of a progressively downhill course. After a thorough assessment that he would be severely impaired and likely to die in the near term, his mother agreed with the team's decision that life support should be removed. Unfortunately, Billy's father worked as a fisherman, and their livelihood depended on his being at sea Monday through Friday of each week. After missing a week's work initially at Billy's birth, he could no longer responsibly stay at the hospital, and therefore his contact with the team was limited to weekends. Billy's mother had become quite attached to the primary care nurse and other members of the team, and although she had assured everyone that Billy's father was informed and in agreement, as the moment came to withdraw life support on a Friday afternoon (so he could be present), he became increasingly agitated and combative. An anesthesia resident on rotation to the NICU was about to turn off the respirator when Billy's father said to him, "If you kill my son, I will kill you. My son is a fighter, and he's going to make it." The psychiatric consultant arrived as Billy's father was aggressively confronting the anesthesia resident.

The immediate intervention was to elicit a promise from the resident and the team that life support would be sustained during the consultation. With that assurance, Billy's father agreed to go to a private setting and discuss his concerns. It became clear that he had not been fully informed, and even though he had heard some of his wife's worries, he continued to believe that his son was "a fighter." He knew his son had suffered severe damage but did not integrate the full implications of the neurological and organ system pathology or prognosis.

The psychiatric consultant asked if the father had ever been in this kind of situation before. After a moment's pause, he replied that the doctors had lied to him about his father. His father suffered from diabetes and had required multiple amputations. He suffered a series of heart attacks and died of congestive failure during Billy's father's mid-adolescence. "The doctor said he would never make it that long." The consultant asked, "How strong was he?" Billy's father replied, "Even though he only had one leg, he could have knocked me out the year before he died, he was a real fighter."

Despite the death of his father a decade ago, Billy's father had only recently mourned the loss of his own father. There had been a long period of drinking and depression that only lifted when he got married 3 years ago.

Billy's father began to cry. He soon saw the connection between denying his father's debilitated state, the consequences throughout his early adolescence, and his denial of the information his wife had been providing. He agreed to meet with the senior physician on the team, and after an explanation that confirmed his wife's understanding, he agreed to remove life supports. One-year follow-up indicated that although the marriage had suffered, they were still together, planning for another child, and there was no return to alcoholism.

As families and pediatric teams face life-and-death situations, denial is among the most difficult defenses to understand and manage. At many points throughout the treatment, some denial is essential. Denial may leave some room for hope and encourages minute-to-minute coping that may be critical to supporting the child. Too much denial interferes with understanding the current circumstances and prognosis as well as, at times, blocks vital decisions that could lead to a definitive diagnosis or positive interventions. Various members of the team, especially those with less experience, may become frustrated by this solution to the parents' needs and use the consultant to "break through" parental denial. The consultant must step back and consider the basis for the denial, what purpose the denial may be serving, the team's investment in "breaking through," and the impact on the health care of the child. Commonly, if there is a decision that needs to be made, especially one that may improve the child's prognosis, then confronting the denial may be appropriate, necessary, and on a tight time frame. Alternatively, if there is no acute medical indication, giving families several days or weeks to come to grips with the full impact of their child's condition may be best for both the child and the family. Although the team may be somewhat unsatisfied by this latter approach, assuring them that the issues should be dealt with in an outpatient setting and giving them some follow-up on how the family is doing 6 months or a year later will both reassure the team and build trust with the consultant.

Establishing a relationship with the parents during a crisis in communication is especially difficult. The consultant initially will need to present himself or herself as neutral and willing to take an objective look at all factors in the child's case. Reviewing medical events, consulting members of the treatment team (including nurses, social workers, and physical and occupational therapists), and assessing pertinent religious and cultural factors are all necessary. The consultant must be able to provide a safe place for the parents to verbalize their concerns. Listening empathically for a history of earlier losses, unresolved grief, or negative past interactions with medical caretakers will often help the consultant to understand the parents' interactions with the team. Helping the family to integrate information, grieve, accept suggestions, and communicate their wishes will often improve the child's care and enhance the parents' sense of contribution (55, 56).

Occasionally, a true impasse between the treating team and the patient or parents may happen. The impasse may occur because of conflicts between the patient's, family's, and team's desires—for example, disagreement about further treatment, withdrawal of life support, or alteration of life-sustaining efforts. Alternatively, there may be dissent within the treatment team. Hospital staff are not always uniformly sensitive to particular family or cultural concerns. These situations need to be addressed quickly and rationally. The central principle guiding decisions in these cases should be the best interests of the child (57), and the decisions should be made by the people who know the children best. Often, a consultant is the person asked to assess the situation and to resolve conflict and mediate difficulties. This may involve clarifying information for the family or patient, communicating a patient's or family's wishes to the treatment team, or meeting individually with team members to assess the degree of conflict within the team.

It is also the consultant's role to assess the extent to which psychopathology may be interfering with a patient's treatment or decision-making capacity and to consult a psychiatrist as needed. Factors that need to be considered include the role of denial, which may be manifest by risk taking and poor compliance with treatment. Clinical depression, whether organic in origin or due to the consequences of the disease process, is extremely common and frequently underdiagnosed and undertreated. Anxiety disorders can cause some children to become noncompliant with procedures or to refuse life-sustaining treatment. Prompt psychological counseling and psychopharmacologic intervention can ameliorate these situations, allowing children to play a more significant role in their care.

Physician and Staff Coping

Life and death issues are considered among the most stressful during a physician's training (58). Pediatrics is probably the specialty least experienced with death both because death is uncommon among children and the field is oriented toward prevention and development. Thus, pediatricians are highly personally invested in each child at risk for dying (59).

Our own history of illness and loss will naturally affect our relationship to these children (60). A study by Woolley and colleagues (61) found significantly increased stress levels in a subgroup of staff at a children's hospice; these staff had either lost a relative or close friend in the past year or showed substantial unresolved grief, or both. Berman and Villarreal (62) found that the use of an educational and support seminar for pediatric interns was rated as helpful in the interns' gaining a better understanding of their own feelings about death, and decreased the stress involved in caring for dying children. Overvaluing one's medical expertise or becoming too much of an authoritative leader of the team can be a defense mechanism indicating an inability to deal with death or the multiple decisions necessary in these situations.

Physicians may unconsciously distance themselves in their communications with seriously ill or dying patients. For example, physicians may falsely reassure a patient that they are sure the patient will have no pain in an effort to be comforting. They may ignore patients' statements of worry and instead focus on dealing with organ systems or unjustifiably exaggerate the significance of small improvements. They may try to alleviate distress by explaining that it is understandable and experienced by others in similar predicaments. Misinformation about a procedure may prevent children from verbalizing their fears; procedures that do not proceed as promised may lead to more profound distrust of caretakers. Physicians who selectively attend to a patient's physical symptoms or who change the subject when a patient raises emotional concerns convey the message that psychological issues should not be freely discussed. Physicians who prematurely speculate about a patient's distress without confirming the patient's actual thoughts can also inhibit further discussion.

Physicians and primary care nurses are at enormous risk of becoming the repository of intense affect and therefore must be especially aware of their own countertransference issues. For example, a physician who promised success, when faced with an imminent death, will have to confront his or her own limitations and sense of inadequacy. A nurse who has taken care of an ill neonate for many weeks becomes attached, and the baby benefits from that caring; if the baby dies, she will need to face her own grief and possibly old angers. Recognition of angry or hopeless feelings facilitates coping through teamwork, consultations, and appropriate investment in the child and family. Inadequate training in and preparation for death and dying issues can leave physicians feeling ineffective and overwhelmed; consequently, seminars and supervision during training are invaluable (63–66). Developing empathy is critical, and it may take considerable experience and effort to understand events that influence a particular family's response to stress and loss.

Physicians also frequently feel guilty, either because their prescribed treatment is not working or because they think they should have discovered something sooner. A particularly stressful time may be when nothing more can be done to keep the child alive. At this time, physicians may emotionally withdraw, feel angry, or even become depressed. Yet, this is the time when children and families need optimum support. Physicians need to acknowledge their personal feelings but not feel so overwhelmed that they turn inward or feel helpless (67). They must be aware of their own particular opinion about a case and yet remain neutral when assessing decisions to be made in the particular child's best interest. Sick children may remind us of painful moments during our childhood or cause us to worry excessively about our own children. Overinvolvement in a case can occur insidiously and be manifest by constant thoughts about the child, entanglement in the personal lives of family members, or alienation from the treatment team.

Consultants may experience denial, which can be both helpful and harmful in coping with the intense emotional experience that occurs with dying children. A certain amount of denial is reasonable if it is based on hope and understanding. However, rigid denial can block treatment decisions and leave a child and parents unprepared for death and unable to deal with difficult emotional issues. Healthcare professionals may underestimate the length of the denial/shock phase that families experience. Families need time to adjust to emotionally wrenching prognoses and decisions; often their denial may be helpful to a child by providing hope and strength. If a child's treatment is not affected, it may suffice to monitor the child and family and help them slowly explore and come to terms with their child's future treatment and the prognosis.

Palliative Care

End-stage management of the dying child is particularly difficult. At this point, hope for recovery or a reprieve is no longer realistic. Medical cure is not possible, but many families continue to hope for a non-medical miracle. The family needs to be told of the need to discontinue treatment and to focus on supportive and palliative care. Many people view this as a hopeless stage in which nothing more can help the patient. However, much can still be done, and palliative care should be viewed as reflecting a philosophy that affirms life (68, 69). The focus changes from curing or prolonging life to improving the quality of life. For this end to be achieved, the patient's and family's fears about the impending death must be addressed. If an image of a caring death can be envisioned, this may permit more living. Mount (70) has described the family assessment issues that are important once the family becomes the unit of care (Table 6–3).

Table 6–3. End-of-life family assessment issues
1. Identity of nuclear family, extended family, and social network (including peers and school)
2. Characteristics of family system: roles, relationships, communication patterns, and past history
3. Presence of concurrent life crises (e.g., unemployment, sibling achievements or needs, financial difficulties)
4. History of coping with past crises (e.g., prior circumstances in a child's course, siblings' and family's previous reactions to illness and loss)
5. Parents' and siblings' values and beliefs about death
6. Response to child's current stage of illness: changes in roles and relationships between siblings and parents
7. Family resources: physical, emotional, financial, social, cultural, and spiritual
8. Immediate and practical family needs (e.g., transportation, funeral arrangements, child care)
9. Long-range family needs (e.g., parent and sibling follow-up, genetic counseling)

Source. Adapted from Mount (40).

Care should be focused on identification and alleviation of symptoms. A flexible care plan that accommodates a patient's changing needs as the disease progresses is essential (71). Adequate pain relief is absolutely crucial. This shifting in therapeutic goals, including the ongoing involvement of a caring physician, helps to support the family and child. It frees them to choose from available options. An increasingly common option today is home care or hospice care for the dying child. Symptoms can be managed as effectively at home as in a hospital (72). Studies have shown that parents of patients in home care programs show less anxiety and depression and fewer somatic and interpersonal problems than do parents of hospitalized patients receiving terminal care (73, 74). Siblings of patients involved in home care programs reported different experiences from those whose brother or sister died in the hospital: they reported being prepared for the death, receiving consistent information and support from parents, feeling directly involved in the care and death, and experiencing closer family relations thereafter (75).

Pediatric hospice care focuses on symptom amelioration and maximizes the current quality of life. Cure is no longer the goal. Hospice care concerns itself with holistic care for patients, friends, and their families, focusing on the alleviation of physical, psychological, spiritual, and social suffering in the context of a meaningful framework (76, 77).

Grief

Parkes (78) described grief as the price we have to pay for having loved someone; the experience of love and joy means that the pain of loss is inevitable. Grief was described by Lindemann (79) as a process encompassing a broad range of feelings, somatic sensations, cognitions, and behaviors that commonly occur after a loss. Feelings can range from sadness to anger and guilt, and physical sensations can include fatigue, decreased energy, and chest or throat tightness. Cognitions may include disbelief, confusion, hallucinations, and behaviors ranging from sleep and appetite disturbances to social withdrawal and preoccupation with the deceased.

Many of the normal manifestations of grief may seem like symptoms of depression. Indeed, prolonged grief can evolve into depression.

Freud distinguished depression from mourning by the presence of angry feelings about an ambivalently loved person that are turned inward (80). In grief, there is not commonly the loss of self-esteem and guilt that accompanies depression.

Grieving for a child encompasses additional stressors. Children are not supposed to die. Most parents wish better lives for their children than they experienced and often have elaborate hopes and fantasies about their children's growth and achievements. Accepting the mortality of one's child means relinquishing these dreams in addition to realizing the unpredictability of life. A critically ill child may produce a level of intimacy and interdependence for which some families may not be fully prepared. Often children are developmentally struggling to find their identity outside of the family system. Their death will mean an irreversible change of the family unit, requiring modification of future plans and goals. One parent may grieve differently from his or her spouse. Validating these differences and helping the couple respect their distinct styles allows them to support each other. Grieving may feel unbearable but should proceed as long as it can be tolerated (81).

In anticipatory mourning, parents withdraw, yielding their emotional attachment to a child prior to the child's death. Reconciliation to the fact of death begins the necessary investment in other relationships. The last phase involves memorialization of the child through a meaningful, mental image (82). Some parents may detach too soon from their children, leaving them alone as they approach death. For example, a child with a critical but longstanding illness may lose support from detached parents too early. Consultants can help parents, staff, and relatives by remaining sensitive to the intense emotions parents experience preparing for the child's death. Angry outbursts, frequent crying, and intense anxiety need to be not only tolerated by hospital staff but also normalized for the grieving individuals.

The bereavement process begins shortly after death and can involve multiple symptoms, including somatic distress, feelings of survivor guilt, disorganization, inability to complete routine tasks, hostility in interpersonal relationships, and preoccupation with images of the dead child (83). All of these symptoms are normal, and families should be prepared by consultants to anticipate these over the first 6 to 8 weeks following the child's death. In cases of unexpected death, parents often are psychologically unprepared. They can experience a surge of intense, intolerable feelings. They frequently experience sadness, depression, loneliness, anxiety, and anger, which can be directed indiscriminately. Encouraging family members to verbalize their feelings in order to understand these intense emotions is critical but may be ignored by physicians and staff who view their work as finished once the child dies.

Sibling grief should not be overlooked. Children in particular try to make sense of difficult experiences and find a variety of ways to deal with memories of deceased loved ones. Normand and colleagues (84) have identified different types of connections maintained by bereaved children with their dead parents. These include maintaining interactive relationships with the deceased in which the deceased may be perceived as active spirits in their lives. Relationships may involve conversing with these spirits, dreaming about them, keeping treasured objects, and/or internalizing the values, goals, personalities, or behaviors of the deceased. These relationships and coping mechanisms may be pertinent in understanding grief suffered by a sibling who has lost a brother or sister.

Consultants should recognize and work through their own grief in order to help children and families with their loss. If consultants do not consciously acknowledge their own grief, they may avoid or reject a family or may discourage the normal show of despair. Indeed, physicians may be tempted to treat physical symptoms of the family's grief with tranquilizers or mood elevators (85). Oversedation represses feelings and prevents parents and siblings from having the opportunity to begin working through their sorrow immediately. We, as consultants, must be able to tolerate painful affects, to provide support appropriately, and to recognize that our assistance does not end with the child. Our role as consultant may entail attending funeral services, spending extra time with the child's siblings or relatives, and allowing the family permission to call us in the first few weeks after the child's death.

Pathologic Grief

The death of a child is profound, and no one has a clear definition of "normal" grieving. However, abnormal or pathologic grief immobilizes people, for many months and years, and prevents them from completing their normal daily tasks. Consultants need to watch for delayed grief reactions (often years after the death of a child), acute changes in the parents' behaviors (such as a sudden increase in somatic symptoms or hyperactivity), or abnormal social adjustment (such as hostility or isolation) (86). Oliver found that 75% of a sample of parents whose children had died in traumatic accidents had pathologic grief. Features of this grief included a lack of a support network beyond the extended family, an avoidant stance to grieving, and a view of God as distant and punitive (87).

Parents may appreciate meeting with the mental health clinician immediately after the death, 2 to 4 days later, and several weeks later. Careful follow-up over time is almost universally welcomed by families, who view such contact as empathic and meaningful. These meetings have the advantage of repeating and clarifying information that the parents may have been unable to process because of their initial shock, and monitoring symptoms to evaluate if parents are beginning to move on with their lives weeks after the death of their child.

Todres and colleagues (88) note that physicians may be reluctant to follow-up with parents after death since they may feel like failures, guilty, or fearful of parental anger. Todres points out that his experience is quite the opposite, noting that parents regard a follow-up with appreciation. He suggests that certain questions be used at 6-, 12-, and 24-month follow-up calls to families after a child's death (Table 6–4). Again, it is best to refer to the child by name (we use "John" in Table 6–4) to emphasize the child as a person.

Conclusion

Children embody our hope, dreams, and deepest sense of ourselves as protectors and nurturers. Separation and loss issues frequently arise in pediatric hospital settings. A child's death calls into question our competence and challenges our role as caregivers. It raises questions concerning life and meaning. But most of all, it can provide a rare privilege to know intimately a child, his or her family, and ourselves. Death gives us the opportunity to be a healer and to relieve suffering, which

Table 6–4. Questions for follow-up call to the family after a child's death

1. An opening remark such as "How are you doing?"
2. How are things going for you since John died?
3. Have you been able to resume your usual routines? [work and recreational]
4. How is your family coping? [e.g., types of support systems, including relatives, counseling, spiritual involvement, etc.]
5. How has John's death affected your relationship with your spouse? [e.g., communication, relatedness and intimacy, future plans]
6. How are your other children [if any] reacting? [e.g., school performance, levels of neediness, peer relationships, aggression or regression]
7. How are you sleeping and eating?
8. Are you enjoying life?
9. Are you able to concentrate?
10. Can I do anything to help?

Source. Adapted from Todres et al. (88).

can be more gratifying than fighting a disease entity. Confrontation with death can foster insight and serve as a profound impetus for psychological growth (89). It gives us a unique chance to assist families with the loss of a child (90) and help them to integrate the experience, such that the family will continue to develop and nurture its members.

References

1. Maguire P: Barriers to psychological care of the dying. BMJ 291:1711–1713, 1985
2. Crain W: Piaget's cognitive-developmental theory, in Theories of Development. New York, Simon & Schuster, 1992, pp 100–133
3. Mahler MS, Pine F, Bergman A: The Psychological Birth of the Human Infant. New York, Basic Books, 1975
4. Benfield DG, Leib SA, Vollman JH: Grief response of parents to neonatal death and parent participation in deciding care. Pediatrics 62:171–177, 1978

5. Geddes S, Pace N: Selectively withholding treatment from newborn babies. Br J Hosp Med 47:281–283, 1992

6. Freund B: Neonatal intensive care and the premature infant: criteria for intervention. Humane Medicine 9:282–288, 1993

7. White MP, Reynolds B, Evans TJ: Handling of death in special care nurseries and parental grief. BMJ 289:167–169, 1984

8. Leikin S: The role of adolescents in decisions concerning their cancer therapy. Cancer 71 (10, suppl):3342–3346, 1993

9. Cincotta N: Psychosocial issues in the world of children with cancer. Cancer 71 (10, suppl):3251–3260, 1993

10. Waechter EH: Dying children—patterns of coping, in Childhood and Death. Edited by Wass H, Corr CA. Washington, DC, Hemisphere, 1984, pp 51–68

11. Gray E: The emotional and play needs of the dying child. Issues in Comprehensive Pediatric Nursing 12:207–224, 1989

12. Wass H: Concepts of death: a developmental perspective, in Childhood and Death. Edited by Wass H, Corr CA. Washington, DC, Hemisphere, 1984, pp 3–24

13. Ettenger RS, Heiney SP: Cancer in adolescents and young adults. Cancer 71 (10, suppl):3276–3280, 1993

14. Cincotta, Psychosocial issues

15. Brock D: Children's competence for health care decision-making, in Children and Health Care. Edited by Kopelman L, Moskop J. Boston, MA, Kluwer Academic, 1989, pp 181–212

16. Leikin S: A proposal concerning decisions to forgo life-sustaining treatment for young people. J Pediatr 115:17–22, 1989

17. Brown PG: Families who have a child diagnosed with cancer: what the medical caregiver can do to help them and themselves. Issues in Comprehensive Pediatric Nursing 12:247–260, 1989

18. Ross-Alaolmolki KR: Supportive care for families of dying children. Nurs Clin North Am 20:457–466, 1985

19. Maguire, Barriers to psychological care

20. Kristjanson LJ, Ashcroft T: The family's cancer journey: a literature review. Cancer Nurs 17:1–17, 1994

21. Worden JW: Grief and Family Systems in Grief Counseling and Grief Therapy. New York, Springer, 1991, pp 117–132

22. Barakat LP, Sills R, LaBagnara S: Management of fatal illness and death in children or their parents. Pediatr Rev 16:419–423, 1995

23. Hersh SP, Wiener LS: Psychosocial support for the family of the child with cancer, in Principles and Practice of Pediatric Oncology. Edited by Rizzo PA, Poplack DG. Philadelphia, PA, JB Lippincott, 1989, pp 1141–1156

24. Benfield et al, Grief response of parents
25. Behnke M, Nackashi JA, Raulerson DM, et al: The pediatrician and the dying child, in Childhood and Death. Edited by Wass H, Corr CA. Washington, DC, Hemisphere, 1984, pp 69–92
26. Wass, Concepts of death
27. Cincotta, Psychosocial issues
28. Behnke et al, Pediatrician and the dying child
29. Worden, Grief and Family Systems
30. Martinson IM, Moldow DG, Armstrong GD, et al: Home care for children dying of cancer. Res Nurs Health 9:11–16, 1986
31. Beresin EV: The difficult parent, in Psychiatric Aspects of General Hospital Pediatrics. Edited by Jellinek M, Herzog D. Chicago, IL, Year Book Medical, 1990, pp 67–75
32. Maguire, Barriers to psychological care
33. Davies B, Eng B: Factors influencing nursing care of children who are terminally ill: a selective review. Pediatric Nursing 19:9–14, 1993
34. Foley GV: Enhancing child-family health team communication. Cancer 71 (10, suppl):3281–3289, 1993
35. Ross-Alaolmolki, Supportive care for families
36. Woolley H, Stein A, Forrest GC, et al: Imparting the diagnosis of life-threatening illness in children. BMJ 298:1626–1628, 1989
37. Spinetta JJ, Rigler D, Karon M: Anxiety in the dying child. Pediatrics 52:841–849, 1973
38. Solnit A, Green MP: The pediatric management of the dying child, Part II: the child's reaction to the fear of dying, in Modern Perspectives in Child Development. Edited by Solnit A, Provence S. New York, International Universities Press, 1963, pp 217–228
39. Cousins N: The head comes first: creating an environment for optimal treatment. Humane Medicine 6:284–288, 1990
40. Mount BM: Care of dying patients and their families, in Cecil Textbook of Medicine, 20th Edition. Edited by Bennett JC, Plum F. Philadelphia, PA, WB Sanders, 1995, pp 6–9
41. Slavin LA, O'Malley JE, Koocher GP, et al: Communication of the cancer diagnosis to pediatric patients: impact on long-term adjustment. Am J Psychiatry 139:179–183, 1982
42. Slavin et al, Communication of the cancer diagnosis
43. Tomlinson T, Brody H: Ethics and communication in do-not-resuscitate orders. N Engl J Med 318:43–46, 1988
44. Ashwal S, Perkin RM, Orr R: When too much is not enough. Pediatr Ann 21:311–317, 1992

45. Fletcher JC, van Eys J, Dorn LD: Ethical considerations in pediatric oncology, in Principles and Practice of Pediatric Oncology. Edited by Rizzo PA, Poplack DG. Philadelphia, PA, JB Lippincott, 1989, pp 1179–1191

46. Nelson RM, Shapiro RS: The role of an ethics committee in resolving conflict in the neonatal intensive care unit. Journal of Law, Medicine and Ethics 23:27–32, 1995

47. LaPuma J, Schiedermayer D, Siegler M: How ethics consultation can help resolve dilemmas about dying patients. [Special Issue: Caring for Patients at the End of Life]. West J Med 163:263–267, 1995

48. Kluge EK: Informed consent by children: the new reality. Can Med Assoc J 152:1495–1497, 1995

49. Leikin, Proposal concerning decisions to forgo life-sustaining treatment

50. Jellinek MS, Catlin EA, Todres ID, et al: Facing tragic decisions with parents in the neonatal intensive care unit: clinical perspectives. Pediatrics 89:119–122, 1992

51. The Hastings Center: Guidelines on the Termination of Life-Sustaining Treatment and the Care of the Dying. Briarcliff Manor, NY, The Hastings Center, 1987

52. Freyer DR: Children with cancer: special considerations in the discontinuation of life-sustaining treatment. Med Pediatr Oncol 20:136–142, 1992

53. Brock, Children's competence

54. Freyer, Children with cancer

55. King NMP, Cross AW: Children as decision-makers: guidelines for pediatricians. J Pediatr 115:10–16, 1989

56. Rowe J, Clyman R, Green C, et al: Follow-up of families who experience a perinatal death. Pediatrics 62:166–170, 1978

57. Howell DA, Martinson IM: Management of the dying child, in Principles and Practice of Pediatric Oncology. Edited by Rizzo PA, Poplack DG. Philadelphia, PA, JB Lippincott, 1989, pp 1115–1124

58. White BD, Hickson GB, Theriot R, et al: A medical ethics issues survey of residents in five pediatric training programs. American Journal of Diseases of Children 145:161–164, 1991

59. Emery JL: Attitudes of parents and pediatricians to a baby's death. J R Soc Med 83:423–424, 1990

60. Benfield et al, Grief response of parents

61. Woolley H, Stein A, Forrest GC, et al: Staff stress and job satisfaction at a children's hospice. Arch Dis Child 64:114–118, 1989

62. Berman S, Villarreal S: Use of a seminar as an aid in helping interns care for dying children and their families. Clin Pediatr (Phila) 22:175–179, 1983

63. Woolley et al, Staff stress

64. Berman and Villarreal, Use of a seminar

65. Whitt JK, Hunter RS, Dykstra W, et al: Pediatric liaison psychiatry: a forum for separation and loss. Int J Psychiatry Med 11:59–68, 1981–1982

66. Gomez CF: A model program in palliative care for residents, in American Board of Internal Medicine, Committee on Evaluation of Clinical Competence: Caring for the Dying: Identification and Promotion of Physician Competency. Philadelphia, PA, American Board of Internal Medicine, 1996, pp 27–30

67. Jellinek MS, Todres ID, Catlin EA, et al: Pediatric intensive care training: confronting the dark side. Crit Care Med 21:775–779, 1993

68. Whittam E: Terminal care of the dying child: psychosocial implications of care. Cancer 71 (10, suppl):3450–3462, 1993

69. Lo B: Improving care near the end of life: why is it so hard? JAMA 274:1634–1636, 1995

70. Mount BM: Care of dying patients and their families, in Cecil Textbook of Medicine, 20th Edition, 1995

71. Wanzer SH, Federman DD, Adelstein SJ, et al: The physician's response toward hopelessly ill patients. N Engl J Med 320:844–849, 1989

72. Martinson IM: Improving care of dying children. West J Med 163:258–262, 1995

73. Mulhern RK, Lauer ME, Hoffmann RG: Death of a child at home or in the hospital: subsequent psychological adjustment of the family. Pediatrics 71:743–747, 1983

74. Brown, Families who have a child diagnosed with cancer

75. Lauer M, Mulhern RK, Bohne JB, et al: Children's perceptions of their sibling's death at home or hospital: the precursors of differential adjustment. Cancer Nurs, February, 1985, pp 21–27

76. Corr CA, Corr DM: Pediatric hospice care. Pediatrics 76:774–780, 1985

77. Whittam, Terminal care of the dying child

78. Parkes CM: Bereavement and mental illness, Part 2: a classification of bereavement reactions. Br J Med Psychol 38:13–26, 1965

79. Lindemann E: Symptomatology and management of acute grief. Am J Psychiatry 101:141–148, 1944

80. Freud S: Mourning and melancholia (1917[1915]), in Standard Edition of the Complete Psychological Works of Sigmund Freud, Vol 14. Translated and edited by Strachey J. London, Hogarth Press, 1957, pp 237–260

81. Davidson GW: Stillbirth, neonatal death, and sudden infant death syndrome, in Childhood and Death. Edited by Wass H, Corr CA. Washington, DC, Hemisphere, 1984, pp 243–257

82. Mount, Care of dying patients and their families

83. Ashwal et al, When too much is not enough
84. Normand CL, Silverman PR, Nickman S: Bereaved children's changing relationships with the deceased, in Continuing Bonds: New Understandings of Grief. Edited by Klass D, Silverman PR, Nickman S. Philadelphia, PA, Taylor & Francis, 1996, pp 87–111
85. Worden, Grief and Family Systems in Grief Counseling and Grief Therapy
86. Lindemann, Symptomatology and management of acute grief
87. Oliver RC, Fallat ME: Traumatic childhood death: how well do parents cope? J Trauma 39:303–308, 1995
88. Todres ID, Earle M, Jellinek MS: Enhancing communication: the physician and family in the pediatric intensive care unit. Pediatr Clin North Am 41:1395–1404, 1994
89. Jellinek et al, Pediatric intensive care training
90. Benfield et al, Grief response of parents

7

End-of-Life Decisions in AIDS

Alexandra Beckett, M.D.

In many respects, AIDS (acquired immunodeficiency syndrome) is not different from other life-
threatening illnesses. Like persons with cancer or severe cardiac
disease, individuals with AIDS battle life-threatening illness and struggle with the ravages of treatment before they reach the end. Persons
with AIDS are no more likely than those with other serious illnesses to
know with certainty when the end is at hand. However, AIDS differs
from other life-threatening medical conditions in significant ways.
Most people living with AIDS in this second decade of the epidemic
have an intimate knowledge of the course of the illness, gleaned
through direct experience with others who have died from the disease.
Furthermore, until very recently, the vast majority of knowledgeable
people have considered AIDS inevitably fatal, whereas cancer or heart
disease, even in their most virulent forms, can sometimes be cured.

These differences become very important with respect to decisions
about whether to continue treatment. What is reasonable to hope for?
If a disease is going to claim one's life swiftly, "quality of life" considerations, rather than mere survival, may become paramount. If, on the
other hand, the potential exists for dramatic improvement in health

and even cure, suffering related to medical therapies may be worth enduring—an unfortunate but inescapable part of the quest for a longer and better life.

The summer of 1996 was a turning point in the world of AIDS research and treatment. At the annual International Conference on AIDS, held in Vancouver in July 1996, researchers announced that they had achieved astonishing success with a new class of antiretroviral drugs, the protease inhibitors. For the first time since the introduction of the antiretroviral drug zidovudine (AZT), scientists had brought about the eradication of measurable virus in the blood of some HIV (human immunodeficiency virus)–infected persons. A milestone in the war on AIDS had been reached: it had became reasonable to hope that, at the very least, AIDS could become a chronic illness like, for example, diabetes. At best, it became reasonable to anticipate a cure for HIV infection through aggressive antiviral therapy.

These changes in the therapeutic options and outcomes in HIV/AIDS therapy have implications for decision making. Patients and doctors are more hopeful regarding the long-term prognosis and see reasons to aggressively treat AIDS-related illnesses that in the recent past might have been allowed to take their course. Doctors are now more hesitant to recommend palliative care, even in the face of considerable illness. Furthermore, patients are likely to forego curative therapy only when they are convinced that a complication is truly untreatable.

The revelations regarding the efficacy of new antiviral treatments have been succeeded by the news that AIDS hospices in many major metropolitan areas have had to close doors because their services are no longer in demand; indeed, death rates from AIDS have plummeted (1). This strengthens the perception of AIDS as a chronic, rather than fatal, illness. It is clear that these remarkable advances in the care of patients with AIDS and the subsequent drop in AIDS deaths engender realistic hopefulness regarding the long-term prognosis for patients with AIDS.

Nonetheless, AIDS continues to be a grave, life-changing diagnosis, and thoughtful persons understand that some HIV-infected persons will not benefit from the new "combination" treatments. A recent article in the *New York Times* (2) identified disappointments that have emerged since the "initial flush of success" of combination treatment involving protease inhibitors. Experts interviewed for the article raised some important questions about the limitations of combination therapy. Although there are many instances in which protease inhibitor therapy has led to remarkable improvement in health, it is also true that compliance with therapy is extremely difficult because of the number of pills that must be taken, the potential for adverse interactions with other drugs, and the physical side effects sometimes experienced. Furthermore, some patients have had no discernible response to combination treatment.

All things considered, it is likely that persons with AIDS will continue to be concerned with the manner in which they will die, all the while hoping to live as long as possible, and to die as well as possible in the natural course of illness. Most individuals with AIDS are aware that things might go badly at the end, as experienced by friends, lovers, and family members who have died of the disease. Many AIDS patients express a wish to define the limits of what they will and will not tolerate in terms of disease complications and, ultimately, with respect to dying. To achieve this level of control requires, at the very least, negotiations with care providers and significant others, the utilization of advanced directives, and the selection of a well-informed healthcare proxy. For some patients, it involves efforts to determine the time of death, whether by forgoing diagnostic evaluation of symptoms, by discontinuing life-prolonging treatments, or through suicide.

Forgoing Treatment

Although persons with AIDS commonly assert that they do not want futile treatments, it is difficult to define futility in the context of AIDS. Wachter and colleagues (3) propose that futile care is that provided to patients with terminal, irreversible illness whose life expectancy is less than 2 weeks. Another, less precise way of conceptualizing futility is that it exists when everyone concurs that no intervention will achieve the desired goal.

In the context of a relatively new disease like AIDS, in which there is rarely a clear short-term prognosis, futility should be understood more in terms of whether the proposed treatment seems worthwhile to the patient. Is there a chance that it will improve his or her quality of life? Will it buy time in the hope for more promising therapies? Or, if the treatment has expectable toxicities, do the potential benefits merit the discomforts?

Despite the often-expressed sentiment against futile treatments in AIDS, a recent report by Goldstone and colleagues (4) identifies a trend toward more aggressive terminal care for AIDS patients in Vancouver, a city with a highly sophisticated system of inpatient and community-based palliative care. A retrospective analysis of AIDS deaths in Vancouver in 1992 found that 19% of individuals were resuscitated before death, notwithstanding the data that demonstrate a zero probability of being discharged alive following resuscitation in advanced AIDS. Another 39% of those who died were aggressively treated to within a mean of 3 days before death, although do-not-resuscitate (DNR) orders were in place. The remainder died while under palliative care.

It is not clear whether this aggressive, end-of-life care was given at the patient's behest or if it occurred because of failures in doctor-patient communication. Investigators in both San Francisco (5) and Boston (6) have found that whereas three-quarters of AIDS patients indicated that they would like to discuss intubation and resuscitation with their doctors, only one-third had done so. Despite the fact that this very important question of whether to use heroic measures is insufficiently addressed, there is a growing trend among patients with AIDS to see themselves as "consumers" who may demand certain treatments and decline others.

According to Miles (7), respect for patient autonomy does not empower patients to oblige physicians to prescribe treatments that are fruitless or inappropriate. Although legislatures and courts are ill suited to determine what treatments are medically appropriate, they have come out strongly in support of the competent individual's right to decline medical care. State courts have upheld the rights of competent patients to refuse treatments, whether or not they are terminally ill, and even if the treatment is lifesaving (e.g., dialysis, surgery, transfusion) (8). As the New Jersey Supreme Court (9) stated, "A young generally healthy person, if competent, has the same right to decline life-saving medical treatment as a competent elderly person who is terminally ill." The patient is protected against "unwarranted bodily intrusions" and is guaranteed personal autonomy in making decisions regarding his or her health and welfare (10).

Clinical Vignette 1:
The Case of D.S.

D.S., a 34-year-old gay man, had been diagnosed with AIDS 2 years earlier and had just recovered from his third episode of Pneumocystis carinii pneumonia (PCP) when he began to feel extremely anxious and depressed. He had always loved his home and community, where he had been active in local politics, but began to think that his neighbors were out to get him and that the FBI was staking out his apartment.

D.S. presented to his doctor in a state of agitation and was admitted to the psychiatric ward. While there, he was treated with fluoxetine and haloperidol and over 2 weeks began to recover to his usual state of mental health. He was able to leave the hospital with a sense of well-being. Following discharge, he met weekly with a psychiatrist, who found D.S. increasingly able to enjoy his family and friends and the outdoor activities that had always been a passion. D.S. returned to the Quaker meeting that he had attended for many years.

Though genuinely happy and serene, D.S. decided to discontinue all antiretroviral and prophylactic medications, reasoning that he had "turned the corner" with his illness, and that he did not wish to die the all-too-familiar and protracted death through which he had nursed several friends. Each time he met with his primary care doctor or psychiatrist, the issue of prophylactic medications was raised; each time D.S. reiterated his position. He maintained his involvement in meaningful activities and described himself as exhilarated with his life.

Nine months later, D.S. developed a high fever and shortness of breath. He notified his doctor, who agreed with D.S.'s assessment that he most likely had PCP, and recommended that he come to the hospital for a definitive diagnosis. D.S. reaffirmed his decision not to be treated and chose to stay home until he became sufficiently uncomfortable, at which time he came to the hospital requesting comfort measures.

The nursing staff, who had known D.S. over the entire course of his illness, were quite attached to him and were extremely reluctant to acquiesce to this request for palliative care in the face of a potentially curable opportunistic infection. His primary nurse was so distressed that she refused to participate in what she characterized as an "assisted suicide."

His psychiatrist was called to evaluate. She found D.S. competent, rational, and at peace with his decision. He was not depressed or otherwise psychiatrically disturbed. Though a hospice bed would soon become available, D.S. did not wish to be transferred to an unfamiliar setting, and wanted to die in the hospital where he had received all his care. He did not wish to go home for fear of burdening his elderly parents, who had come from out-of-state to be with him.

Despite the conflict among the hospital staff, and after another nurse signed off the case citing ethical concerns, D.S. remained in the hospital on oxygen and intravenous morphine. He slipped into a coma and died 3 days later with his parents at his side.

The controversy surrounding D.S. illustrates the problems encountered by competent patients who wish to forgo treatments that are not heroic. Although on paper the patient is protected against "unwarranted bodily intrusions" and is guaranteed personal autonomy in making decisions regarding his or her health and welfare, it may be extremely difficult to stand by while a beloved person like D.S. chooses to let himself die of a treatable infection. It is in such situations that psychiatrists are often consulted to assess whether the patient is depressed, delirious, demented, or otherwise mentally impaired. The question, implicitly, is one of competence.

The law affirms the patient as decision-maker, provided he or she has the capacity to reason and make judgments, that his or her decisions are voluntary and uncoerced, and that he or she understands clearly the nature of the disease, its prognosis, and the consequences of his or her choices. Nevertheless, there is a powerful inclination to question whether it is ever rational for a person to desire death. Psychiatrists have come to see a wish for death as a psychopathological symptom that will disappear with appropriate treatment.

It is commonly held that a depressed person is not capable of making a rational choice to die. Sullivan and Youngner (11) have pointed out that psychiatry has inappropriately extended its views on suicide in the medically well to the case of treatment refusal by the seriously medically ill. Although these authors acknowledge that depressed individuals may be able to understand facts yet fail to appreciate their personal importance, they argue that a diagnosis of depression is neither necessary nor sufficient to conclude that an individual's decision-making capacity is impaired.

To date, there are no systematic studies of the wish to die and its relation to psychopathology among individuals in the terminal stages of AIDS. Fogel and Mor (12) studied care preferences among 817 outpatients with AIDS and found a correlation between depression and unwillingness to accept nursing home placement or intubation. On reinterview, some subjects who were no longer depressed had changed their minds and were now willing to accept such interventions in order to prolong life. Among patients with cancer, studies suggest that the wish for death is, in fact, associated with depression. In one study of 44 terminally ill cancer patients, 11 wished for death to come early, and all 11 were found to suffer from clinically significant depressive illness (13). A more recent investigation involving 200 terminally ill cancer patients in a hospice setting (14) found that *occasional* desires for death were common—44.5% of subjects acknowledged having had such desires—though transient. A *serious* desire for death was expressed by 8.5% of the subjects and was highly correlated with measures of pain, family support, and depression.

Is there a difference between AIDS and cancer with respect to wishes for death and choices to forgo treatment? In the author's experience with hospitalized patients, both patients with AIDS and patients with cancer assert that there is a quality of life that is not worth living. Those with AIDS are more likely to be able to describe such a state in detail and to specify what they might do in such a situation. It is not possible to know whether such stated preferences are predictive of future actions.

Do differences in physician attitudes influence patient choices in end-of-life matters? Wachter and colleagues (15) discovered that house staff discussed DNR orders significantly more often with patients who had AIDS or lung cancer than with patients who had cirrhosis or heart failure despite a generally similar prognosis among the four groups. Furthermore, they were very much more likely to write DNR orders for the former two groups. Although this may reflect a nihilistic attitude toward treatment of AIDS and cancer, it seems more probable that it reflects the physicians' impression that patients with these illnesses are more prepared to discuss such weighty matters.

Suicide in HIV/AIDS

Most patients with AIDS view their illness as inevitably fatal, and some argue that choosing to die sooner rather than later should be seen as something other than suicide. Rabkin and her coauthors (16) conceive of such a choice as "self-determined" or "accelerated" death. In their book *Good Doctors, Good Patients: Partners in HIV Treatment*, Rabkin et al. write, "We believe that people who are about to die have the right to determine the timing of their deaths." Some social activists within the AIDS community believe that this right to determine the timing of death conveys an obligation to healthcare providers to assist patients in committing suicide.

Thoughts of Suicide Among Persons With HIV/AIDS

Rabkin and colleagues interviewed 53 men with AIDS who had survived 3 or more years after AIDS diagnosis, and discovered that one-quarter of them had made arrangements to end their lives if necessary (17). These individuals cited debilitating illness, pain, dementia, and incontinence as potential reasons for suicide.

Suicidal ideation has been documented across the spectrum of HIV-related illness. HIV serologic testing itself is a critical event that is often accompanied by psychological distress (18). Perry and colleagues (19) questioned people undergoing HIV testing at the New York Blood Bank and found the rate of suicidal ideation before the test (as measured by a single item on the Beck Depression Inventory) was 30.2%. Two months after testing, suicidal ideation persisted in 16.3% of those who were seropositive and in 15.9% of those who were seronegative. The majority of subjects had passive suicidal thoughts without intent.

Several investigators have studied suicidal ideation among men at high risk for HIV infection. Joseph and colleagues (20) found that 18.8% of a large cohort of gay men in the Chicago Multicenter AIDS Cohort Study reported suicidal ideation during three or more visits. In the Los Angeles Multicenter AIDS Cohort Study (21), 27% of 778 gay and bisexual men with unknown serostatus reported suicidal ideation during the preceding 6 months. These thoughts were associated with bereavement following the loss of a partner, recent diagnosis of AIDS-related complex (ARC), and having multiple close friends with ARC. High suicide intent on the Beck Scale for Suicide Ideation (22) was similarly correlated with having multiple close friends with AIDS, having a partner with ARC or AIDS, and having ARC.

Interestingly, McKegney and O'Dowd (23) reviewed inpatient psychiatric consultations with 322 AIDS patients and 82 HIV-seropositive patients without AIDS and found that the AIDS patients had no more suicide ideation than the 1,086 control subjects with negative or unknown HIV status. In contrast, the seropositive patients without AIDS had significantly more suicide ideation.

Although suicide rates in HIV/AIDS have been shown to be significantly elevated over those in the general population (24), suicide is still a rare event. Suicidal thoughts, on the other hand, are common and may have a particular calming or soothing function in the face of serious illness.

Clinical Vignette 2:
The Case of P.D.

P.D., a 32-year-old gay man, started psychotherapy in 1988, a few months after testing positive for HIV. Because he had engaged in prostitution during college, he was not particularly surprised at his test result. He was quite anxious about how he was going to cope with HIV and with the sense that he had so many other unresolved problems.

P.D. described long-standing difficulties with intimate relationships and said that he wanted most of all to be able to love and be loved in a healthy relationship. He was a bright, creative man who had grown up in a working class family in a rural town. The youngest of seven children, P.D. was 13 when his mother died of cancer. During the ensuing years, his father sank deeply into alcoholism and was frequently physically assaultive, especially to P.D.

The one adult to show interest in him was his parish priest, who sexually molested P.D. beginning at the time of P.D.'s mother's death. In therapy, P.D. often wondered whether he had brought this on himself because he was gay, or whether he was gay as a result of the experience.

He began to understand that this early, exploitative experience was fundamentally related to his years of prostitution and to his inability to experience genuine intimacy.

During the next five years, P.D. continued in twice-weekly psychotherapy and joined a support group for HIV-seropositive men. He became quite successful in his career as a graphic artist and began a serious relationship with a man. His attempts to deepen his connection to his family were met with indifference, and even hostility, after he disclosed his HIV status to them, but he found himself more at peace having done so.

By 1993 P.D.'s CD4 count had declined to 70, and he was hospitalized for the first time with PCP. He suffered a series of AIDS-related complications that rendered him progressively weaker. A painful peripheral neuropathy made it impossible to walk more than a few blocks. In 1994 he underwent an extensive diagnostic evaluation for severe abdominal pain, fevers, and weight loss. In the midst of his medical workup, his doctor admitted to a strong suspicion that the symptoms were related to lymphoma. P.D. asked for a barbiturate prescription that he said he might use "down the road" if his condition became intolerable.

Although inclined to grant the request, his doctor first consulted with P.D.'s psychiatrist. She agreed that P.D. was of sound mind and that he was not depressed. Furthermore, P.D. had spoken many times over the years about the possibility of "rational suicide." After weighing the evidence, his doctor wrote the prescription.

Despite the exhaustive medical evaluation, no explanation was found for P.D.'s symptoms. His symptoms persisted, and he became essentially bedridden. He decided to proceed with suicide in 3 months' time if his condition failed to improve. When the date arrived, P.D. postponed his suicide another month, during which time his health started to improve. He determined that his life was again worth living.

One year later, P.D. is working part-time. He continues to derive comfort from knowing that the barbiturates are available should he need them in the future.

Although thoughts of suicide—and to a lesser extent, making suicide preparations—are not uncommon in the setting of AIDS, the vast majority of those who make such preparations, like P.D., never act. In such cases, the suicide arrangements constitute a means toward gaining a sense of control in the face of the extraordinary physical and psychological assault of the illness. Reserving the "right" to commit suicide—and for some individuals, acquiring the means to do so—can provide comfort without necessarily increasing the risk of actual self-destruction.

We lack data to compare the incidence of suicidal thoughts across illnesses. In an ongoing study at Beth Israel Deaconess Medical Center in Boston, persons with AIDS are significantly more likely than persons with cancer to regard suicide as an option at some future point, though there is no difference between these subject groups with respect to whether they believe in the right of terminally ill patients to commit suicide. The majority of these subjects are not depressed according to a structured diagnostic interview or on a self-report scale, nor do they rule in for suicidality on the Beck Scale for Suicide Ideation (to rule in for suicidality, a subject must score at or above the cut-off on a scored, multiple-choice self-report questionnaire) (25). This suggests that these thoughts of suicide are not correlated with psychopathology or with a likelihood of suicide within the next month. Without careful longitudinal follow-up, it is not possible to know whether these thoughts have any correlation with eventual suicide.

Attempted Suicide in HIV/AIDS

Although there are no prospective studies of attempted suicide among individuals with HIV/AIDS, the psychiatric literature contains several case reports (26–28). In 1992 Rundell and colleagues (29) reviewed the United States Air Force (USAF) experience with HIV-seropositive personnel and found 15 suicide attempts—an attempt rate 16 to 24 times higher than that among USAF personnel in general. Factors correlated with suicide attempt included social isolation or perceived lack of social support; HIV-related interpersonal or occupational problems; a current psychiatric diagnosis of adjustment disorder, personality disorder, or alcohol abuse; and a past history of depression. Two-thirds of these attempts occurred within the first year of having been diagnosed seropositive, and nearly half within the first 3 months. More than half of the persons who attempted suicide acknowledged alcohol use at the time of the attempt.

These impulsive suicide attempts occurred in a context of psychopathology and profound psychosocial stress. Although the crisis of HIV seropositivity was a precipitant, these attempts do not at all resemble the "rational" suicide of persons in the throes of severe medical illness. Such attempts warrant aggressive psychiatric and psychosocial intervention. They indicate an urgent need for the patient to develop coping skills and to recognize that it is possible to have a satisfying and meaningful life despite having an HIV-seropositive status.

Completed Suicide in HIV/AIDS

The association between medical illness and suicide is well known, and it is likely that reported rates of suicide in the medically ill are lower than the actual rates, if death results from a nontraumatic cause such as medication overdose. Among substance abusers with AIDS, suicide by drug overdose is very likely to be erroneously classified as accidental death. Among persons with AIDS, medication overdose is increasingly the mode of suicide, accounting for 16% of suicides in New York City in 1985 and for more than half in 1987 (30).

Estimated suicide rates among persons with AIDS range from 7.5 times that of the general population (31) to an astounding 36 times that of age-matched control subjects and 66 times that of the general population found by Marzuk's group (32). Other illnesses have been associated with elevated suicide rates; among persons with cancer, for example, the suicide rate is 1.5 to 4 times higher than those of the general population (33, 34), and among persons with Huntington's disease the rate is from 6 to 23 times higher than that of the general population (35, 36). It is noteworthy that both Huntington's disease and AIDS can be predicted before their onset by a laboratory test and that both disorders are slow in onset and affect the central nervous system, with consequent deterioration in motor control and cognitive ability. In addition, both Huntington's and AIDS patients are likely to have witnessed the death of at least one friend or relative with the disease.

Clinical Vignette 3:
The Case of E.B.

E.B., a 37-year-old artist, was urgently referred to a psychiatrist from her doctor's office. She had just been informed that she was both pregnant and HIV-positive and that her symptoms of nausea and fatigue were due to active hepatitis C. On hearing this news, E.B. became panicked and began to sob uncontrollably, stating that she didn't know if she could cope.

There was a remote history of polysubstance abuse, including a brief period when E.B. injected heroin and cocaine with a boyfriend. But E.B. had been sober for 8 years and, up until the last month, was in excellent health. During a stay in a halfway house when she first stopped using, she had asked a physician whether she should be tested for HIV. He assured her that her risk for infection was quite low and advised against testing because of the "high risk of false positives." She had been married just a few months, and although they had not planned this pregnancy, E.B. was hoping to have a child soon.

When she arrived at the psychiatrist's, E.B. was profoundly agitated. She felt that her HIV infection was a punishment for her "badness" and for seven abortions she had had since the age of 16. She was certain that her husband would be better off without her. Though extremely distraught, she denied having suicidal ideation and agreed to return to see the psychiatrist 3 days later.

At the next visit, E.B. was still considerably distraught, obsessed with worries that she had infected her husband with hepatitis and HIV, and grief-stricken over the plight of her unborn child. She acknowledged fleeting suicidal thoughts but insisted that such an act would be cowardly and unacceptable to her. Though unable to sleep or eat, psychotropic medications were contraindicated because of her pregnancy.

One week later, E.B. was considerably more composed. She and her husband had just met with the gynecologist to discuss their situation. Despite the data suggesting a reasonable chance of delivering an uninfected child, they had decided to terminate the pregnancy so that E.B. could receive interferon for her active hepatitis. Though they were both appropriately sad, E.B. was visibly relieved. A therapeutic abortion was planned for the next day.

The following evening the psychiatrist received a call from the emergency room. E.B.'s husband had returned from work at midday to accompany her to the abortion. He found an empty vodka bottle and a suicide note. After several frantic hours, E.B. was found in a local park. Despite aggressive resuscitation efforts, she was pronounced dead an hour after arriving at the emergency room.

There can be no question that E.B.'s suicide was a tragic act that one would want to avert at all costs. Her situation was devastating and, coupled to her profound sense of culpability, left her no psychological space in which she could manage. The final trauma—another abortion, the loss of another child—was ultimately more than she could bear.

Suicide Risk Factors in HIV/AIDS

What are the reasons for the elevated suicide rates in AIDS? Suicide among persons with HIV/AIDS is associated with the same demographic, psychosocial, and psychopathological factors that elevate suicide risk in the general population (37). Furthermore, it is likely that certain AIDS-specific factors convey additional risk. As one enumerates these factors, it becomes increasingly apparent that persons with AIDS are often multiply at risk for suicide.

Demographics

Demographic factors associated with suicide include male gender, Caucasian race, and homosexuality. Although blacks and Hispanics constitute a disproportionately large segment of those with HIV/AIDS, in the United States and Europe the disease still overwhelmingly strikes gay white men, the demographic group at highest risk for suicide.

Psychopathology

Studies have consistently found that the vast majority of persons who commit suicide do so while mentally ill (38) and that these individuals are observably disturbed prior to their suicide (39). Depressive illness is identified in almost half, alcoholism in about 20%, and schizophrenia in 10% of completed suicides (40).

Hopelessness has an even higher predictive value for eventual suicide than does depression (41–43). Although hopelessness is often a feature of depression, it may exist in the absence of psychopathology. For example, an individual with an incurable illness may feel hopeless about the possibilities for recovery, or may realistically anticipate inexorable physical deterioration, without having other symptoms of psychiatric illness.

Research indicates elevated rates of depression among persons with HIV/AIDS. Brown's cohort of largely asymptomatic HIV-infected USAF personnel (44) had elevated rates of mood disorders, both antedating and subsequent to seroconversion, in comparison to population base rates. The lifetime prevalence of major depression among the USAF cohort was almost double that of the general population, and a current diagnosis of major depression was made three times as often. Belkin and colleagues (45) interviewed 831 HIV-infected individuals, most of whom had AIDS, and found that 42% were depressed. The likelihood of depression increased with the number of self-reported AIDS-related physical symptoms, including weakness or numbness, fever, chills, night sweats, shortness of breath, diarrhea, weight loss, and difficulty with cognition.

Substance Abuse and Dependence

The evidence linking alcohol and suicide is extremely strong (46, 47), and the coexistence of alcoholism and depression elevates suicide risk beyond that of either disorder alone (48). Alcohol use, with or without alcoholism, occurs in up to 30% of all suicides (49). Alcohol is also significant in attempted suicide; studies have found that up to 64% of those attempting suicide consume alcohol before the attempt (50). In Brown's USAF cohort of HIV-seropositive persons, the lifetime rate of alcohol abuse was 29%, nearly double the population base rate. Of note, a study of randomly selected USAF personnel (51) found a significant increase in new-onset alcohol abuse disorders after a diagnosis of HIV seropositivity.

Intravenous Drug Use

We lack reliable data on completed suicide among intravenous drug users, though an increased suicide attempt rate has clearly been found in this population. In one study, the use of intravenous drugs was associated with an eightfold increase in suicide attempts compared with no drug use, when the presence of comorbid disorders was controlled (52). As with alcoholism, comorbidity with psychiatric disorders is common.

Organic Mental Disorders

There have been some reports (53, 54) linking HIV-related dementia with suicide. HIV-infected persons with organic mental disorders should be considered to be at increased risk because of the impulsivity, lability, impaired judgment, and disinhibition that are associated with these disorders. Furthermore, the loss of cognitive abilities and a fear of dementia are often cited by healthy HIV-infected persons as potential reasons to consider suicide in the future.

Assisted Dying

Although assisted suicide and euthanasia in the United States are virtually underground activities, it is estimated that 3% to 37% of American doctors help their patients commit suicide despite the potential legal ramifications (55). Among a sample of San Francisco physicians, 23% indicated that they would grant an AIDS patient's request for assisted suicide (56), and public attitude surveys generally demonstrate, as was found in one survey, that 65% of Americans support voluntary active euthanasia (57).

In The Netherlands, where euthanasia can be administered without legal consequences provided certain conditions are met (58), at least 21% of those granted euthanasia suffer from AIDS, and an astounding 35% of patients with AIDS in Amsterdam die by euthanasia (59). This rate is 10 times higher than the rate among patients with any other illness. Another 45% of patients with AIDS have discontinued treatment and received life-shortening pain medication at the time of death.

It is extremely important to understand the reasons for these startling statistics. Do they reveal a prejudice on the part of physicians that a life with AIDS is not worth living, culminating in an overwillingness to prescribe euthanasia? Do they suggest a frightful suffering associated with AIDS, well beyond that experienced in other fatal illnesses? If so, have we given the necessary attention to the possibilities for palliation? Is it possible to conjecture that these statistics reflect that something right is going on in The Netherlands?

While it is clear that a majority of Americans believe in the "right to die" for persons with incurable illness, and that a sizable number endorse the principle of physician assistance in expediting death under such circumstances, we are still a great distance from a consensus over whether, when, and how physician-assisted suicide and euthanasia might be administered. As delineated earlier, the courts have strongly endorsed our right to refuse treatment, but not to assistance in dying. What if there is no life-sustaining treatment to refuse, and thereby no legally sanctioned means to hasten death? Under the law, there is a critical difference between withdrawing or withholding life-prolonging treatments and acting to bring about a patient's death. Quill points out that although medical ethicists make a very clear distinction between passive participation in a patient's death (e.g., by withholding treatment) and active participation, in the clinical world this distinction is often much less distinct (60). He further maintains that the ethical distinction is not compelling, provided the appropriate conditions are met.

Clinical Vignette 4:
The Case of J.M.

J.M., a 43-year-old gay white man, had been living with AIDS for 4 years at the time he began to plan for his suicide. He was an accomplished documentary filmmaker whose latest project, which had been completed a few months earlier, was to be shown on public television in 3 months time. He had just received a prestigious award for accomplishments in his field. It was midwinter, and he looked forward to the opening baseball game, for which he had tickets along the third baseline. He decided that he would take his life at the end of April.

For the last two years, J.M. had been in treatment with a psychiatrist who specialized in HIV/AIDS. He grappled with the effects of AIDS on his personal and work life, and explored the impact his illness had on his parents, Holocaust survivors who had each lost entire families to the death camps. J.M. had experienced periods of despondency, generally precipitated by acute illness, and for the last year had remained on an antidepressant that had been quite effective in stabilizing his mood. J.M. had been aggressive in seeking out experimental treatments and was very much committed to holistic therapies.

From time to time, J.M. spoke about his conviction that certain AIDS-related complications would be unacceptable to him. Having lost more than 30 friends and acquaintances to AIDS, he could describe in detail those whose deaths he viewed as grueling and senseless. A former lover with AIDS died suddenly while on vacation in the tropics, and J.M.

often imagined that he had committed suicide. J.M. was frightened of going blind and worried about becoming physically limited to the extent of being homebound.

Over the 6 months prior to his decision to end his life, J.M. had been increasingly compromised by a variety of ailments, including cytomegalovirus retinitis, from which he was slowly losing his vision, and chronic vertigo that had proved refractory to any treatments except those that put him to sleep. He told his psychiatrist that his life held less and less pleasure for him and that time weighed heavily. He found himself longing for it all to be over, and except for the showing of his film and opening day at the ballpark, he did not look forward to anything. Although he did not believe himself to be depressed, J.M. agreed to a trial of another antidepressant, first alone and then in combination with a psychostimulant, but did not find that it altered his wish to die.

It was at this point that J.M. assembled his six closest friends, among them his twin sister, to discuss his suicide plans. Initially, there was considerable distress regarding J.M.'s intentions, particularly at his request that the group assist him in taking his life. His sister was especially upset and even angry, concerned with the pain she felt his suicide would cause their parents.

The group met weekly with J.M. for a period of 2 months. His sister sought counseling and ultimately concluded that given the inevitability of his death, J.M.'s wish to take his life was acceptable to her, provided their parents were never told about it. In the end, the group accepted J.M.'s decision, and four members agreed to be with him at the time of suicide. J.M. had one last meeting with his psychiatrist during which he reiterated his reasons for choosing suicide, and his view that nothing short of a cure for AIDS would change his mind. Although his psychiatrist was sad and somewhat disturbed, he had consulted with several colleagues, all of whom concurred that in the absence of a treatable psychiatric or medical condition, there were no grounds to intervene.

At the end of April, as planned, J.M. took the lethal medications that his physician had prescribed 6 months earlier with the knowledge that they might be used for suicide. J.M. died 21 hours later.

A "Rational" Suicide?

How is one to understand J.M.'s suicide? Given the terminal nature of his illness, the presence of unremitting symptoms, his long-standing involvement in psychiatric treatment, and the considerable time between his initial thoughts and his ultimate act, might J.M.'s be considered a "rational" suicide? According to Siegel (61), a rational suicide is one in which there is a realistic understanding of one's condition and an absence of treatable psychiatric illness, and in which a majority of uninvolved observers from the individual's community would find the decision acceptable.

In their proposed clinical criteria to guide physician-assisted suicide, Quill, Cassel, and Meier (62) build upon Siegel's definition of rational suicide, listing the following as elements necessary to the process:

1. The request to die must be uncoerced and freely, clearly, and repeatedly made.
2. The patient's judgment must not be impaired.
3. The patient's condition must be incurable and associated with severe, unrelenting, intolerable suffering.
4. The suffering and the request must not result from inadequate hospice care.
5. Physician-assisted suicide should only be carried out in the context of a meaningful doctor-patient relationship.
6. Another experienced physician should be consulted.
7. There should be clear documentation proving that the above conditions were met.

J.M. believed that his quality of life was unlikely to improve appreciably, and he dreaded its decline. His assessment of his medical situation was corroborated by his doctors. Far from impulsive, he deliberated long and hard before effecting his suicide plan. If Siegel's criteria constitute the essence of rational suicide, then J.M.'s death could be viewed as such. Were physician-assisted suicide legal and governed by the conditions proposed by Quill et al., J.M. would probably have been granted assistance in dying.

It is important to ask in what way psychological factors distinguish J.M. from numerous others who have suffered a similar course with AIDS but have not chosen suicide—and moreover, whether a psychological formulation would elicit a different response to J.M.'s wish to be helped to die. J.M. was a perfectionist, with a powerful need to be in control. He was quick to find fault and extremely demanding of others. He was narcissistic, proud of his talents, and certain that his ill health would render him unable to take on further projects. Although he had suffered depression in the past, he had responded well to medications and was not depressed at present.

In Quill's formulation, rational suicide is undertaken by persons who would not want to die under other circumstances but have reached a point at which they would rather die than continue to live under the conditions imposed by their illness. And although most notions of suicide would consider a person's essence to be destroyed in the act, Quill argues that "[f]or patients for whom recovery is impossible, and for whom further disintegration of their person is all that lies in the future, the motive in choosing death is to preserve what remains of their personhood" (63). This is the essence of J.M.'s wish to die. His personality was such that he believed himself entitled to enlist others in his quest for a good death.

Psychiatrist Herbert Hendin, executive director of the American Suicide Foundation, warns against the "marketing" of assisted death through the presentation of case histories like J.M.'s, designed to show the necessity of assisted suicide or euthanasia in a particular instance (64). He believes the clamor for legalized assisted suicide and euthanasia is symptomatic of "our failure to develop a better response to death and the fear of intolerable pain or artificial prolongation of life." In his view, Hendin echoes that of Ivan Illich (65), that patients have lost faith in their ability to die naturally and have therefore made the right to be "professionally killed" into a major issue.

Assisted Dying and HIV/AIDS

It is widely believed among clinicians working with the HIV/AIDS population that many AIDS suicides are assisted, whether by a physician, nurse, care provider, lover, family member, or friend—or more commonly, by a group of such individuals. Two newspaper reports in June 1994 underscored this fact and the associated perils. Social worker Russel Ogden, as reported in the *New York Times* (66), discovered that half of 34 assisted suicides among men with AIDS in Vancouver were bungled and that the failed attempts resulted in greater suffering for the patient and those who tried to assist. Ogden attributed these suicide failures to inadequate medical knowledge and insufficient availability of appropriate drugs. In another *New York Times* story (67), reporter Gina Kolata described the horrifying emotions of the intended victim's friends when instructed by him to cover his head with a dry-cleaning bag if he failed to die within 6 hours of taking an overdose.

Conclusion

Is there a limit to what we can or should do to prevent suicide? Is there such a thing as a rational suicide? This question confronts psychiatry at the very limits of its therapeutic tradition. According to Sullivan and Youngner (68), "for the intractably suffering, terminally ill patient, activities providing pleasure may no longer be available. One may be unable to help oneself or others in any meaningful way. Intolerable symptoms may in fact persist for the short remainder of one's life. One may have no real future."

When there is no medical or psychiatric condition to treat, we may find ourselves in the uncomfortable position of validating a patient's request to die. But how are we to do this? How far should such validation extend? Do we advise about suicide techniques? caution against engaging loved ones in activities that might traumatize, such as suffocation? Do we write a prescription, or bid others to do so?

Unless or until we have mutually agreed on guidelines, we are left to our own devices. In the era of AIDS, these problems are too complex for clinicians to bear alone. They are also too common to be ignored. How we formulate a response to these challenges constitutes a central task for the coming years.

References

1. Altman LK: Deaths from AIDS decline sharply in New York City. New York Times, January 25, 1997, A1
2. Altman LK: With AIDS advances, more disappointment. New York Times, January 19, 1997, A1

3. Wachter RM, Juce JM, Lo B, et al: Life-sustaining treatment for patients with AIDS. Chest 95:647–652, 1989

4. Goldstone I, Kuhl D, Johnson H, et al: Patterns of care in advanced HIV disease in a tertiary treatment centre. AIDS Care 7 (suppl 1):S47–S56, 1995

5. Steinbrook R, Lo B, Moulton J, et al: Preferences of homosexual men with AIDS for life-sustaining treatment. N Engl J Med 314:457–460, 1986

6. Haas J, Weissman J, Cleary P, et al: Discussion of preferences for life-sustaining care by persons with AIDS: predictors of failure in patient-physician communications. Arch Intern Med 153:1241–1248, 1993

7. Miles SH: Informed demand for "non-beneficial" medical treatment. N Engl J Med 325:512–515, 1991

8. Emmanuel EJ: A review of the ethical and legal aspects of terminating medical care. JAMA 84:291–301, 1988

9. In re Claire C Conroy, 98 NJ 321 (1985)

10. Bopp J: Choosing death for Nancy Cruzan. Hastings Cent Rep 20(1):42–44, 1990

11. Sullivan MD, Youngner SJ: Depression, competence, and the right to refuse life-sustaining treatment. Am J Psychiatry 151:971–978, 1994

12. Fogel BS, Mor U: Depressed mood and care preferences in patients with AIDS. Gen Hosp Psychiatry 15:203–207, 1993

13. Brown JH, Helteleff P, Barakat S, et al: Is it normal for terminally ill patients to desire death? Am J Psychiatry 143:208–211, 1986

14. Chochinov HM, Wilson KG, Enns M, et al: Desire for death in the terminally ill. Am J Psychiatry 152:1185–1191, 1995

15. Wachter RM, Luce JM, Hearst N, et al: Decisions about resuscitation: inequities among patients with different diseases but similar prognoses. Ann Intern Med 111:525–532, 1989

16. Rabkin J, Remien R, Wilson C: Good Doctors, Good Patients: Partners in HIV Treatment. New York, NCM Publishers, 1994, pp 139–140

17. Rabkin JG, Remien RH, Katoff LS, et al: Resilience in adversity among long-term survivors of AIDS. Hospital and Community Psychiatry 44:162–167, 1993

18. Catalan J: Psychiatric manifestations of HIV disease. Baillieres Clin Gastroenterol 4:547–562, 1990

19. Perry S, Jacobsberg L, Fischman B: Suicidal ideation and HIV testing. JAMA 263:679–682, 1990

20. Joseph JG, Caumartin SM, Tal M, et al: Psychological functioning in a cohort of gay men at risk for AIDS: a three-year descriptive study. J Nerv Ment Dis 178:607–615, 1990

21. Schneider SG, Taylor SE, Kemeny ME, et al: AIDS-related factors predictive of suicidal ideation of low and high intent among gay and bisexual men. Suicide Life Threat Behav 21:313–328, 1991

22. Beck AT, Kovacs M, Weissman A: Assessment of suicidal intention: the Scale for Suicide Ideation. J Consult Clin Psychol 47:343–352, 1979

23. McKegney FP, O'Dowd MA: Suicidality and HIV status. Am J Psychiatry 149:396–398, 1992

24. Marzuk PM, Tierney H, Tardiff K, et al: Increased risk of suicide in persons with AIDS. JAMA 259:1333–1337, 1988

25. Beck et al, Assessment of suicidal intention

26. Frierson RL, Lippmann SB: Suicide and AIDS. Psychosomatics 29:226–231, 1988

27. Rundell JR, Wise MG, Ursano RJ: Three cases of AIDS-related psychiatric disorders. Am J Psychiatry 143:777–778, 1986

28. Stern RA, van der Horst CM, Hooper SR, et al: Zidovudine overdose in an asymptomatic HIV seropositive patient with hemophilia. Psychosomatics 33:454–457, 1992

29. Rundell JR, Kyle KM, Brown GR, et al: Risk factors for suicide attempts in a human immunodeficiency virus screening program. Psychosomatics 33:24–27, 1992

30. Marzuk PM: Suicidal behavior and HIV illnesses. International Review of Psychiatry 3:365–371, 1991

31. Cotée TR, Biggar RJ, Dannenberg AL: Risk of suicide among persons with AIDS: a national assessment. JAMA 268:2066–2068, 1992

32. Marzuk et al, Increased risk of suicide in persons with AIDS

33. Fox BH, Stanek EJ III, Boyd SC, et al: Suicide rates among cancer patients in Connecticut. Journal of Chronic Diseases 35:89–100, 1982

34. Marshall JR, Burnett W, Brasure J: On precipitating factors: cancer as a cause of suicide. Suicide Life Threat Behav 13:15–27, 1983

35. Blumenthal S. Suicide: a guide to risk factors, assessment, and treatment of suicidal patients. Med Clin North Am 72:937–971, 1988

36. Schoenfeld M, Myers RH, Cupples LA, et al: Increased rate of suicide among patients with Huntington's disease. J Neurol Neurosurg Psychiatry 47:1283–1287, 1984

37. Beckett A, Shenson D: Suicide risk in HIV infection and AIDS. Harvard Review of Psychiatry 1:27–35, 1993

38. Black DW, Winokur G: Suicide and psychiatric diagnosis, in Suicide Over the Life Cycle: Risk Factors, Assessment, and Treatment of Suicidal Patients. Edited by Blumenthal SJ, Kupfer DF. Washington, DC, American Psychiatric Press, 1990, pp 135–153

39. Barraclough B, Bunch J, Nelson B, et al: A hundred cases of suicide: clinical aspects. Br J Psychiatry 125:355–373, 1974
40. Clark DC, Fawcett J: An empirically based model of suicide risk assessment for patients with affective disorder, in Suicide and Clinical Practice. Edited by Jacobs D. Washington, DC, American Psychiatric Press, 1992, pp 55–73
41. Beck AT, Steer RA, Kovacs M, et al: Hopelessness and eventual suicide: a 10-year study of patients hospitalized with suicidal ideation. Am J Psychiatry 142:559–563, 1985
42. Beck AT, Steer RA: Clinical predictors of eventual suicide: a 5- to 10-year prospective study of suicide attempters. J Affect Disord 17:203–209, 1989
43. Kovacs M, Beck AT, Weissman A: Hopelessness: an indicator of suicidal risk. Suicide 5:98–103, 1975
44. Brown GR, Rundell JR, McManis SE, et al: Prevalence of psychiatric disorders in early stages of HIV infection. Psychosom Med 54:588–601, 1992
45. Belkin GS, Fleishman JA, Stein MD, et al: Physical symptoms and depressive symptoms among individuals with HIV infection. Psychosomatics 33:416–427, 1992
46. Kessel N, Grossman G: Suicide in alcoholics. BMJ :1671–1672, 1961
47. Kendall RE. Alcohol and suicide. Substance and Alcohol Actions/Misuse 4:121–127, 1983
48. Fowler RC, Liskow BI, Tanna VL: Alcoholism, depression, and life events. J Affect Disord 2:127–135, 1980
49. Clark MA, Campagnari KD, Jones LM: The major causative role of ethanol and the minor of other drugs in the deaths of military personnel in San Diego County, California. Mil Med 150:487–491, 1985
50. Roizen R: Estimating alcohol consumption in serious events, in Alcohol Consumption and Related Problems (Alcohol and Health Monograph). Washington, DC, National Institute on Alcohol Abuse and Alcoholism, 1982
51. Pace J, Brown GR, Rundell JR, et al: Prevalence of psychiatric disorders in a mandatory screening program for infection with human immunodeficiency virus: a pilot study. Mil Med 155:76–80, 1990
52. Dinwiddie SH, Reich T, Cloninger CR: Psychiatric comorbidity and suicidality among intravenous drug users. J Clin Psychiatry 53:364–369, 1992
53. Alfonso CA, Cohen MA: HIV-dementia and suicide. Gen Hosp Psychiatry 16:45–46, 1994
54. Tostes M: Psychiatric emergencies in HIV infection: high risk of suicide in organic mental syndromes. International Conference on AIDS 8(2):B222 (abstract no PoB3788), 1992

55. Ruling favors doctor who aided in suicides. New York Times, February 18, 1992, A20

56. Slome L, Moulton J, Huffine C, et al: Physicians' attitudes toward assisted suicide in AIDS. J Acquir Immune Defic Syndr Hum Retrovirol 5:712–718, 1992

57. Painton P, Taylor E: Live or let die. Time, March 19, 1990

58. de Wachter MA: Active euthanasia in The Netherlands. JAMA 262:3316–3319, 1989

59. van der Wal G, van Eijk JT, Leenen HJ, et al: Euthanasia and assisted suicide by physicians in the home situation, I: diagnoses, age and sex of patients. Neth J Med 135:1593–1598, 1991

60. Quill TE: Physician-assisted death: progress or peril? Suicide Life Threat Behav 24:315–325, 1994

61. Siegel K: Rational suicide: considerations for the clinician. Psychiatr Q 54(2):77–84, 1982

62. Quill TE, Cassel C, Meier D: Care of the hopelessly ill: proposed clinical criteria for physician-assisted suicide. N Engl J Med 327:1380–1384, 1992

63. Quill, Physician-assisted death, p 319

64. Hendin H: Selling death and dignity. Hastings Cent Rep 25(3):19–23, 1995; see p 19

65. Illich I: Limits to Medicine—Medical Nemesis: The Expropriation of Health. London, Penguin, 1976, p 111

66. Farnsworth CH: Vancouver AIDS suicides botched. New York Times, June 14, 1994, C12

67. Kolata G: AIDS patients seek solace in suicide but many find pain and uncertainty. New York Times, June 14, 1994, C1

68. Sullivan and Youngner, Depression, competence, and the right to refuse life-sustaining treatment, p 976

8

Evaluating Patient Requests for Euthanasia and Assisted Suicide in Terminal Illness: The Role of the Psychiatrist

Susan D. Block, M.D.

J. Andrew Billings, M.D.

The issue of physician-assisted suicide (PAS) has been the focus of intensive public attention and discussion over the past 5 years. The debate about PAS is taking place in living rooms, ethics committees, professional organizations, the media, state legislatures, and the courts. In 1997, the United States Supreme Court struck down two lower-court decisions, ruling that there is no constitutional right to PAS, and returned this contentious debate to the states. At the same time, in the view of constitutional

This chapter is a revision of Block SD, Billings JA: "Patient Requests for Euthanasia and Assisted Suicide in Terminal Illness." *Psychosomatics* 36:445–457, 1995. Used with permission.

scholars, the Supreme Court decision affirmed a constitutional right to appropriate palliative care. In November 1997, the people of the state of Oregon affirmed their support of the Oregon Death with Dignity Act by a substantial majority, legalizing PAS under specified conditions. As a result of these decisions, the debate about PAS has now moved into a new phase. The state of Oregon is struggling to develop appropriate processes for the implementation of PAS. Several other states are considering PAS legislation. The Supreme Court decision has focused increased attention on the need for enhanced palliative care services. The role of psychiatric assessment and treatment in the optimal management of patients who request assisted suicide is central to this next phase of the debate.

Although there has been tremendous growth in the literature about the ethics of euthanasia and assisted suicide over the past 10 years (1–4), very little has been written about the psychiatric aspects of requests by terminally ill patients for accelerated death and the role of the psychiatrist (5–7). Research has shown that psychiatrists tend to be more supportive than other physicians of legalizing assisted suicide and euthanasia (8). A recent survey of the attitudes of Oregon psychiatrists toward assisted suicide showed that two-thirds believed that physicians should have the option, under certain circumstances, of prescribing medication the sole purpose of which would be that of hastening death, and that more than half supported Oregon's Ballot Measure 16. Only 6% expressed high levels of confidence that they could adequately evaluate the possible impact of a psychiatric diagnosis on the patient's judgment in a single evaluation (9). In contrast to the situation in psychiatry, in which we are beginning to learn more about the views of psychiatric clinicians on these issues, we know little about attitudes and views of other mental health professionals about PAS.

If mental health clinicians are to participate in shaping the policies currently being addressed through legislation, we must become educated about the issues and take on the responsibility of advocating for appropriate mental health care for patients requesting PAS. If PAS is legalized, it is critical that psychiatrists, as clinicians with expertise in the dynamics of suicide, the interface between psychological well-being and medical illness, and the impact of physical and organic factors on psychological functioning, contribute to the development of appropriate clinical standards for evaluation and management of such patients.

In this chapter we provide an overview of the critical issues in assessing and managing a patient's request for hastened death, delineate the role of the mental health expert, and argue that psychiatric consultation should be a mandatory part of any procedure whereby PAS is legally permitted. In a previous paper (10) we addressed the management in primary care of requests for accelerated dying. As the issue of PAS moves further into the mainstream of clinical concern, it is critical that we better describe the roles of mental health clinicians in these complex situations.

Although recent developments in the care of the terminally ill, such as the growth of hospice services and the increasing use of advance directives, aim to promote a sense of comfort and control during the dying process, many patients still fear pain and loss of control and distrust the healthcare system's ability to ease their passage to death (11–13). Indeed, Dr. Kevorkian's well-publicized activities have fostered a view among the public that PAS is a reasonable response to terminal illness. Some patients may view euthanasia and assisted suicide as the sole alternatives to prolonged suffering.

> J.A., a 68-year-old woman with pancreatic cancer, broached the issue of euthanasia with her oncologist after an escalation in symptoms of pain and nausea while receiving chemotherapy. The oncologist asked for a psychiatric consultation. The psychiatrist learned that J.A. had been wanting to stop chemotherapy for some time but felt that she would alienate her oncologist if she suggested this course. She anticipated that her physician would be unable to control her pain and that her suffering would be disregarded. These expectations led her to opt for "an early out." The psychiatrist, struck by the patient's hopelessness and helplessness, suggested that J.A. might benefit from treatment with a psychostimulant and encouraged J.A. to discuss her concerns about discontinuing chemotherapy and about pain relief with her oncologist. J.A. began treatment with methylphenidate and then negotiated discontinuance of her chemotherapy, entry into a hospice program, and initiation of an aggressive program of pain and symptom control. Her depression improved, and she died comfortably 1 month later.

As this case illustrates, requests for hastened death can be a focal point for a variety of problems that arise in the care of patients with terminal illness: fear about irremediable physical suffering, the impact of depression on the sense of control in terminal illness, difficulties in physician-patient communication, lack of knowledge about options for care, and lack of empowerment to express one's wishes. Problems in these areas are cited as frequent contributors to desires for early death (14). The case also demonstrates that appropriate attention to these problems can result in dramatic improvement in patients' quality of life.

Background

Little direct information exists about the frequency of requests for hastened death among terminally ill persons. Such requests are described by oncologists and acquired immunodeficiency syndrome (AIDS) care providers as regular but infrequent phenomena. Chochinov and colleagues found that 44.5% of terminally ill patients reported occasional wishes for death to come soon and that 8.5% expressed a severe and pervasive desire for early death. Nearly two-thirds of those who expressed a desire to die met the criteria for a major depression. In follow-up interviews conducted on six patients 2 weeks after an initial interview, four reported a decrease in their desire to die, and two demonstrated a sustained wish to die (15).

Breitbart and colleagues, in a study of ambulatory HIV-infected patients, found that 55% had considered PAS as an option for themselves and that psychological distress and experience with the terminal illness of a relative or friend were the two best predictors of interest in PAS (16).

In another study, about two-thirds of oncology patients believed that PAS was an acceptable practice for the treatment of patients with unremitting pain; PAS was viewed as least acceptable in situations in which the patient was viewed as a burden on his or her family or when he or she viewed life as meaningless. More than 25% of this population of patients had considered PAS or euthanasia seriously. These beliefs were more prevalent among patients with psychological distress (17).

In The Netherlands, where euthanasia and PAS under specified conditions are not prosecuted, 2.9% of all deaths are associated with active interventions to end life (1.8% voluntary euthanasia, 0.3% assisted suicide, and 0.8% euthanasia without explicit and persistent patient request) (18).

Multiple sources of additional but indirect data about the prevalence of wishes for hastened death add to our understanding of such requests. Although about 25% of cancer patients develop depression during the course of their illness, and about 6% meet the criteria for major depression (19), suicidal thoughts are rather common (20). In the late stages of illness, the incidences of depression and suicide have been noted to increase significantly (21–25). Although many patients desire that the options of euthanasia and assisted suicide be available (26), only a very small proportion, according to The Netherlands data, actually choose to exercise these options. It appears, however, that there has been a progressive increase in suicide risk among cancer patients between 1971 and 1986 (27).

In a study of family members of patients who had recently died, Jacobson and colleagues found that among respondents who reported that they understood the preferences of their relative, 21% believed that their relative would have wanted assistance in dying, if it had been offered, and that they, the family members, would have wanted assisted dying for their relative at even higher rates (28).

Among AIDS patients, studies demonstrate markedly elevated suicide rates (29, 30) (see also Chapter 7, this volume). In a study of medical inpatients with AIDS, about 35% cited a "wish to die," and 17% had active suicidal wishes (31). Within the culture of the gay community, assisted suicide and euthanasia are widely seen as reasonable alternatives to a "living death" with AIDS (32).

Practitioners report anecdotally that recent attention to legislative proposals for legalization of PAS, the 1997 United States Supreme Court PAS decision, the publication of *Final Exit* (a suicide guide for the terminally ill), and widely reported cases of assisted suicide appear to be associated with increased frequency of such requests. Clinicians report that the increasing media attention to PAS has also accelerated patients' interest in, and willingness to talk about, PAS with their physicians. These impressionistic data are reinforced by the evidence of recent increase in suicide rates among Danish patients (33) and by a study that documented an increase in the frequency of suicide by asphyxiation, as recommended in *Final Exit*, following the book's publication (34).

Although these studies lay a critical foundation for our understanding of the psychological issues involved in patient requests for hastened death, there are significant limitations in all of them. More research on these issues is essential to better define the prevalence of desires for hastened death among different populations of terminally ill persons, the natural history of desires for hastened death, the impact of different models of care on desires for PAS, and the attitudes of family members about PAS.

The Setting of Care

Hospitals and nursing homes are still the major loci of care for the dying (35, 36), although it appears that the numbers dying in hospice programs are increasing. No studies address how the setting of care affects the desire for hastened death and its expression, or how patients and healthcare workers act on the request. Hospice programs have suggested that provision of palliative care services "treats" the wish to hasten death, but no systematic data are available. We noted persistent requests for hastened death in 2 of 400 consecutive hospice patients (S. D. Block and J. A. Billings, unpublished data, 1994). We hypothesize that the rates of such requests would be higher in settings that do not adequately address the full spectrum of physical, psychosocial, and existential/spiritual concerns and needs of patients.

The Clinical Approach to Patient Requests for Accelerated Death

The primary clinical approach to requests for hastened death should be one of prevention. Although there are no systematic data on this issue, it is clear that fear of loss of control over decisions about care at the end of life is a major impetus for patients to consider PAS. One way of preventing the issue of hastening death from arising is for physicians to discuss the patient's values about and wishes for care throughout the course of a serious or life-threatening illness and to reassure the patient and his or her family members of the ready availability of good pain and symptom control and psychological support and of the physician's firm commitment to alleviating suffering. In particular, fear of pain and other severely distressing symptoms (e.g., choking) should be explored and addressed, with reassurances that effective comfort measures will be utilized. Although limited in their effectiveness in preventing unwanted medical treatment (37), advance directives and healthcare proxies offer patients an opportunity to express their desires for care to their physician and other family members. Discussion of care preferences often builds the patient's confidence and trust that his or her wishes will be respected, improves understanding about available care options, and returns a sense of control to the patient, reducing the impetus for consideration of PAS.

Even with the best of preventive efforts, however, fleeting thoughts about hastening death occur frequently among terminally ill patients in all settings. Sustained requests are distinctly unusual, especially when patients are receiving palliative care services. Most dying patients face their illnesses with remarkable equanimity, hanging on to whatever time they have left despite devastating difficulties. Requests to hasten death should be viewed as falling outside the usual spectrum of responses to terminal illness and as requiring special attention. Full evaluation of patient requests for assistance in dying demands an in-depth psychosocial assessment with an expanded focus on existential or spiritual issues. Although parts of the assessment of the patient can and should involve nonpsychiatric mental health clinicians—especially in the areas of family dynamics and spirituality—the psychiatrist's competencies complement those of the primary physician (and, ideally, other interdisciplinary team members) in carrying out a comprehensive evaluation of the clinical issues involved in the patient's desire for accelerated death. The mental health clinician should focus on the following major areas:

1. Physical suffering
2. Psychological suffering
3. Decision-making capacity
4. Social suffering
5. Existential/spiritual suffering
6. Dysfunction in the physician-patient relationship

Physical Suffering

Although treatment of physical symptoms is not usually the responsibility of the psychiatrist or other mental health professional, physical suffering has such a profound effect on psychological well-being that all professionals need to advocate for effective symptom palliation as the first element of an overall treatment plan. Undertreatment of pain is common, because of deficiencies in health professionals' education about pain management as well as concerns about addiction among patients, family members, and clinicians (38–43).

Although infrequently the main reason for requests for assisted dying in The Netherlands (44), uncontrolled pain is a major risk factor for suicide among cancer patients (45, 46). Sixty percent to 90% of cancer patients experience pain during the last year of life; 10% to 20% endure pain that is difficult to control (47–49). In The Netherlands, an estimated 85% of patients withdraw their requests for hastened death after receiving better symptom palliation (50). More than 90% of patients with cancer pain respond to simple analgesic measures (51, 52). The remaining 10% of patients, however, may require sophisticated treatment approaches, including additional pharmacologic interventions (antidepressants, anxiolytics, anticonvulsants, antiarrhythmics, corticosteroids), psychotherapy, and cognitive and behavioral strategies, as well as neurosurgical or anesthetic procedures.

Major depression, anxiety disorders, somatoform disorders, and some personality disorders may contribute to intractable symptoms (53, 54); psychiatric expertise is invaluable in diagnosis and management. Psychiatric input may also be useful when substance abuse disorders complicate management of symptoms in the terminally ill (e.g., when a patient with a history of heroin addiction has difficult-to-manage cancer pain). Many common psychopharmacologic agents can be used for symptom control in the terminally ill (benzodiazepines for anxiety and insomnia; anticonvulsants and tricyclic antidepressants for pain; psychostimulants for depression and sedation; and antipsychotics for nausea, anxiety, and agitation). The psychiatrist's familiarity with these agents and their clinical use complements the knowledge base of primary physicians and may lead to enhanced effectiveness of pharmacologic interventions. In addition, behavioral treatments can be highly effective for commonly encountered symptoms such as anxiety, nausea, and insomnia. These treatments can be offered by a variety of types of mental health professionals.

Psychological Suffering

Grief

The terminally ill patient faces an array of losses that commonly give rise to psychological pain severe enough that hastening death may seem desirable. In addition to the anticipated loss of relationships because of death, the patient loses current relationships as illness progressively narrows the individual's interpersonal world. Also, often lost are independence, control over one's body, hopes and expectations for the future, social and occupational roles, and sexual desire (55). The patient's request for hastened death may be a cry for help in feeling valued, a plea for someone to share in the grief, or a protest against unbearable suffering.

Most patients manage to cope with these losses on their own, through relationships with family and friends, and, sometimes, through relationships with mental health clinicians, other physicians, the clergy, and volunteers. Some patients, however, lack such supports and/or have psychiatric disorders—depression, anxiety, organic mental disorders, and personality disorders—that complicate the process of adapting to dying. These disorders can be difficult for primary physicians to diagnose and differentiate from normal grieving and may contribute to a desire for hastened death (56). Many of these patients may benefit from psychotherapy, which can be carried out competently by nurses, social workers, and psychologists, as well as by psychiatrists. The psychiatrist, however, often has additional expertise in the diagnosis of psychiatric disorders and of dysfunctional grieving in the setting of serious medical illness.

Depression

Major depression tends to be underrecognized and undertreated and is a major source of unnecessary suffering among the terminally ill. Contrary to popular and nonpsychiatric professional opinion, depression is *not* a normal feature of terminal illness.

An array of somatic symptoms that overlap with symptoms of depression—pain, insomnia, fatigue, loss of sexual interest—regularly accompany terminal illness. Medication-induced depressive symptomatology and depression-like symptoms of normal grief also make for difficulty in establishing the diagnosis of major depression in advanced terminal illness (57–61). A high level of clinical skill is required to make clinically important distinctions. Rarely are primary care physicians adequately trained to carry out this task. In addition, nonpsychiatric mental health clinicians do not generally have the extensive experience in diagnosing psychiatric illness in the context of serious medical illness, a situation that is commonly encountered in patients requesting hastened death. Because of the high prevalence of depression in the terminally ill (and especially in terminally ill patients who desire euthanasia or assisted suicide), its treatability, and the difficulty of diagnosis, a psychiatrist should be involved in evaluating all patients who request hastened death. The psychiatrist's role extends through assessment and treatment to a point at which either the patient's symptoms have improved or sufficient approaches have been tried to suggest that the depression is not ameliorable.

R.T. is a 63-year-old divorced Puerto Rican truck driver with far-advanced esophageal cancer who had a gastrostomy and cervical esophagostomy for palliation. He is living at home with hospice support. During his four months in the hospice program, R.T. has reported constant pain in his abdomen that does not respond to high doses of narcotics and has experienced intolerable side effects from multiple medications. He describes continual discomfort and odors from his ostomy, which, on multiple inspections, appeared to be functioning well and to have no odor. His interactions with the hospice staff are often hostile. He denies depression. He states that he considers himself to be Catholic but wants no contact with the clergy.

Since coming to the United States 40 years ago, R.T. has worked steadily and raised five children. He is living with a devoted girlfriend and is often visited by his children and grandchildren. He gets out of bed only to use the bathroom, sleeps most of the time, and refuses to watch the World Series, despite a lifelong love of baseball. Members of his family attribute his distress to his cancer and the effects of his medications.

Hospice staff describe to the psychiatric consultant their frustrations with R.T. They do not feel he is depressed, expressing the view that his disease, the difficulties caused by his ostomy, and his pain sufficiently explain his mental status. The psychiatrist evaluates R.T., determines that he is depressed, and recommends treatment with dextroamphetamine 2.5 mg twice a day. Four days later R.T. is watching baseball and building a model in the living room with his 9-year-old grandson. His family expresses relief that he seems to be "back to his old self."

Further education of patients, physicians, nurses, and social workers practicing in terminal care settings is needed to counter prevailing beliefs about the normality of depression among patients with terminal illness and its consequent undertreatment. Additionally, psychiatrists should promote the appropriate use of antidepressants in the care of depressed terminally ill patients. In informally polling several groups of clinicians, we found that, although they are aggressive in the treatment of physical symptoms, antidepressants for the treatment of depression are utilized at a rate that is considerably below what would be expected based on the reported rates of depression in this population. Inappropriate medication choices are common, including the underutilization of psychostimulants, inappropriate dosing, and the reliance on tertiary-amine tricyclics with needlessly high rates of toxicity. Psychostimulants are effective agents in the treatment of depression in the terminally ill because they work quickly and have a lower incidence of side effects than tricyclics among patients with medical illness (62–64). The selective serotonin reuptake inhibitors (SSRIs) are highly effective in this setting and well tolerated by medically ill patients. (See Chapter 3, this volume, for discussion of diagnosis and treatment of depression in this population.)

Anxiety Disorders

Anxiety is a common accompaniment of terminal illness, growing out of uncertainty about the future, apprehension about symptoms and their treatments, concerns about caretaking arrangements, and fear about the process of dying and how it will be handled. Anxiety is frequently amplified by pain, physical symptoms (especially dyspnea), metabolic abnormalities, hormone-secreting tumors, and medications

(65). Anxiety may be manifested as agitation, restlessness, anger, or other psychological responses that are difficult to evaluate. Differentiation among these sources of anxiety often requires psychiatric expertise because of the complex interplay among medical, pharmacological, and psychological issues. The psychiatrist's familiarity with the use of psychotropics, as well as interpersonal and cognitive-behavioral approaches to anxiety reduction, complements the expertise of other professionals involved in the care of the terminally ill.

Organic Mental Disorders

Organic mental disorders frequently cause cognitive disturbances, suspiciousness, anxiety, and impulsivity that can contribute to desires for accelerated death. Especially among AIDS patients, organic mental disorders are risk factors for suicide attempts (66, 67). Even subtle cognitive impairments may contribute to suicidal ideation and requests for accelerated death. Nonpsychiatric physicians frequently fail to recognize, diagnose, and appropriately treat these disorders (68). All patients who raise the question of hastening death should be evaluated for the presence of organic mental disorders; the psychiatrist is usually the best-equipped professional for this clinical task. Psychiatrists are also needed to educate physicians and other health professionals who care for the dying regarding the diagnosis of organic mental disorders.

Substance Abuse Disorders

As in nonmedical settings, preexisting substance abuse disorders among cancer patients are associated with increased suicide rates (69). Among the factors likely to increase suicide risk among substance abusers are impulsivity, inadequate coping skills, intolerance of affect, and depression. In addition, intravenous drug abusers who develop cancer or AIDS-related pain are especially likely to have analgesics withheld (70); undertreated physical pain may represent an additional factor that predisposes them to request hastened death. Psychiatrists have an important role in the management of patients with substance abuse disorders—as educators about the pharmacokinetics of opioids in patients with histories of substance abuse, as resources in the management of substance abuse, and as advocates for effective analgesia in this population of stigmatized patients, whose needs for analgesia are often minimized and labeled as drug-seeking behavior.

Personality Style and Personality Disorder

Some patients may describe their wishes for euthanasia or assisted suicide as growing out of ideas about self-determination and "death with dignity." Nonpsychiatric clinicians may take such expressions at face value, failing to explore the individual meanings of these abstract ideas. Why is this patient at this time feeling afraid of losing control and dignity? What is the nature of this patient's suffering such that death is preferable to loss of control and loss of an intact self? Exploration of these questions often identifies and highlights personality characteristics such as self-reliance, perfectionism, self-control, rigidity, and the tendency to respond judgmentally. These defensive styles may have been highly adaptive in many spheres of life. However, in the setting of terminal illness, self-reliance may be expressed as difficulty in trusting others, accepting help, and being dependent; perfectionism, as frustration with personal weakness and neediness; self-control, as intolerance of the noncontrollable vicissitudes and uncertainties of illness; the tendency to be judgmental, as self-criticism and self-blame over being ill and incapacitated. Giving up control, accepting dependency, and tolerating physical deterioration may be so intolerable that hastening death becomes a way to preserve the self.

Individuals with these personality traits may be highly successful professionals who have prided themselves on their accomplishments and ability to control their lives. Often, little is remediable about their experience and feelings, and they make a convincing case for assisted death. Mental health intervention may help such patients reframe their experience; alternative expressions of control and of living up to high personal standards of behavior include forbearance in the face of uncertainty and difficulty, capacity to model grace in confronting impending annihilation, and allowing oneself to receive help as a means of permitting others to master their feelings of loss.

A.L. is a 46-year-old former Marine officer in the terminal phase of lung cancer. His wife sought psychiatric assistance after her husband told her that he planned to use one of his large collection of military weapons to kill himself. Mr. L. had joined the military at age 18 and had risen through the ranks through "gritting my teeth, shutting up, and doing what had to be done." He said that he found it unbearable to feel weak and preferred to die before he "stopped being a man." Mr. L. told the psychiatrist that he had discussed his wish for assisted suicide with his physician, who had declined to help him. Following that, he felt his only option was to kill himself. He stated that he was not in pain but that he could not bear to watch his wife suffer through his dying. He said that he had not spoken about his feelings about his illness and death with his wife because he felt she could not tolerate them. In a joint meeting, Ms. L. described her increasing isolation from her husband and beseeched him to talk with her. Initially, Mr. L. refused, but he gradually came to redefine his task in dying in terms that he found acceptable: "It takes a strong man to look death in the face and talk about it" and "A good man takes care of his wife for as long as he can."

In a more extreme form, self-reliance, perfectionism, self-control, rigidity, and the tendency to be judmental may be conceptualized as part of a narcissistic or obsessive-compulsive personality disorder. In our experience, these are the most common personality configurations seen in patients whose physical, psychosocial, and spiritual problems are well managed and who persistently seek hastened death. While the patient's request for accelerated death may be framed as an issue of "rights" and "autonomy," it also may reflect deep emptiness and conflict over dependency. Clinicians sometimes perceive such patients as cold, ungrateful, demanding, demeaning, or help-rejecting (71), and may be troubled by the discrepancy between the patient's description of intolerable suffering and the medical realities of the patient's situation.

Ms. B. is a 52-year-old woman with metastatic cancer who insists on receiving immediate help in accelerating her death and is referred for psychiatric evaluation at home by her hospice nurse. The psychiatrist is met at the door of the patient's elegant apartment by the patient's two grown sons. They describe their mother's precipitous decline over the past few weeks and request that her wishes for help in dying be honored as soon as possible. The patient, seeming impatient about having to speak with another physician, articulates her urgent wish for help in dying. She says that she is physically comfortable but anticipates future deterioration. She states that she is angry that no one will help her, and plans to throw herself out of her forty-seventh-floor window in the next 2 days if she cannot be helped to die.

Ms. B. is convinced that this may be her last chance to control the end of her life because of her increasing weakness. Her rapid decline suggests to the psychiatrist that she is likely to be unable to get out of bed very soon. Having been a successful academic, she finds the prospect of "having my sons wipe my ass" intolerably humiliating. She describes herself as a strong, independent woman who has surmounted considerable adversity in her life, including the loss of a parent when she was 15 and her own divorce. Although she has many supportive and involved family members and friends, she does not want them to have to take care of her. She describes herself as "vain" and "concerned about appearances" and states that several years of intensive psychotherapy have not changed these characteristics. She feels that the losses of bodily functions and attractiveness are unbearable insults to her "core self." As the psychiatrist leaves, Ms. B. demands to know when she can expect help.

One of her sons calls the next day to say that the follow-up appointment scheduled will not be necessary because his mother had died in her sleep. No further information is divulged by the family.

As this example indicates, patients with narcissistic or obsessive-compulsive personality disorders may ask for or demand help in hastening death in a setting and manner that health professionals find difficult to understand or tolerate. By making the patient's behavior comprehensible to members of the healthcare team, the psychiatrist helps his or her colleagues to remain involved with the patient instead of withdrawing, to set limits on the patient's demands when appropriate, to tolerate the patient's oscillations between intense dependency and anger, and to redefine the goals of treatment to reflect the likelihood that the patient's dysphoria and anger will continue regardless of the team's actions. This "impossible" patient thus becomes manageable, and the team retains its cohesiveness and ability to provide compassionate professional services despite the patient's difficult behavior.

Self-destructive patients with borderline personality disorder may also seek physician-assisted death. Self-destructive patients may be unconsciously seeking a physician to hurt or abuse them in order to confirm their views of themselves as damaged and unworthy. These patients often have significant associated depressions and impaired decision-making capacity. Such patients can generate great distress within the caregiving team. By helping the team understand the patient's defenses, relationships, vulnerabilities, and personality, the psychiatrist enables care providers to manage the difficulties that are arising in providing care and to resist the intense pressures to either accede to the patient's request or abandon the patient.

Decision-Making Capacity

As described previously, depression and organic mental disorders are commonly encountered among patients who request assistance in dying. These disorders can both impair patient autonomy and coexist with autonomous wishes for hastened death. Because of the irrevocability of hastening death, decisions about competency must be especially rigorous. Determination of competence in this setting is often extraordinarily challenging, requiring subtle evaluations of thought processes and complex assessments of the patient's cognitive understanding, affective and emotional appreciation, and characterologic limitations in understanding the implications of alternative choices (72–76). Very rarely are nonpsychiatric clinicians adequately prepared to address this broad concept of competence, so psychiatric input is essential. The issue of determining competence in patients seeking hastened death is dealt with more comprehensively by Youngner in Chapter 2 of this volume.

Social Suffering

Difficulties in interpersonal relationships commonly trigger requests for accelerated death. Dying patients may channel anger, disappointment, and the wish to avoid the pain of a slow separation from loved ones into a request for hastened death. They also may fear that they will overburden their caretakers with the physical tasks of care, deplete financial resources intended for others, or encumber loved ones with painful memories. Decisions about desired care at the end of life are heavily influenced by the desire to avoid burdening others, especially children (77). The SUPPORT study documented that the economic burden of serious illness is significant enough to influence patients' care preferences in the direction of comfort-oriented over life-prolonging care (78). Although there are many reasons to be concerned about the impact of financial coercion on end-of-life decision making, it is important that patients' wishes—for example, to leave a financial legacy for family members, to avoid forcing an adult child to give up a job to provide medical care—be understood and respected. Requests for hastened death are sometimes designed to test love and the commitment of family members to providing care. In saying that he or she wants to die, the patient may be asking for reassurance that he or she is still valued and that others want him or her to go on living. The skills of mental health clinicians in exploring and understanding personal meanings and experience, as well as nuances and tensions in interpersonal relationships, are valuable resources for the primary physician or interdisciplinary team caring for terminally ill patients.

> M.T., a 62-year-old man with metastatic lung cancer, began speaking of his desire for euthanasia at a time when his symptoms were relatively stable. The physician sought psychiatric consultation to evaluate further the patient's state of mind. The psychiatrist learned that the patient and his wife had been fighting constantly over recent weeks, an intensification of their long-term dysfunctional relationship. On further exploration it became clear the patient viewed accelerating his death as a way of retaliating against his wife, stating, "I want her to believe that she made me do this."

Particular attention should be devoted to exploration of meanings of loss of control and dependency, both to the self and in relationship with significant others. Among the common social themes that arise in exploring patients' desires to hasten death are loss (or anticipated loss) of support from a spouse, distrust of family members' ability and willingness to provide care, anger related to perceived disappointments, and inability to relinquish the role of caretaker.

Existential/Spiritual Suffering

In saying that he or she wants to die, the patient may be asking to be given a reason to live or for help in finding a reason to carry on.

Conscious patients who are facing death confront questions of meaning that may give rise to existential/spiritual suffering. Grieving entails a process of life review, remembering, and reckoning with earlier experiences. Clinicians must appreciate that religious and spiritual despair may contribute to desires for hastened death. Common themes that arise are guilt over past actions, anger at God, fear of punishment, and anxiety about lack of meaning. Exploration of the patient's current and past religious and spiritual identity, affiliations, and beliefs is an important first step in understanding such concerns. Further discussion of the patient's feelings about the sources of meaning in his or her life, beliefs about why he or she became ill, and expectations about what happens after death can help identify whether the patient might benefit from pastoral care or other forms of spiritual counseling.

Dysfunction in the Physician-Patient Relationship

Difficulties in the patient's relationship with the primary physician may also contribute to desires for hastened death. The wish to hasten death often grows out of fears about how death will be handled: Will I be given adequate pain relievers? Will I be alone? Will I be able to express my wishes and be listened to? The patient often feels more in control and more confident in caregivers when the primary physician is able to explore these concerns, reassure the patient about his or her ongoing involvement, and educate the patient about what is likely to happen and about options for care. However, because of the intense emotions surrounding discussions of death, communication between patient and physician may be problematic. Patients are often unclear about what the implications of their wishes and requests might be, and have been shown to misunderstand information they receive about such emotionally loaded issues as cardiopulmonary resuscitation (79). Additionally, physicians' concerns about upsetting or frightening patients in the course of discussions of wishes for care at the end of life may lead to euphemistic or incomplete discussions (80). Since ambivalence is such a universal aspect of discussions about death, it is all too easy for the physician to hear only one side of the patient's feelings, ignoring or minimizing the opposite side (81, 82). In seeking a quick and painless end to living, a patient may simultaneously be hoping for a cure of the underlying medical disorder, remission of symptoms, lifting of a depression, or alleviation of the social and economic burdens of illness. In expressing a wish to separate from the living, a patient may be searching for a relationship that counters loneliness and frustration.

For many physicians, a dying patient represents a personal failure. Some physicians, in response to this sense of failure, withdraw from their patients as a way of reducing their own distress about the patient's deteriorating condition (83, 84). Sensing the physician's withdrawal, the patient may then become more needy or withdrawn, or even come to view hastening death as a way to control the feelings of abandonment. The psychiatrist may be a useful consultant in exploring these issues with the patient and physician and in identifying problematic dynamics in the physician-patient relationship that may impede the patient's ability to express feelings and wishes fully and clearly.

The request to hasten death itself often generates a strong emotional response in the physician. The primary physician may find it painful and difficult to endure a patient's sustained and escalating plea for help and may respond with depression, avoidance, anger, denial, or guilt. These emotional responses must be understood and addressed in developing an optimal care plan for the patient. Unfortunately, few settings legitimize discussions of physicians' emotional reactions to patients and the impact of these responses on care.

> Dr. M. sought out a colleague at a conference on euthanasia to talk about a patient whose death he had assisted several years ago. Dr. M. described in depth his long-standing relationship with the patient and his wife, the patient's illness, and the events that led to his administering a lethal dose of barbiturates to the patient. Dr. M. acknowledged that he thought about the case nearly every day but had never talked about it with anyone. He described it as the most significant and difficult situation he had encountered in his professional life. He wondered how his own unresolved feelings about this event influenced his care of dying patients in the present.

Clinicians who have encountered requests to hasten death and have allowed themselves to enter into the patient's dilemma often describe such experiences as wrenching and disturbing. Psychiatrists can play an important role in helping to create a nonjudgmental setting for these issues to be discussed, modeling an accepting and inquiring openness to these feelings, and using the physician's emotional response in the service of dealing effectively with the situation.

A physician's refusal to participate in accelerating death often creates a crisis in the physician-patient relationship. The patient may feel rejected, abandoned, criticized, or controlled by the physician's decision. The patient's feelings may cause the physician to respond by withdrawing from the patient, with the patient left feeling abandoned. The psychiatrist can help the primary physician find a way to maintain connection with the patient, bear the burden of the patient's anger and despair, and tolerate the conflict and guilt engendered by the decision not to participate in hastening death. In this situation physicians are sometimes tempted to withhold medication that might be needed for symptom control because of fear that the patient will use it for suicide. Primary physicians must be encouraged to avoid this understandable response and to accept the risk that a patient will use medication prescribed for symptom control to accelerate death.

Working With the Patient Who Persistently Requests Hastened Death: Clinical and Collegial Issues

On rare occasions clinicians encounter patients who are receiving excellent symptom palliation, are not depressed or psychologically impaired, have supportive social networks, and have fully and comfortably discussed with their physicians their personal values, priorities, and choices about dying. Yet their suffering remains profound and intractable, and they explicitly request assistance in hastening death.

> L.T. was a 47-year-old gay psychologist with far-advanced AIDS. Throughout his illness, he had planned to kill himself before the disease "took over," and had many discussions with a large network of devoted friends and with his physician about his wishes. He had nursed his lover through the end stages of the disease, which included central nervous

system involvement and invasive procedures; that experience had a powerful impact on his own feelings about how he wanted his life to end. He feared loss of control and loss of dignity.

L.T. had seen a psychiatrist for psychotherapy at several times during his illness to help him deal with feelings of depression, grief, and loss of control. He had also tried several different antidepressants because he wondered whether his mood might improve with medication. Medication had not been helpful, but psychotherapy had. His depression improved, although he was still often sad.

Although he was in no pain, L.T. had been experiencing more frequent infections and had lost 40 pounds. He had a taste disturbance that made him aversive to nearly all foods, and he was increasingly confined to his home by fatigue and weakness. As his illness progressed, L.T.'s central focus became his spiritual growth and coming to terms with his death within the framework of his faith. Although he had been raised as a Catholic, in recent years he had become a Buddhist, and he expected a life after death.

As he became sicker, L.T. stopped working because he could no longer concentrate. He felt unburdened by the end of these professional reponsibilities but also missed his work. Although his relationships with friends remained important, he found himself less eager for their companionship and for the pushes and pulls of human interaction. Small things—an open window that made the room chilly, a visitor who came late—bothered him greatly, and L.T. was disturbed by his disproportionate reactions to these events. Although he did not feel depressed, the constriction of his world and the preoccupation with sickness diminished his sense of meaning and connection. At this point, he asked his physician to assist him in suicide, and a psychiatrist was consulted.

The psychiatrist evaluated the patient and concluded that 1) the patient did not have a major depression; 2) his current thinking was not irrationally distorted by the trauma of his lover's death; 3) he had a full cognitive and affective understanding of his situation and the implications, for himself and his friends, of hastening his death; and 4) he felt a strong and reassuring connection with his primary care physician. In fact, the psychiatrist was impressed by L.T.'s clear understanding of his situation, by his ironic appreciation of both the preciousness and the intolerability of his life, and by his personal warmth, vivacity, and connectedness.

The primary care physician and the psychiatrist talked extensively about L.T.'s situation and about what it would mean to the physician to honor or to refuse L.T.'s request. The primary care physician then decided to help L.T. end his life by prescribing a lethal dose of barbiturates and attending his suicide.

Although this case raises difficult ethical and legal issues that have been extensively discussed in the literature (85–88), we will address here only the psychiatrist's clinical and collegial role. Although the practice of PAS has now been legalized in the state of Oregon, it is unlikely that a consensus about the moral and ethical implications of PAS can be reached. What we can do, and where psychiatry has a unique and critical contribution to make, is to clarify the key psychiatric and psychosocial issues that must be addressed to provide optimal care to a suffering patient.

In assessing a patient who requests hastened death, the psychiatrist performs several different functions:

- Offering a second opinion on the patient's psychological status
- Asking probing questions of the patient, creating opportunities for a deeper level of self-reflection and self-understanding
- Providing a sophisticated evaluation of the patient's mood and decision-making capacity
- Validating that no treatable disorder is being missed
- Assessing the patient's important relationships, including the state of the primary physician–patient relationship
- Helping create a setting in which the primary physician and the team can formulate a thoughtful decision about how to respond in the best interests of the patient

In order for the primary physician to be comfortable turning to the psychiatrist, the two parties ideally will have a history of working with each other in difficult situations, and a degree of trust in each others' clinical and moral judgment. Such a relationship develops most readily when the psychiatrist is part of an interdisciplinary team with a shared history and set of values. While not always achievable, this ideal is a goal to strive for in caring for patients with terminal illness. Often the psychiatrist pulls together input from other mental health professionals who may know the patient, presenting it to the team that is making the clinical decision about how to respond. Psychiatrists must continue to define their roles in the settings in which terminally ill patients receive care (i.e., general hospitals, cancer centers, oncology units, and nursing homes). In addition, psychiatrists should become much more involved with the hospice and palliative care programs—inpatient, outpatient, and home based—that are a growing locus of care for the dying.

We believe that assisted suicide and euthanasia should be options of last resort. Prevention of PAS and euthanasia is an important human and social goal and can be accomplished through improvements in communication about desires for end-of-life care, better access to palliative care services, and provision of high-quality psychiatric care to patients with terminal illness.

Conclusion

The appropriate response to the rare case of a competent, terminally ill adult patient who is experiencing suffering he or she considers unbearable, like L.T. in the case example above, is likely to remain a source of contention and disagreement. However, increasing understanding of the dynamics of requests for PAS over the past few years has made it clear that psychiatrists and other mental health clinicians have an essential role in assessing individual patients, educating other healthcare professionals about psychiatric aspects of palliative care, carrying out research on psychosocial dimensions of palliative care, and developing procedural safeguards for PAS legislation. Patients will continue to request PAS and to require a sophisticated and psychologically informed assessment of the meanings of their wishes. Their physicians will continue to be troubled by these requests and will benefit from opportunities to discuss these difficult clinical dilemmas with clinicians who understand the psychological issues, both for patients and for physicians, involved in responding to requests for PAS.

New attention to education about palliative care has created opportunities for psychiatrists to be involved in educating other healthcare professionals about the diagnosis and treatment of depression in the terminally ill, the experiences of suffering and loss, the relationship between pain and psychological distress, the process of bereavement, the assessment of decision-making capacity in the terminally ill, and other essential topics. Psychiatrists and other mental health clinicians are playing an important role in shaping the emerging discipline of palliative care, designing and implementing essential research on decision making, communication, and diagnosis and treatment of end-of-life psychological distress.

The Oregon experience with legalization of PAS will bring new challenges and dilemmas into the PAS discussion and stimulate further change. The finding, for example, that fewer than 10% of psychiatrists are confident that they would be able to carry out an appropriate assessment in one session of the impact of psychiatric diagnosis on a patient's judgment raises significant questions about how well a requirement for mental health consultation will work in practice, and certainly suggests a need for additional training of mental health professionals in clinical assessment of this population. The next phase of psychiatric involvement in the issue of PAS, we believe, will require professional assessment in all of these areas, as well as close collaborations with colleagues in other disciplines and advocacy for comprehensive palliative care for all patients with terminal illness.

References

1. Wolf SM: Holding the line on euthanasia. Hastings Cent Rep 19 (1, suppl):13–15, 1989
2. Singer PA, Siegler M: Euthanasia—a critique. N Engl J Med 322:1881–1883, 1990
3. Gaylin W, Kass LR, Pellegrino ED, et al: Doctors must not kill. JAMA 259:2139–2140, 1988
4. Quill TE: Death and dignity—a case of individualized decision making. N Engl J Med 324:691–694, 1991
5. Baile WF, DiMaggio JR, Schapira DV, et al: The request for assistance in dying: the need for psychiatric consultation. Cancer 72:2786–2791, 1993
6. Huyse FJ, van Tilburg W: Euthanasia policy in The Netherlands: the role of consultation-liaison psychiatrists. Hospital and Community Psychiatry 44:733–738, 1993

7. Conwell Y, Caine ED: Rational suicide and the right to die—reality and myth. N Engl J Med 325:1100–1103, 1991

8. Cohen JS, Fihn S, Boyko EJ, et al: Attitudes toward assisted suicide and euthanasia among physicians in Washington State. N Engl J Med 331:89–94, 1994

9. Ganzini L, Fenn DS, Lee MA, et al: Attitudes of Oregon psychiatrists toward physician-assisted suicide. Am J Psychiatry 153:1469–1475, 1996

10. Block SD, Billings JA: Patient requests to hasten death: evaluation and management in terminal care. Arch Intern Med 154:2039–2046, 1994

11. Humphry D: Final Exit. Eugene, OR, The Hemlock Society, 1991, pp 109–113

12. Levin DN, Cleeland CS, Dar R: Public attitudes toward cancer pain. Cancer 42:1385–1391, 1985

13. Owens C, Tennant C, Levi J, et al: Suicide and euthanasia: patient attitudes in the context of cancer. Psycho-oncology 1:79–88, 1992

14. Wanzer SH, Federman DD, Adelstein SJ, et al: The physician's responsibility toward hopelessly ill patients. N Engl J Med 320:844–849, 1989

15. Chochinov HM, Wilson KG, Enns M, et al: Desire for death in the terminally ill. Am J Psychiatry 152:1185–1191, 1995

16. Breitbart W, Rosenfeld BD, Passik SD: Interest in physician-assisted suicide among ambulatory HIV-infected patients. Am J Psychiatry 153:238–242, 1996

17. Emmanuel EJ, Fairclough DL, Daniels ER, et al: Euthanasia and physician-assisted suicide: attitudes and experiences of oncology patients, oncologists, and the public. Lancet 347:1805–1810, 1996

18. van der Maas PJ, van Delden JJM, Pijnenborg L, et al: Euthanasia and other medical decisions concerning the end of life. Lancet 338:669–674, 1991

19. Breitbart W: Suicide, in Handbook of Psychooncology. Edited by Holland JC, Rowland JH. New York, Oxford University Press, 1989, pp 291–299

20. Brown JH, Henteleff P, Barakat S, et al: Is it normal for terminally ill patients to desire death? Am J Psychiatry 143:208–211, 1986

21. Chochinov HM, Wilson KG, Enns M, et al: Prevalence of depression in the terminally ill: effects of diagnostic criteria and symptom threshold judgment. Am J Psychiatry 151:537–540, 1994

22. Breitbart W: Suicide in cancer patients. Oncology 1:49–54, 1987

23. Weisman AD: Coping behavior and suicide in cancer, in Cancer: The Behavioral Dimensions. Edited by Cullen JW, Fox BH, Isom RN. New York, Raven, 1976, pp 331–358

24. Bolund C: Suicide and cancer, I: demographic and social characteristics of cancer patients who committed suicide in Sweden, 1973–1976. Journal of Psychosocial Oncology 3:17–30, 1985

25. Bolund C: Suicide and cancer, II: medical and care factors in suicides by cancer patients in Sweden, 1973–1976. Journal of Psychosocial Oncology 3:31–52, 1985
26. Owens et al, Suicide and euthanasia
27. Storm HH, Christensen N, Jensen OM: Suicides among Danish patients with cancer: 1971 to 1986. Cancer 69:1507–1512, 1992
28. Jacobson JA, Kasworm EM, Battin MP, et al: Decedents' reported preferences for physician-assisted death: a survey of informants listed on death certificates in Utah. J Clin Ethics 6:149–157, 1995
29. Marzuk PM, Tierney H, Tardiff K, et al: Increased risk of suicide in persons with AIDS. JAMA 259:1333–1337, 1988
30. Cot TR, Biggar RJ, Dannenberg AL: Risk of suicide among persons with AIDS. JAMA 268:2066–2068, 1992
31. Snyder S, Reyner A, Schmeidler J, et al: Prevalence of mental disorders in newly admitted medical inpatients with AIDS. Psychosomatics 33:166–170, 1992
32. Frierson RL, Lippman SB: Suicide and AIDS. Psychosomatics 29:226–231, 1989
33. Storm et al, Suicides among Danish patients with cancer
34. Marzuk PM, Tardiff K, Hirsch CS, et al: Increase in suicide by asphyxiation in New York City after the publication of Final Exit. N Engl J Med 329:1508–1510, 1993
35. McCusker J: Where cancer patients die: an epidemiologic study. Public Health Rep 98:170–176, 1983
36. Sager M, Easterling D, Kindig D, et al: Changes in the location of death after passage of Medicare's prospective payment system. N Engl J Med 320:433–439, 1989
37. The SUPPORT Principal Investigators: A controlled trial to improve care for seriously ill hospitalized patients. JAMA 274:1591–1598, 1995
38. Foley KM: The relationship of pain and symptom management to patient requests for physician-assisted suicide. J Pain Symptom Manage 6:289–297, 1991
39. Marks RM, Sachar ES: Undertreatment of medical inpatients with analgesics. Ann Intern Med 78:173–181, 1973
40. Hanks GW, Justin DM: Cancer pain: management. Lancet 339:1031–1036, 1992
41. Cleeland CS: Barriers to the management of cancer pain. Oncology 1 (2, suppl):19–26, 1987
42. Max MB: Improving outcomes of analgesic treatment: is education enough? Ann Intern Med 113:885–889, 1990

43. Jacox A, Carr DB, Payne R, et al: Management of Cancer Pain (Clinical Practice Guideline No 9) (AHCPR Publ No 94-0592). Rockville, MD, Agency for Health Care Policy and Research, U.S. Department of Health and Human Services, March 1994
44. van der Maas et al, Euthanasia and other medical decisions
45. Breitbart W: Cancer pain and suicide, in Advances in Pain Research and Therapy. Edited by Foley KM, Bonica JJ, Ventafridda V. New York, Raven, 1990, pp 399–412
46. Helig S: The San Francisco Medical Society euthanasia survey: results and analysis. San Francisco Medicine 61:24–34, 1988
47. Twycross RG, Lack SA: Symptom Control in Far Advanced Cancer: Pain Relief. London, Pitman Publishing, 1984
48. Cleeland CS: The impact of pain on patients with cancer. Cancer 54:235–241, 1984
49. Portenoy RK: Cancer pain: pathophysiology and syndromes. Lancet 339:1026–1031, 1992
50. Admiraal P: Personal communication. Cited in Lo B: Euthanasia—the continuing debate. West J Med 149:211–212, 1988
51. Ventafridda V, Tamburini M, Caraceni A, et al: A validation study of the WHO method for cancer pain relief. Cancer 59:350–356, 1987
52. Grond S, Zech D, Schug SA, et al: Validation of World Health Organization guidelines for cancer pain relief during the last days and hours of life. J Pain Symptom Manage 6:411–422, 1991
53. Bukberg J, Penman D, Holland JC: Depression in hospitalized cancer patients. Psychosom Med 46:199–212, 1984
54. Massie MJ, Holland JC: The cancer patient with pain: psychiatric complications and their management. Med Clin North Am 71:243–258, 1987
55. Block SD: Coping with loss, in Outpatient Management of Advanced Cancer. Edited by Billings JA. Philadelphia, PA, JB Lippincott, 1985, pp 195–235
56. Kathol RG, Noyes R, Williams J, et al: Diagnosing depression in patients with medical illness. Psychosomatics 31:434–440, 1990
57. Plumb NM, Holland JC: Comparative studies of psychosocial function in patients with advanced cancer, I: self-reported depressive symptoms. Psychosom Med 39:264–276, 1977
58. Plumb NM, Holland JC: Comparative studies of psychological function in patients with advanced cancer, II: interviewer-rated current and past psychological symptoms. Psychosom Med 43:243–254, 1981
59. Lindemann E: Symptomatology and management of acute grief. Am J Psychiatry 101:141–148, 1944

60. Brown JT, Stoudemire A: Normal and pathological grief. JAMA 250:378–382, 1983

61. Clayton P: Mourning and depression: their similarities and differences. Can J Psychiatry 19:309–312, 1974

62. Woods SW, Tesar GE, Murray GB, et al: Psychostimulant treatment of depressive disorders secondary to medical illness. J Clin Psychiatry 47:12–15, 1986

63. Masand P, Pickett P, Murray GB: Psychostimulants for secondary depression in medical illness. Psychosomatics 32:203–208, 1991

64. Burns MM, Eisendrath SJ: Dextroamphetamine treatment for depression in terminally ill patients. Psychosomatics 35:80–83, 1994

65. Massie MJ, Holland JC: The cancer patient with pain: psychiatric complications and their management. J Pain Symptom Manage 7:99–109, 1992

66. MacKenzie TB, Popkin MK: Suicide in the medical patient. Int J Psychiatry Med 17:3–22, 1987

67. Breitbart, Suicide, in Handbook of Psychooncology

68. Levine PM, Silberfarb PM, Lipowski ZJ: Mental disorders in cancer patients: a study of 100 psychiatric referrals. Cancer 42:1385–1391, 1978

69. Breitbart et al, Interest in physician-assisted suicide

70. Macaluso C, Weinberg D, Foley KM: Opioid abuse and misuse in a cancer pain population (abstract). J Pain Symptom Manage 3(suppl):S54, 1988

71. Groves JE: Taking care of the hateful patient. N Engl J Med 298:883–887, 1978

72. Appelbaum PS, Grisso T: Assessing patients' capacities to consent to treatment. N Engl J Med 319:1635–1638, 1988

73. Bursztajn HJ, Harding HP, Gutheil TG, et al: Beyond cognition: the role of disordered affective states in impairing competence to consent to treatment. Bull Am Acad Psychiatry Law 19:383–388, 1991

74. Culver CM, Gert B: The inadequacy of incompetence. Milbank Q 68:619–643, 1990

75. Drane JF: Competency to give an informed consent. JAMA 252:925–927, 1984

76. Sullivan MD, Youngner SJ: Depression, competence, and the right to refuse lifesaving medical treatment. Am J Psychiatry 151:971–978, 1994

77. Zweibel NR, Cassel CK: Treatment choices at the end of life: a comparison by older patients and their physician-selected proxies. Gerontologist 29:615–621, 1989

78. Covinsky KE, Landefeld S, Teno J, et al: Is economic hardship on the families of the seriously ill associated with patient and surrogate care preferences? Arch Intern Med 156:1737–1741, 1996

79. Amchin J, Perry S, Manevitz A, et al: Interview assessment of critically ill patients regarding resuscitation decisions. Gen Hosp Psychiatry 11:103–108, 1989

80. Miller A, Lo B: How do doctors discuss do-not-resuscitate orders? West J Med 143:256–258, 1985

81. It's over Debbie. JAMA 259:272, 1989

82. Bursztajn H, Gutheil TG, Warren MJ, et al: Depression, self-love, time and the "right" to suicide. Gen Hosp Psychiatry 8:91–95, 1986

83. Schulz R, Aderman D: How the medical staff copes with dying patients: a critical review. Omega 7:11–21, 1976

84. Nuland S: How We Die. New York, Alfred Knopf, 1994

85. Singer PA, Siegler M: Euthanasia—a critique. N Engl J Med 322:1881–1883, 1990

86. Gaylin et al, Doctors must not kill

87. American Geriatrics Society, Public Policy Committee: Voluntary active euthanasia. J Am Geriatr Soc 39:826, 1991

88. American Medical Association, Council on Ethical and Judicial Affairs: Decisions near the end of life. JAMA 267:2229–2233, 1992

9

Legal Aspects of End-of-Life Decision Making

Alan Meisel, J.D.

Alittle more than two decades ago, doctors lost their innocence about their role in hastening the death of patients. Until that time the codes among doctors—both the informal code and the formal codes of medical ethics—held that it was not permissible for doctors to participate in hastening death. Although Hippocrates might not have been the first to admonish doctors "to give no deadly medicine to anyone if asked" (1), his admonition is historically the best known. Until relatively recent times, giving a "deadly medicine" was usually the only way for a doctor to hasten death. Withholding or withdrawing treatment—now the predominant option— was rarely an option until well into the twentieth-century because so little treatment had any lifesaving effect. Whatever efforts doctors or others made to hasten the death of a patient were usually covert. The reason is obvious: mercy killing or assisting in suicide was a crime.

All of this changed, literally overnight—the night of April 15, 1975—when a 21-year-old unconscious woman named Karen Ann Quinlan was brought to the emergency room of a New Jersey hospital.

This set in motion a series of events leading to a ruling by the New Jersey Supreme Court, little less than a year later, allowing doctors to terminate the life support that was keeping this now permanently unconscious woman alive (2).

There were some precursors to *Quinlan,* some of which even made the news, but because most never reached an appellate court, they never became legal precedent. Thus, although *Quinlan* did not spring full grown from the New Jersey Supreme Court the way Athena did from the head of Zeus, it did represent a significant paradigm shift. Moreover, *Quinlan* broke the ice of secrecy; it gave permission for the open discussion of issues that were previously either taboo or so infrequent as not to require public discussion and debate. *Quinlan* began a public debate that continues unabated to this day and is unlikely to become quiescent anytime soon, though its form and content have changed considerably.

The Consensus About End-of-Life Decision Making

The significance of *Quinlan* extended beyond the social ramifications described above. The case spawned progeny in the form of other court cases and legislation, which, taken together, have yielded a consensus about end-of-life decision making. Legislatures in all states have enacted statutes recognizing the validity of one or more forms of advance directives. Many have also enacted surrogate decision-making statutes and do-not-resuscitate (DNR) statutes, and recently a few have enacted statutes intended to promote the use of analgesic medications for the terminally ill. More important in creating this consensus, however, have been the opinions of slightly more than half of the states' appellate courts. Frequently writing lengthy treatises on the subject, the courts managed, over the course of about 15 years, to reach a fairly high degree of agreement about the law governing end-of-life decisions.

Competent Patients' Right to Refuse Treatment

The bedrock of the consensus about end-of-life decision making is that patients who possess decision-making capacity have a right to refuse treatment. This is not a particularly novel legal proposition. What is novel is its application in a context in which the patient will certainly, or almost certainly, die if the treatment in question is refused. For if that happens, can it be said that the doctor's termination of treatment killed the patient, thus exposing the doctor to possible criminal liability?

Consent to Medical Treatment

Beginning with *Quinlan,* the courts concluded that the forgoing of life-sustaining medical treatment, whether by withholding or with-drawing, does not subject doctors to criminal liability. The route to this conclusion was long in developing. Beginning near the end of the nineteenth century and continuing through the beginning of the twentieth century (3, 4), courts began to formally recognize a right to refuse medical treatment, based on the law of battery that had developed in English law beginning centuries ago. This early movement culminated in 1914 with the Schloendorff case, in which Judge Benjamin Cardozo, then on the New York Court of Appeals and later a member of the United States Supreme Court, announced, in a phrase that is repeated in virtually every medical decision-making case, that "[e]very human being of adult years and sound mind has a right to determine what shall be done with his own body . . ." This requirement of consent to medical treatment was gradually transformed over the course of the next half-century into the doctrine we now know as *informed consent.* Under this doctrine, not only do patients have the right to refuse medical treatment, they also have the right to be provided with adequate information about their medical options to exercise that right in an intelligent fashion.

Informed Consent

By the early 1970s (5, 6), informed consent was a well-established and almost thoroughly explicated doctrine, and it was ripe for use in end-of-life decision-making cases. However, in a somewhat odd twist, the New Jersey Supreme Court chose in the Quinlan case to base the right to refuse treatment not on the common-law doctrine of informed consent, but on the relatively newly enunciated constitutional right of privacy. Yet, within a relatively short time, most courts—and eventually the New Jersey Supreme Court (7)—came to plant the right to die in the common-law right of informed consent rather than the constitutional right of privacy. As will be seen, however, the constitutional basis for end-of-life decision making is once again in the forefront of discussion in the efforts to establish a constitutional right to physician-assisted suicide.

Application When Refusal Leads to Death

We should not overlook the fact that *Quinlan* involved a patient who lacked decision-making capacity—a situation that creates special problems, which will be discussed later. However, within 2 years of the *Quinlan* decision, the Florida courts considered the case of a competent patient who wished to forgo life-sustaining treatment. This case, *Satz v. Perlmutter*, involved a man in his 70s who was dying of amyotrophic lateral sclerosis (ALS) and wished to have his ventilator turned off because of the unbearable suffering he was experiencing. (The court quoted him as saying, "I'm miserable, take it out," and that death "can't be worse than what I'm going through now" [8].)

   A straightforward application of the principles of battery law, not to mention informed consent, should have easily led to the conclusion that Mr. Perlmutter had a right not to be treated without his consent. However, although the courts eventually granted Mr. Perlmutter's request, the process by which the result was reached was not so simple, because the result of his refusing treatment was that it would cause his death.

Countervailing State Interests

Long before *Quinlan*, a small body of case law had developed from the refusal of blood transfusions by Jehovah's Witnesses. The courts in these cases recognized in principle that competent adult patients have a right to refuse treatment, even if its refusal would lead to death; but they were loath to apply the principle and found a variety of ways to circumvent it and order the administration of a blood transfusion (9–11).

   Borrowing from the blood transfusion cases, the court balanced Mr. Perlmutter's right to refuse medical treatment against interests that society has in keeping people alive—so-called countervailing state interests. Four such interests had been enunciated only a year earlier by the Massachusetts Supreme Judicial Court (12), though drawing on more than a decades' worth of blood transfusion cases: 1) the preservation of life, 2) the prevention of suicide, 3) the protection of third parties, and 4) the maintenance of the ethical integrity of the medical profession.

The Florida court determined that there was little or no weight to be accorded to any of these state interests in Mr. Perlmutter's case. Although the preservation of life is an important interest in general, it is far less compelling when a patient is terminally ill. As to suicide, the court concluded that the withdrawing of life support would not constitute suicide for three reasons. First, death would occur from natural causes (in this case, ALS) rather than from Mr. Perlmutter's own actions (or more properly his authorization for others to act). Second, Mr. Perlmutter did not actually wish to die but wished to end his suffering. Unfortunately, given the nature of his condition, the former was a necessary route to the latter. And, finally, the underlying cause of his suffering—ALS—was not "self-induced." This reasoning is not without some difficulties, as will become clear when we consider physician-assisted suicide.

The state's interest in protecting third parties also presented no barrier to the termination of Mr. Perlmutter's treatment. In the Jehovah's Witnesses cases, the patients were parents of young children, and the courts gave as one reason for overriding the refusal of treatment the state's interest in assuring that these children would not be abandoned. Mr. Perlmutter, by contrast, had no young children. In fact, his adult children were supportive of his wishes.

The final state interest, the maintenance of the ethical integrity of the medical profession, was dealt with by the Florida court by quoting from the year-old *Saikewicz* case in Massachusetts:

> Prevailing medical ethical practice does not, without exception, demand that all efforts toward life prolongation be made in all circumstances. Rather, as indicated in Quinlan, the prevailing ethical practice seems to be to recognize that the dying are more often in need of comfort than treatment. Recognition of the right to refuse necessary treatment in appropriate circumstances is consistent with existing medical mores; such a doctrine does not threaten either the integrity of the medical

profession, the proper role of hospitals in caring for such patients or the State's interest in protecting the same. It is not necessary to deny a right of self-determination to a patient in order to recognize the interests of doctors, hospitals, and medical personnel in attendance on the patient. (13)

Patients Who Are Not Terminally Ill

In retrospect, the Perlmutter case was a simple one because Mr. Perlmutter was terminally ill. Inevitably, more difficult cases arose in which competent patients were not conventionally thought of as being terminally ill, but rather severely disabled by illness or injury. These people would have a long life expectancy if treatment were continued. Perhaps the most renowned of these cases—but also the most problematic because of her uncertain mental state—involved Elizabeth Bouvia, a woman in her early thirties, suffering from severe cerebral palsy, with a life expectancy of decades if she received proper medical and nursing care (14).

Courts have decided a few other similar cases, all involving otherwise healthy, cognitively intact young men who were quadriplegics as a result of an accident and who needed a ventilator or feeding tube to maintain their lives (15–17). As in the Perlmutter case, all four courts weighed the state's interests against the individual's interest in self-determination and bodily integrity and concluded that because the patients were competent, the states' interests should be accorded little or no weight, and each court proceeded to uphold the right to refuse treatment. Thus, in an incremental fashion, the courts moved from permitting competent terminally ill patients to hasten their deaths by forgoing life-sustaining treatment to applying the right to refuse life-saving medical treatment to patients who were not terminally ill.

Jehovah's Witness Cases Revisited

As mentioned above, the courts traditionally honored the right of Jehovah's Witnesses to refuse blood transfusions more in the breach than the observance. But eventually the progeny of *Quinlan* began to work important changes in the judicial analysis and outcome of Jehovah's Witness cases. Especially after *Perlmutter* and the cases involving nonterminally ill patients, courts have been far more willing to respect and enforce the refusal of blood transfusions by Jehovah's Witnesses.

Interestingly, the basis for upholding this right has not been the fact that the refusal was motivated by religious belief, but the more general common-law right of all individuals to refuse medical treatment. For example, the Massachusetts Supreme Judicial Court held that the Jehovah's Witness mother of a young child, who was the child's primary caretaker and who had a bleeding ulcer, could refuse a blood transfusion even if the refusal would lead to her death. In addressing the legal basis for the holding, the court observed the following:

> We do not think it is necessary, however, to decide whether Ms. Munoz has a free exercise [i.e., a religious-based] right to refuse the administration of blood or blood products, since we have already held that she has a common law and constitutional privacy right to refuse a blood transfusion. Also, we need not decide whether a patient's right is strengthened because the objection to the medical treatment is based on religious principles. (18)

Summary: An Absolute Right to Refuse Treatment?

Although it might be risky to say that there is an absolute right of a competent person to refuse any medical treatment, the net effect of the cases—especially those involving nonterminally ill patients—has been to bring the right to refuse treatment about as close to absolute as anything ever gets in law. The four countervailing state interests are routinely intoned by courts but so rarely given any effect that they have become a vestigial part of these cases (19).

End-of-Life Decision Making for Incompetent Patients

The development of the law governing end-of-life decision making for competent patients has been relatively straightforward in comparison with that for incompetent patients. The law of battery and the law of informed consent—the legal basis for end-of-life decision making—are both premised on the assumption that the patient possesses decision-making capacity. Self-determination, the moral foundations for these two doctrines, also assumes that actors possess decisional capacity. What then to do when a patient lacks decision-making capacity?

One solution is to prohibit the forgoing of life-sustaining medical treatment when patients lack decision-making capacity. However unsatisfying this might be from an intuitive and practical perspective, it does have the virtue of respecting autonomy because it requires that any decision be based on an individual's articulated wishes. For the most part, however, the law has rejected this approach. Almost without exception, courts have instead acknowledged that incompetent patients have the same substantive legal rights that competent patients have, but that the manner of exercising them must, of necessity, be different. Courts and legislatures have staked out a wide and varying middle ground that attempts to respect patients' wishes while acknowledging that such wishes are difficult, and sometimes impossible, to discern.

The law governing end-of-life decision making for incompetent patients has two components: procedural and substantive. The procedural component addresses the issues of where end-of-life decisions are to be made and by whom; the substantive one considers the question of what criteria the decision-maker—regardless of who makes end-of-life decisions and how and where the decision is made—is to use in making the decision for the incompetent patient.

Procedural Aspects

Where Decisions Are to Be Made

The question arose very early in the legal development of end-of-life decision making about whether such decisions required judicial supervision and/or approval. The courts squared off on this issue in the first two right-to-die cases. In 1976, the New Jersey Supreme Court concluded that decisions of this sort are best made between the patient's family and the patient's physician with the approval of the hospital's ethics committee but without any judicial involvement. Its pithy conclusion was that judicial involvement would be "a gratuitous encroachment upon the medical profession's field of competence . . . [and would be] impossibly cumbersome" (20).

However, the following year, the Massachusetts Supreme Judicial Court rejected this conclusion because

> questions of life and death seem to us to require the process of detached but passionate investigation and decision that forms the ideal on which the judicial branch of government was created. Achieving this ideal is our responsibility . . . , and is not to be entrusted to any other group purporting to represent the "morality and conscience of our society," no matter how highly motivated or impressively constituted. (21)

Yet, within about 3 years, the Massachusetts courts did a significant, though subtle, about-face (22). By 1984 the debate about judicial involvement in end-of-life decision making was all but over when the Washington State courts did a much more explicit about-face. After holding in 1983 that a judicial hearing was required to terminate life support for an incompetent patient (23), it reversed itself only a year later (24).

It is now well-accepted law in all states that have had a major right-to-die case in the courts that judicial involvement in end-of-life decision making is ordinarily not required. It is accepted practice in the other states for there not to be routine judicial involvement. As many courts have said, judicial involvement is not routinely required, but "[t]he courts . . . are always open to hear these matters if request is made by the family, guardian, physician, or hospital" (25). A judicial proceeding should be initiated if there are any serious questions about whether the patient possesses or lacks decision-making capacity or about who the appropriate person is to make decisions for the patient, when there is insoluble conflict among the patient's next-of-kin about what should be done or between the patient's family and the healthcare team, or when there is a serious conflict of interest between the family and the patient. Otherwise, end-of-life decision making does not require, nor should it ordinarily have, judicial involvement.

By Whom Decisions Are to Be Made

The term ordinarily used to refer to the person who has the legal authority to make decisions for one who lacks decision-making capacity is a *surrogate*. A surrogate may be appointed by the patient and referred to as a *proxy* (see discussion of healthcare powers of attorney later in this chapter) or be appointed by a court and referred to as a *guardian*. Or there may be a statute designating who the surrogate is to be.

In the absence of a patient-appointed surrogate or a statute designating the surrogate, most courts that have considered the question have concluded that end-of-life decisions for incompetent patients are to be made by the patient's "family" or "next-of-kin." This simple statement of the problem raises some difficult issues. First, it must be determined who the patient's "family" is and, closely related, who is to decide if the patient has no family? Second, to say that the family is to decide begs the question of how—or by what standards—they are required to make decisions.

Because of the uncertainty engendered by court decisions about who the family is, about two-thirds of the states have now enacted "surrogate decision making" or "family decision making" statutes; these statutes contain a list of the order in which family members have authority to make medical decisions for a patient who lacks decision-making capacity and recommendations as to how to resolve disputes among family members (26). In states without such statutes, it is generally accepted that there should be a consensus among close family members, and it will be readily apparent if such a consensus exists. If it does not—if there is strong disagreement even by one family member, not even necessarily a "close" family member—efforts should be made through in-hospital dispute-resolution mechanisms such as an ethics consultation, pastoral counseling, social work intervention, or even mediation to achieve a consensus. Otherwise, judicial involvement will be necessary.

Substantive Aspects

To say that close family members are generally accorded the legal authority to make end-of-life decisions for patients lacking decision-making capacity—indeed, to say that judges have this authority—fails to address the question of what standard is to be used in making the decision. This has been the core issue in end-of-life decision making for incompetent patients. Although a consensus has clearly been reached, there are reasons to believe that this consensus is somewhat fragile and still evolving. Further, almost half of the states still have not addressed and resolved this issue, and it is somewhat risky to predict what the courts in these states will do when a case arises posing it.

There are three generally accepted standards for making end-of-life decisions for incompetent patients. The consensus arranges these standards in a hierarchy reflecting the dominant value of patient self-determination. The preferred standard, based on the patient's *actual* wishes, is that which is most consistent with self-determination; the second standard, based on a patient's *probable* wishes, accords self-determination less value; and the lowest priority standard, the *best-interests* standard, is not based on self-determination at all.

Clear and Convincing Evidence—Actual Wishes

A few courts insist that to forgo life-sustaining treatment for a patient who lacks decision-making capacity there be clear and convincing evidence of the patient's "actual" wishes. This standard offers no compromise with the root premise of self-determination. Even those courts that accept the looser substituted judgment standard prefer to rely on the patient's actual wishes if they can be ascertained rather than the patient's probable wishes.

New York State has taken the lead in the rejection of the substituted judgment standard, entirely prohibiting its use. Michigan, Missouri, and Wisconsin reject it in some kinds of cases. (Maine rejects the *terminology* of the substituted judgment standard but seems to apply it in substance.) These courts reason that because decision making for competent patients rests on the moral principle of autonomy, decisions for incompetent patients must be similarly based. Thus, when decisions are being made for incompetent patients in these states, a standard variously referred to as a *clear and convincing evidence standard*, a *subjective standard*, or an *actual intent standard* is used.

What is the difference between the probable- and actual-wishes standards? The states that require the use of the actual-wishes standard limit the evidence to be considered to statements made by the patient. They prohibit the surrogate from inferring what the patient would have wanted from other, less direct evidence of the patient's wishes. Not all of the patient's written or oral statements may be taken into account. Only if they are "solemn pronouncements and not casual remarks" may they be considered (27). Thus, "reactions to the unsettling experience of seeing or hearing of another's unnecessarily prolonged death" is not the kind evidence that may be used under this standard. The reason for requiring this strict standard is that "[n]othing less than unequivocal proof will suffice when the decision to terminate life supports is at issue."

Of the three states applying this standard, only New York's adherence to it is absolute. Its application by the Missouri Supreme Court led to the first right-to-die case in the United States Supreme Court—the Cruzan case (28)—in 1990. The Missouri Supreme Court imposed an actual-wishes standard, holding that the parents of a woman who had been in a persistent vegetative state for 5 years did not have the legal right to authorize the termination of tube feeding and allow their daughter to die in the absence of clear and convincing evidence that the patient, herself, had made this decision prior to losing decision-making capacity. The parents claimed that such a requirement infringed their daughter's constitutional rights—specifically, the right not to be deprived of liberty without due process of law guaranteed by the Fourteenth Amendment to the constitution. In Cruzan the United States Supreme Court held that an actual-wishes requirement is constitutional. However, this decision does not require that all states use an absolute wishes standard; it merely permits them to do so if they choose.

In a later case, the Missouri courts backtracked some on Cruzan. In Warren (29) the Missouri Court of Appeals allowed life-sustaining medical treatment to be withheld on the basis of a much less stringent standard: the best-interests standard (see discussion later in this chapter). Although the Missouri Supreme Court had held in Cruzan that an actual-wishes standard must be applied, the Court of Appeals interpreted this requirement as applying only if the treatment to be forgone was artificial nutrition and hydration, and the Warren case involved the withholding of cardiopulmonary resuscitation (CPR). Warren was not appealed to the Missouri Supreme Court, and thus there is no final word as to whether the Cruzan holding should be limited in this fashion.

Finally, in 1996, the Michigan Supreme Court required the application of the actual-wishes standard in a case—Martin v. Martin—involving an incompetent patient who was severely brain damaged but conscious (30). A prior decision of the Michigan Court of Appeals, a lower appellate court in Michigan, had approved the use of the substituted judgment standard in the case of a permanently unconscious patient. The Michigan Supreme Court approved this decision in the Martin case, but distinguished it from the Martin case itself because of the fact that Mr. Martin was neither permanently unconscious nor terminally ill. Consequently, although the appropriate decision-making standard in Michigan is not free from doubt, it appears as if the substituted judgment (or probable-wishes) standard may be used if a patient is terminally ill or permanently unconscious, but the actual-wishes standard must be used otherwise.

Substituted Judgment—Probable Wishes

Most states employ a standard for decision making for incompetent patients known as *substituted judgment,* a term with potentially seriously misleading connotations. The phrase might be thought to suggest that the surrogate is to substitute his or her judgment for that of the patient, who because incompetent—indeed, in many cases unconscious—has no judgment at all. This is not, however, what the term is intended to mean. Rather, under the substituted judgment standard, the surrogate is charged with attempting to determine what decision the now-incompetent patient would make if he or she were not incompetent. In effect, the surrogate's responsibility is to arrive at a determination of the patient's probable wishes, and thus a better, less misleading—though also less frequently used—term for this standard is the *probable-wishes* standard (31).

In determining what the patient's probable wishes would be, courts have mentioned a host of factors for the surrogate to consider, some of them conflicting with each other, and some not entirely consistent with the core notion of attempting to ascertain what the *patient's* wishes would be. Nonetheless, with little doubt we can say that the surrogate's task is to provide evidence, preferably in the form of statements made by the patient, before losing decision-making capacity, that would shed light on what he or she would now decide if capable of doing so.

The primary consideration is any statement(s), written or oral, that the patient made about forgoing life-sustaining treatment. These statements might include formal documents such as living wills, serious oral statements about the same subject, and reactions to the treatment of others. Other factors that courts have cited include the following (32):

- Patient's age
- Probable side effects of treatment
- Chance of producing a temporary or permanent cure
- Likelihood that treatment will cause suffering, such as a continuing state of pain and disorientation
- Patient's ability to cooperate with the treatment (because an uncooperative patient would have to be physically restrained to administer treatment, which would compound pain and fear)
- Patient's religious beliefs
- Consistent pattern of conduct by the patient with respect to prior decisions about his or her own medical care
- When there is a "close-knit" family, the decision of the family, particularly when in accord with the recommendation of the attending physician
- Life expectancy with or without the contemplated procedure
- Extent of the patient's physical and mental disability and degree of helplessness
- Patient's statements, if any, that directly or impliedly manifest his or her views on life-prolonging measures
- Quality of the patient's life with or without the procedure (i.e., the extent, if any, of pleasure, emotional enjoyment, or intellectual satisfaction that the patient will obtain from prolonged life)
- Type of care that will be required if life is prolonged as contrasted with what will be actually available
- Patient's prognosis, both with and without treatment
- Impact on the patient's family
- Nature of the prescribed medical assistance, including its benefits, risks, invasiveness, painfulness, and side effects
- Sentiments of the family or intimate friends
- Patient's "value system"

Best Interests

Although some courts have insisted on a more stringent standard for forgoing life-sustaining treatment than the substituted judgment standard, others have permitted the use of a *less* stringent standard when the substituted judgment standard cannot be met. In many cases, there is no evidence of a patient's actual or probable wishes. Many of these cases have involved children and mentally retarded individuals, but others have involved formerly competent adults about whom not enough was known to infer their wishes. In some of these cases, the courts have applied the substituted judgment standard, but doing so has stretched that standard to its breaking point. Other courts, in a more intellectually honest fashion, have simply acknowledged that the only options were either to maintain treatment or to employ another standard, and at least a handful, but not all, have chosen the latter course.

The standard that they use is referred to as the *best-interests* standard. Its basis is not patient autonomy, because the patient's wishes are unknown and unknowable, and there is not even any evidence from which the patient's wishes could be inferred with any reasonable possibility of being accurate. Rather, it is based on the *parens patriae* power of the state: the power, and indeed the obligation, to do what is best for individuals who lack the capacity to look out for their own welfare. The best-interests standard is disfavored by courts in end-of-life decision making because it is not based on the patient's wishes and because in practice it can afford the surrogate a tremendous latitude.

When applying the best-interests standard, surrogates must weigh the burdens and benefits of various courses of action. In general, a treatment may be forgone if it is more burdensome than beneficial to a patient (33), though some courts have insisted that the disparity between burdens and benefits be more substantial than a mere preponderance of the former over the latter (34).

Role of Advance Directives in Decision Making for Incompetent Patients

It is now well accepted in all states that written documents can play an important role in meeting the actual-wishes or probable-wishes standard.

The two generally accepted documents are commonly referred to as *living wills* and *healthcare powers of attorney,* and collectively as *advance directives.* Most states have enacted statutes recognizing the validity of advance directives; however, even in the very few states that have not done so—Massachusetts, Michigan, and New York lack living will statutes—there is little doubt that advance directives are legally valid documents, and the practice among healthcare professionals is to view them as such. Either kind of advance directive must be executed by an individual who is presently in possession of decision-making capacity with the intent that they become effective at some future time if the person loses decision-making capacity and an important medical decision (though not necessarily an end-of-life decision) then needs to be made.

Living Wills

In a living will, an individual gives instructions about the kind of treatment that he or she would wish to have withheld or withdrawn (although living wills may also be used to give instructions about kinds of treatment a patient would wish to have *administered*), and this is why living wills are sometimes referred to as "instruction directives" (35).

There are serious difficulties inherent in living wills. They require, especially in states using the *actual-wishes* standard, that people be able to predict the circumstances under which they will die and the kinds of treatments that might be administered in those circumstances. Thus, living wills are likely to be either underinclusive or overinclusive; that is, it would be very simple for an individual to fail to give instructions about some treatment he would not wish to have if he were able to make a contemporaneous decision about it, and it would be just as simple for someone to anticipatorily reject a treatment which she might well wish to have if she were able to decide about it at the time it was to be administered.

Healthcare Powers of Attorney

Because living wills cannot be adequately "fine tuned," healthcare powers of attorney have become increasingly popular. In a healthcare power of attorney, rather than giving instructions about future treatment, an individual appoints another person, referred to as a *proxy* (or *agent*), to make decisions for him in the event of future decision-making incapacity. Thus, healthcare powers of attorney are also sometimes referred to as *proxy directives* (36). A healthcare proxy is a type of surrogate, specifically one appointed by the patient himself or herself.

Combination Directives

The existence of a proxy permits the kind of fine-tuning absent from living wills but does not provide any serious assurance that the proxy will follow the patient's wishes or even have the slightest surmise about what those wishes might be. As a result, individuals can either use both documents or combine the two, appointing a proxy and giving him or her at least general instructions about what kind of medical treatment the patient might or might not want. For purposes of reducing potential conflict between the two types of advance directives, it is preferable for them to be coordinated in a single document, though this is not a legal requirement.

Advance directives have been touted as providing the best assurance to patients that their wishes will be honored in the future if they are in a situation in which they are unable to make decisions for themselves. Unfortunately, the legislation that has been adopted in most states places some serious limitations on advance directives, in addition to the previously mentioned practical ones. Almost all state legislation requires that a patient be either terminally ill or permanently unconscious before the advance directive may go into effect. In many instances, this requirement will not create a limitation. In the case of a slow-onset disease such as Alzheimer's, however, many patients may be neither terminally ill (at least not as defined in the advance directive statute) nor permanently unconscious. Had an individual specifically contemplated living in that condition, he or she might have issued specific instructions not to have his or her life prolonged through medical treatment such as CPR or feeding tubes. Most state statutes also prohibit the forgoing of life-sustaining treatment if the patient is pregnant, even if he or she is terminally ill or permanently unconscious, but as a practical matter, this provision has a far less wide-reaching impact.

Nonstatutory Advance Directives

It is important to emphasize that advance directives do not need to conform to statutory requirements.

Oral nonstatutory advance directives. The most important implication of the fact that advance directives do not need to conform to statutory requirements is that advance-directive statutes do not preclude the enforcement of orally expressed wishes or the oral designation of a proxy. Needless to say, there can be serious problems associated in determining what a patient's wishes are if they were orally expressed, and it can be difficult for courts, let alone healthcare professionals, to sort out conflicting claims by different people who profess to know what the patient wanted.

Written nonstatutory advance directives. Another important implication of the fact that advance directives need not conform to statutory requirements is that individuals are free to write advance directives specifically requesting treatment to be forgone even if the patient is not permanently unconscious or terminally ill, or to give a proxy authority to make medical decisions if the patient is not permanently unconscious or terminally ill. Advance-directive statutes state that they are intended to preserve and supplement existing common-law and constitutional rights and not to supersede or limit them. Advance-directive statutes were enacted not to create legal rights, but merely to provide a mechanism for implementing rights that already exist—namely, the right of individuals to implement their wishes about life-sustaining medical treatment once they lacked the capacity to do so contemporaneously (37). About the only possible disadvantage of using a nonstatutory advance directive is that it might not be as recognizable to many healthcare professionals, and thus they might be more reluctant to honor it.

Patient Self-Determination Act. The difficulties inherent in advance directives are only one of the reasons that a relatively small fraction of the adult population is estimated to have one. Another important barrier to the creation of advance directives is the lack of awareness of what they are. To address this problem, Congress enacted legislation in 1990 popularly known as the Patient Self-Determination Act. This legislation requires that institutional healthcare providers—hospitals, nursing homes, hospices, HMOs, and home health agencies—provide patients with information about their rights under state law to create an advance directive.

Actively Hastening Death

A bedrock assumption on which the consensus about forgoing life-sustaining treatment is grounded is that there is a fundamental distinction between a patient's death resulting from, on the one hand, forgoing treatment and, on the other, actively hastening death. The courts have demonstrated an unflagging insistence on establishing and maintaining a bright line between active euthanasia and passive euthanasia, even when it seriously strains reasoning to do so (38). So intent have courts been on maintaining this distinction that they have avoided using the term "euthanasia" except when condemning it. Out of fear of confusing the two, or because the unmodified term "euthanasia" for some people has acquired connotations of active euthanasia, involuntary euthanasia, or both, courts refer to passive euthanasia as *forgoing life-sustaining treatment* or *terminating life support* or *refusing treatment,* and to active euthanasia as *killing* or *mercy killing,* or *suicide* or *assisted suicide.*

In the mid-1980s, and certainly since 1990, the bright-line distinction between actively and passively hastening death has begun to fade. Dr. Kevorkian, Dr. Quill, and the unsuccessful voter initiatives in California and Washington followed by the successful referendum in Oregon to legalize physician-assisted suicide have all been integral to this process. Ironically, Justice Scalia of the United States Supreme Court—who is on record as being a strong opponent of a federal constitutional right to die—pointed out in the Court's first foray into end-of-life decision making in the Cruzan case in 1990 that this line has never really been very bright. Whether a patient's death is hastened by self-administered means or by a lethal injection by a physician on the one hand, or by withholding or withdrawing life-sustaining medical treatment on the other, "the cause of death in both cases," Justice Scalia remarked, "is the suicide's conscious decision to 'pu[t] an end to his own existence'" (39).

Because of the great perceived difference between actively and passively hastening death, it was widely thought that little would come of the efforts to bridge the chasm. Thus, it was a tremendous surprise in 1996 when two federal courts of appeals ruled that first the Washington and then the New York statutes making assisted suicide a crime violated the United States Constitution. In the first case, *Compassion in Dying v. Washington* (40), the United States Court of Appeals for the Ninth Circuit ruled that competent, terminally ill patients have a fundamental right, based on the due process clause of the Fourteenth Amendment to the Constitution, to determine the "time and manner" of their death, and that the Washington statute violated this right by imposing criminal penalties on individuals who assist others in committing suicide. The holding in the other case, *Quill v. Vacco* (41), was narrower. The Court of Appeals for the Second Circuit declined to find that there was a fundamental right to assistance in actively hastening death. Rather, the court held that because New York permits competent, terminally ill adults to end their lives passively by forgoing treatment, they are denied equal protection of the laws, also guaranteed by the Fourteenth Amendment, by the New York statute that penalizes the active hastening of death involved in physician-assisted suicide.

The United States Supreme Court agreed to review both of these cases and issued its opinions a little more than a year after the rulings by the Courts of Appeals. In decisions that were widely expected, the Supreme Court reversed both of these rulings. It held that there is no fundamental right to physician-assisted suicide, so that the due-process clause is not violated by state statutes that criminalize assisted suicide (42), and that there is a rational difference between actively and passively hastening death, so that neither do these statutes violate the equal protection guarantee (43). The Court did, however, leave the door open for each state, by legislation or state court ruling, to legalize physician-assisted suicide. Thus, the Supreme Court's decisions do not invalidate the Oregon referendum legalizing physician-assisted suicide, nor would they prohibit a state court from ruling that laws penalizing assisted suicide violate the state's constitution (44).

Moreover, the Supreme Court's decision approved of two related practices in the care of dying patients that come precariously close to—indeed, they may even exceed—physician-assisted suicide: terminal sedation and the use of adequate pain medication even if the unintended effect of that medication is to hasten the patient's death (the so-called principle of double effect). In approving these practices, the Court approved of doctors' hastening death through their own ministrations rather than by providing the patient with a lethal substance—that is, the Court approved of active euthanasia. The Court went beyond the approval of physician-assisted suicide in yet another way. Physician-assisted suicide is limited to competent patients; terminal sedation and double effect can be, and are, used with patients who no longer possess decision-making capacity and whose surrogates make decisions for them to hasten death.

Indeed, as the Supreme Court was deliberating about these cases, a trial court in Florida ruled that that state's law against assisted suicide violated the Florida constitutional right of privacy. However, within a month of the United States Supreme Court's rulings, the Florida Supreme Court reversed this trial court's ruling and held that the Florida constitutional right of privacy did not guarantee the right to physician-assisted suicide (45).

This decision was less widely expected than those of the United States Supreme Court and in some respects constitutes even more of a setback to proponents of physician-assisted suicide. Although it does not prohibit courts in other states from finding that laws against physician-assisted suicide violate their state constitutions, because the Florida constitutional right of privacy has traditionally been given broad sway in end-of-life decision-making cases, it seems unlikely, at least in the foreseeable future, that courts in other states will be inclined to strike out where the Florida Supreme Court refused to tread.

Conclusion

The New Jersey Supreme Court legalized the passive hastening of death in the Karen Ann Quinlan case on March 31, 1976. Nearly two decades later, on March 6, 1996, the United States Court of Appeals for the

Ninth Circuit legalized the active hastening of death through physician-assisted suicide, a decision that was followed a month later by a similar decision in federal court in New York. Although the United States Supreme Court formally reversed these two decisions in 1997, the Court's decisions approved of terminal sedation and double effect, two practices that come preciously close to actively hastening death.

The path to the legalization of actively hastening death will likely be long and circuitous, as has been the path to legalizing passively hastening death. But its legalization is virtually a certainty. People do not want the government dictating how they will die, and they do not want doctors doing so either. As more and more people experience the protracted, painful, and undignified death of a loved one, they are likely to become more supportive of means of avoiding such deaths. Improved palliative care will provide such a means for many people, but not for all. For the latter, the only way to avoid an undignified death will be through self-administration, or administration by a doctor, of a lethal substance.

References

1. Quoted in Katz J: Experimentation With Human Beings. New York, Russell Sage Foundation, 1972, p 311
2. In re Quinlan, 355 A2d 647 (NJ 1976)
3. State v Housekeeper, 16 A 382 (Md 1889)
4. Pratt v Davis, 79 NE 562 (Ill 1906)
5. Canterbury v Spence, 464 F2d 772 (DC Cir), cert denied, 409 U.S. 1064 (1972)
6. Cobbs v Grant, 502 P2d 1 (Cal 1972)
7. In re Conroy, 486 A2d 1209 (NJ 1985)
8. Satz v Perlmutter, 362 So2d 160, 161 (Fla Dist Ct App 1978)
9. In re President & Directors of Georgetown College, 331 F2d 1000 (DC Cir 1964)
10. United States v. George, 239 F Supp 752 (D Conn 1965)
11. John F Kennedy Memorial Hospital v Heston, 279 A2d 670 (NJ 1971)
12. Superintendent of Belchertown State School v Saikewicz, 370 NE2d 417 (Mass 1977)
13. Satz v Perlmutter, 362 So2d 160, 163 (Fla Dist Ct App 1978)
14. Bouvia v Superior Court, 225 Cal Rptr 297 (Ct App 1986)

15. State v McAfee, 385 SE2d 651 (Ga 1989)
16. McKay v Bergstedt, 801 P2d 617 (Nev 1990)
17. Thor v Superior Court, 855 P2d 375 (Cal 1993)
18. Norwood Hospital v Munoz, 564 NE2d 1017, 1022 (Mass 1991)
19. Meisel A: The Right to Die, 2nd Edition. New York, Wiley, 1995, §8.14
20. In re Quinlan, 355 A2d 647, 669 (NJ 1976)
21. Superintendent of Belchertown State School v Saikewicz, 370 NE2d 417, 435 (Mass 1977)
22. In re Spring, 405 NE2nd 115 (Mass 1980)
23. In re Colyer, 660 P2d 738 (Wash 1983)
24. In re Hamlin, 689 P2d 1372 (Wash 1984)
25. John F Kennedy Memorial Hospital v Bludworth, 452 So 2d 921, 926 (Fla 1984)
26. Orentlicher D: The limits of legislation. Maryland Law Review 53:1255-1305, 1994
27. In re Westchester County Medical Center (O'Connor), 531 NE2d 607, 612, 614 (NY 1988)
28. Cruzan v Director, 497 U.S. 261 (1990)
29. In re Warren, 858 SW2d 263 (Mo Ct App 1993)
30. Martin v Martin, 538 NW2d 399 (Mich 1995)
31. National Center for State Courts: Guidelines for State Court Decision Making in Life-Sustaining Medical Treatment Cases, 2nd Edition. National Center for State Courts, 1992, pp 36–37
32. Meisel, The Right to Die, 2nd Edition, §7.9
33. Barber v Superior Court, 195 Cal Rptr 484 (Ct App 1983)
34. In re Conroy, 486 A2d 1209 (NJ 1985)
35. President's Commission for the Study of Ethical Problems in Medicine and Biomedical and Behavioral Research: Deciding to Forgo Life-Sustaining Treatment. Washington, DC, U.S. Government Printing Office, 1983
36. President's Commission, Deciding to Forgo Life-Sustaining Treatment
37. Meisel, The Right to Die, 2nd Edition, §10.10
38. Rachels 1975
39. Cruzan v Director, 497 U.S. 294 (1990)
40. 79 F3d 790 (9th Cir 1996)
41. 80 F3d 716 (2d Cir 1996)
42. Washington v Glucksberg, 117 S Ct 2258 (1997)
43. Vacco v Quill, 117 S Ct 2293 (1997)
44. Lee v Harcle Road, 118 S Ct 328 (1997)
45. McIver v Krischer, 697 So2d 97 (Fla 1997)

10

Termination-of-Treatment Decisions: Ethical Underpinnings

David Mayo, Ph.D.

The ethics of dying is more complex than it was a half-century ago. Two developments responsible for this are the availability of new treatment options and the abandonment of medical paternalism. Before, most people died only after all available treatment options had been exhausted, but today most Americans die in intensive care unit (ICU)–equipped hospitals where high-tech life-prolonging therapies are readily available. Often these treatments may be so burdensome as to outweigh their marginal benefits to patients near the end of life. Increasingly, people die following decisions to forgo some treatment that could probably delay the moment of death, at least briefly. Moreover, medical paternalism has given way to the doctrine of informed consent. Thus, termination-of-treatment decisions are no longer made by physicians alone but also by patients and their families.

In what follows I first explore the history and the ethical underpinnings of the right to informed consent. I then turn attention to the application of this principle to end-of-life decisions, chronicling the evolution of the "right to die" from cases in which patients refuse life-sustaining therapy in order to avoid treatments that promise more burden than benefit, through a progression of cases that begin to resemble suicide. Finally, I examine the ethical issues surrounding physician-assisted suicide, the legalization of which strikes many observers as imminent. I suggest that physician-assisted suicide will pose a special challenge to psychiatry, since, by all accounts, optimal implementation of any policy permitting physician-assisted suicide will often require the involvement of psychiatrists in competence assessments of patients who wish to end their lives. Such involvement, in turn, will require a major change in attitude toward suicide on the part of a profession that has traditionally been inclined to hold that only a troubled mind would opt for suicide.

The Right to Informed Consent

The most dramatic change in medical ethics in the last 40 years has been the repudiation of medical paternalism in favor of the patient's right to informed consent. Today, it is understood that competent patients have both the moral and the legal right to be informed and to decide for themselves whether to undergo or refuse recommended medical treatments.

It was not always so. Katz (1) has effectively documented that throughout most of the history of Western medicine, treatment decisions were made by physicians who regarded their sick patients as incapable of understanding or deciding on their own behalf. Thus, the Hippocratic oath held it was the physician's duty "to follow that regimen which, *according to my ability and judgement, I consider* for the benefit of my patient" (2). Katz points out that Hippocrates's only explicit reference to informing patients occurs in *Decorum*, where he indicates physicians should be cheerful, solicitous, and comforting, while all the while "concealing most things from the patient . . . revealing nothing of the patient's future or present condition" (3). Katz documents that as late as 1961 a dentist who had extracted all the teeth of an aesthetized patient who had insisted extractions be only partial could testify as follows in his own defense:

A: . . . I think you should strive to do for the patient what is the best thing over a long period of time for the patient. We tried to abide by that.

Q: Isn't that up to the patient?

A: No, I don't think it should be. If they go to a doctor they should discuss it. He should decide.

Q: Isn't this up to the patient? . . . If I want to keep these teeth can't I do it?

A: You don't know whether they are causing you trouble.

Q. That is up to me, isn't it?

A: Not if you came to see me, it wouldn't be . . . (4)

The doctrine of medical paternalism has its appeal. Optimal decision making requires both a full understanding of the situation and the options at hand, and clearheadedness about one's authentic values. Neither of these may be attainable by a patient suffering pain, panic, despair, hopelessness, and/or dependency. Even as Anna Freud advised aspiring physicians against treating patients paternalistically, she also warned them that "every adult who is ill, who has fever, who is in pain, or who expects an operation, returns to childhood in some way. He feels small and helpless" (5).

Nevertheless, the legal right of the competent patient (or, in the case of an incompetent patient, a suitable proxy) to be informed and then to give or withhold consent, even to treatment necessary to prolong life, has been firmly established in the courts in this country during the last 40 years, and the doctrine of medical paternalism has been unequivocally repudiated. Today, the American physician who withholds important information from patients, or makes important medical decisions on their behalf without their consent, does so at his or her legal peril (6).

Both medical paternalism and the doctrine of informed consent that has supplanted it are deeply rooted in Western political and ethical traditions. At its core, medicine is driven by moral imperatives that are basic to any credible vision of how we should live: the promotion of life, health, and human flourishing, and the minimizing of illness and pointless suffering. For Aristotle human flourishing (*eudaimonia*) was the ultimate good; for the Utilitarians, from Epicurus to Mill, it was happiness, understood as a preponderance of pleasure over pain. (John Stuart Mill was at pains to stress the "higher pleasures" of the sentiments and intellect [7].) In earlier times, when respect for authority was greater than it is today, and medicine had little more than comfort and placebo reassurances to offer most critically ill patients, the Hippocratic oath quite plausibly urged physicians to use their own judgment to promote the welfare of their patients as they saw fit.

The historical, political, and philosophical roots of the doctrine of informed consent trace back as far as the Renaissance and the first sparks of skepticism regarding religious authority. In science, appeal to authority began to yield during that period to reason and empirical enquiry. Nature, like man, began to be seen as intelligible apart from its teleological role in the Divine Plan (8). Beginning in the seventeenth century, England, America, and France all saw political upheavals in which governments claiming to speak with divine authority gave way to representative forms of government. Jefferson echoed the political theories of Hobbes, Rousseau, Montesquieu, and Locke when he wrote in the Declaration of Independence, "Governments are instituted among men, and derive their just powers from the consent of the governed." Moreover, the political theories played out in the American and French revolutions postulated a fundamental moral equality among persons. The notion of rights, and analysis of the nature of such rights, emerged for the first time as prominent features of political and ethical theories. Rights came to be seen, by Mill and other rights theorists (9), as legal or moral claims of individuals, with respect to which the individual was entitled to protection by society. (As we will see, this is precisely what has happened with the right to informed consent in the courts during the last 40 years.) High on the list of human rights described as "fundamental" or "natural" was the right to self-determination. Jefferson's phrase "life, liberty and the pursuit of happiness" was borrowed from John Locke's reference to a person's God-given natural right to "preserve his property, that is, his life, liberty and estate" (10).

This emphasis on self-determination was seconded in the less political writings of other eighteenth- and nineteenth-century ethical theorists. Although he did not speak in terms of rights, Immanuel Kant, one of the giants of Western philosophical thought, argued for a vision of morality that has at its core the notion of respect for autonomy (11). According to Kant, all rational beings owe each other mutual respect by virtue of the capacity each bears for autonomous choice—that is, for governing his or her own life by rules, principles, or values that are genuinely one's own ("self-authored" and not imposed by others). Thus, in Kant's view, we each manifest our personhood precisely when we govern our own lives and each allow others to govern theirs. Mill, who differed with Kant on many other points, agreed on the need for each person to respect others' capacities to decide personal matters for themselves. In *On Liberty*, a brilliant defense of classic liberalism, Mill argues that paternalistic policies will be counterproductive of happiness in the long run because they must proceed by general principles that will inevitably be insensitive to what each person knows better than anyone else about his or her own idiosyncratic preferences and life plans.

One hundred thirty years later this same argument is advanced by Katz in connection with medical decision making (12). Katz argues that optimal medical decision making must be based on the values of the patient, who after all is the one who must live with the consequences of the decision and whose values may well differ from those of the physician. Thus, the emergence of the doctrine of informed consent over medical paternalism parallels the earlier emergence of constitutional democracies and respect for self-determination over the notion that people owe unquestioning allegiance to higher and wiser authorities.

Katz has chronicled the emergence of the legal doctrine of informed consent in this century. Traditionally, the law protected patients against unwanted surgeries, which amounted to "unwanted touching" or battery. In 1914 Justice Benjamin Cardozo rendered his famous pronouncement in such a case: "Every human being of adult years and sound mind has a right to determine what shall be done with his own body; and a surgeon who performs an operation without his patient's consent, commits an assault, for which he is liable in damages" (13). This sweeping statement notwithstanding, legal recognition of a patient's right to the information necessary for a rational decision about whether to permit a surgical procedure—that is, information about risks, benefits, and possible alternatives—had to wait until a series of cases in the 1950s. And even then, Katz argues, "Judges were hesitant to intrude on [paternalistic medical] practices. . . . Their impulse to foster individual self-determination collided with an equally strong desire to maintain the authority of the profession . . ." (14).

The case for the right to informed consent to medical treatment gained ground as philosophers and other ethicists began to turn their attention to healthcare decision making in the 1960s and 1970s. Formal recognition of the right to informed consent began to appear in the 1970s in the form of policies and even legislation promoting "patient's bills of rights."

In 1982 the President's Commission for the Study of Ethical Problems in Medicine and Biomedical and Behavioral Research issued its first report, *Making Health Care Decisions: The Ethical and Legal Implications of Informed Consent in the Patient-Practitioner Relationship* (15). In the spirit of both Kant and Mill, the Commission held that the right to informed consent was grounded in the promotion of two values: personal well-being and self-determination. Moreover,

> to ensure these values are respected and enhanced, the Commission finds that patients who have the capacity to make decisons about their care must be permitted to do so voluntarily and must have all relevant information regarding their condition and alternative treatments, including possible benefits, risks, costs, other consequences, and significant uncertainties surrounding any of this information. (16)

Only a short chapter of the report was devoted to arguments in defense of the values underlying this doctrine. These were now taken as a given. As its title implies, the bulk of the report was concerned with its ethical and legal implications, including the central role of patients' values (rather than physicians' values) in shaping individual healthcare decisions, the danger of trying to restrict the right to "well-educated, articulate, self-aware individuals," and the special problems that arise when proxies must decide for patients who are clearly incompetent to make decisions on their own behalf.

Termination-of-Treatment Decisions

All of these considerations apply to end-of-life termination-of-treatment decisions. These decisions, and their implications for conflicts that may occur between physicians' and patients' treatment preferences, were the focus of a subsequent Presidential Commission report, *Deciding to Forgo Life-Sustaining Treatment: Ethical, Medical, and Legal Issues in Treatment Decisions,* issued in 1983 (17). This report began with the recognition that "death is less of a private matter than it once was. . . . Death [is now] more a matter of deliberate decision. For almost any life-threatening condition, some intervention can now delay the moment of death" and hence that "matters once the province of fate have now become a matter of human choice" (18). The first recommendation of this report was a direct application of the key recommendation of the first report:

> The voluntary choice of a competent and informed patient should determine whether or not life-sustaining therapy will be undertaken, just as such choices provide the basis for other decisions about medical treatment. Health care institutions and professionals should try to enhance patients' abilities to make decisions on their own behalf and to promote understanding of the available treatment options. (19)

Nevertheless, the potential for conflict was recognized in the second recommendation, that "health care professionals serve patients best by maintaining a presumption in favor of sustaining life." This, however, was to remain a *presumption* and not an *overriding principle,* to be made "while recognizing that competent patients are entitled to choose to forgo any treatments, including those that sustain life" (20).

By the time of these reports it was clear that the preservation of life was an important goal of medicine but that it was by no means an absolute goal that invariably trumped other considerations. Moreover, it was also clear that critically ill patients (or their proxies) were morally and legally entitled to refuse life-prolonging therapies, even when that meant death. Interest in advanced directives of one sort or another surged following this report: living-will legislation was passed in most states, followed in many states by legislation that recognized durable powers of attorney for healthcare decisions. This culminated in 1990 in the federal Patient Self-Determination Act, the aim of which is to enhance patient self-determination by requiring that all patients entering healthcare institutions receiving Medicare and Medicaid funding be asked whether they have advance directives.

Granting patients the right to refuse any recommended treatment had implications for end-of-life decisions beyond what many had initially recognized. Subsequent developments have begun to reveal how far this right may go in the direction of empowering patients who wish to end their own lives. In 1996 both the Ninth and the Second Circuit Federal Courts of Appeals went so far as to find Constitutional grounds for a right to physician assistance in suicide for competent, terminally ill patients. Both of these court decisions grounded their arguments not only in the right to self-determination as embodied in the doctrine of informed consent, but also in subsequent developments in accepted medical practice. These rulings were both appealed to the U.S. Supreme Court. Although the Supreme Court overturned both of these rulings in June 1997, they were careful to indicate that part of their reason for doing so was to encourage the ongoing national debate and to allow citizens to decide the issue on a state-by-state basis.

My concern in the remainder of this chapter is to illuminate the far-reaching implications of the right to refuse treatment, by exploring the moral significance of two distinctions. The first is the distinction between a death that is merely foreseen and a death that is intended. The second is the distinction between "passively" allowing a patient to die and "actively" killing. Both of these distinctions have been invoked in attempts to draw a sharp moral line delineating what physicians may and may not do in helping patients who decide they have suffered enough. In what follows, I argue that neither distinction can bear the moral weight put on it by those who would use it to draw such a line. I then amplify this point in connection with "double-effect deaths." There I argue that these distinctions are sometimes finessed to justify what is indistinguishable in practice from intentionally killing patients whose suffering is judged to be so great that an earlier death is viewed as a net benefit. I conclude by considering briefly one implication the legalization of physician-assisted suicide would have for psychiatry.

Merely Foreseen Versus
Intended Consequences

The morality of an action can depend on not only what an agent accomplishes but also what the agent aims or intends to accomplish. We are inclined to view helpful actions admiringly, but this would change if we were to learn a helpful agent's intention was to ingratiate himself or herself for some personal gain. A person who unintentionally offends someone with a crude joke is less blameworthy than someone who would tell the same joke with the intention of giving offense. Likewise, patients (and physicians) may act with a variety of intentions when they are making end-of-life decisions, and these may influence moral assessment of their actions. Patients may refuse therapies that could offer some benefit in order to avoid burdens associated with the treatment. Alternatively, a terminally ill patient wanting to die as quickly as possible may refuse even a minimally burdensome life-prolonging therapy with the intention of hastening his or her own death.

The most uncontroversial reason a terminal patient might have for refusing life-prolonging therapy would be to avoid the burdens of a treatment that outweigh any expected benefits. High-tech interventions that have at least some potential to prolong life can impose various sorts of burdens: they can be invasive, painful, and expensive, and near the end of life they may promise only marginal benefits. Consequently, as the President's Commission pointed out, most Americans now die following a decision to forgo some possible life-prolonging treatment that is deemed to offer only marginal benefits that are outweighed by associated burdens.

The notion of withholding life-prolonging treatments with associated burdens that outweigh their anticipated benefits can be traced back to at least the sixteenth century, when Catholic theologians designated such treatments "extraordinary"—that is, extraordinarily burdensome—and argued that the duty each person had to preserve his or her life did not extend so far as to require subjecting himself or herself to undertakings involving pain or anguish "extraordinarily disproportionate to one's state in life" (21). (At that time major surgeries were horribly painful and rarely successful, and surgical chambers were commonly thought of as torture chambers. A typical case might have involved someone accepting certain death from gangrene rather than undergoing amputation of an infected limb without benefit of anaesthesia or antiseptic, and with only a very slim hope of survival.)

When patients exercise their right to forgo treatments without which they will die, they usually do so with the intention of avoiding extraordinary burdens associated with those treatments. Sometimes, however, patients exercise the right to forgo life-prolonging treatment with quite different intentions. One might intend to honor religious proscriptions on certain treatments, for instance, or to spare themselves or loved ones the suffering, or the expense, associated with a protracted terminal illness. A Jehovah's Witness may forgo a needed blood transfusion even though she would like to survive. A frail elderly person with an easily treatable pneumonia may refuse an antibiotic so that the pneumonia will end his suffering. Some patients with acquired immunodeficiency syndrome (AIDS) eventually decide to forgo the pentamidine mist treatments that have kept pneumocystis pneumonia at bay so that they will die of pneumonia before any further deterioration of their general quality of life results from the ravages of other opportunistic infections.

The underlying distinction at issue here is between a death that is merely foreseen but unintended and a death that is intended. Some patients would prefer to live, but refuse life-prolonging therapies in order to avoid the extraordinary burden associated with them, even though death is foreseen as the outcome. Other patients do not merely foresee death as the consequence of refusing treatment, but refuse treatment precisely because they intend to precipitate their death.

Both of these reasons for patient refusal of life-sustaining treatment can sometimes be troubling for their healthcare providers. Patients facing invasive procedures that might restore them to health may be terrified of such procedures out of all proportion to the pain or risk their physicians realize the procedures actually involve. (The converse may also be true: patients who have actually experienced chemotherapy, for instance, may understand better than their physicians the burdens involved.) Sometimes healthcare workers strongly committed to the preservation of life are even more troubled by patients who reject nonburdensome treatments with the intention of ending their lives. This was highlighted in the 1983 case of Elizabeth Bouvia. Bouvia, an institutionalized 26-year-old woman so disabled with cerebral palsy she had to be spoon-fed, decided to end her life by starving herself to death. Bouvia's decision to refuse spoon-feeding was controversial precisely because her avowed intention seemed to be to commit suicide—that is, to end her life. When her healthcare providers told her that unless she consented they would have her declared incompetent and a danger to herself, she sought a court order to prevent this from happening. The court ruled first that her right to refuse treatment did imply a right to refuse artificial nutrition. However, it also ruled that she had no right to dictate the terms of her other treatment and to demand that others care for her while she starved to death. Thus, it denied her request. (Subsequently, in 1986, after she had been moved to another institution, she was back in court and obtained a favorable ruling for the removal of a nasogastric tube that had been inserted against her will.) (22)

Some people hold a deep conviction that although healthcare workers must acquiesce to a patient's refusal of treatment, they must never intentionally hasten patients' deaths. Bonnie Steinbock, for instance, has argued that although physicians may sometimes withhold a life-prolonging therapy, either because the patient has refused the treatment or because they themselves consider it to be extraordinarily burdensome, they must never do so with the intention of hastening death (23). Steinbock holds that withholding treatment in order to hasten the death of a patient would amount to passive euthanasia, which would be in violation of American Medical Association (AMA) policy forbidding "the intentional termination of the life of one human being by another" (24). In the same spirit, recent policy statements by the AMA (25), American Nurses Association (26), American Geriatrics Society (27), and National Hospice Organization (28) all denounce the intentional hastening of a patient's death by a healthcare worker.

Notwithstanding the depth of the conviction some people have that a sharp moral line is to be drawn at the intentional hastening of death of a terminal patient that they never overstep, there are reasons to doubt that such a line is always respected in practice, or even that it can be drawn sharply. The difference between a death that is intended and one that is not intended but merely foreseen is often not a black-and-white distinction. This is true whether the intentions at issue are those of the patients or those of others such as family, physicians, or other healthcare providers. A suffering, terminally ill patient may weary of both treatment and life at the same time. Choices, after all, must be made from among available alternatives, and a patient who understands that some ongoing treatment (e.g., ventilation) is a precondition of remaining alive may well conceptualize the choice as one between death and life-on-these-terms. Having done so, the patient may decide the suffering is so great that death is the preferred option, without bothering to address the purely academic question of whether life *would* be worth it if the terms could be otherwise.

Moreover, compassionate second parties may empathize completely with such a patient and share the patient's analysis of the situation. If that second party is the attending physician, and the physician also happens to hold the view (as many do) that physician-assisted suicide (or even active euthanasia) would sometimes be morally justified in order to cut short pointless suffering, it seems disingenuous at best to suggest that in honoring the patient's refusal and withholding treatment, the physician does not *intend* the patient's death. Moreover, it seems absurd to insist, as current AMA policy does, that he or she *must* not.

Of course the situation is rarely quite that simple. As a critically ill patient's condition fails to improve or continues to deteriorate, everyone involved, including patient, family, and healthcare providers, typically feels ambivalence about the possibility of impending death, and hence about whether treatment should be discontinued. But if all these parties witness a patient's continuing deterioration, and come to know the patient's values, they all may come to share the patient's view that since further treatment can at best only prolong an unwanted, marginal existence, "it's no longer worth it." In such cases a physician may well understand and agree fully with a patient's decision to refuse some non-burdensome treatment with the intention of cutting short the burden of life. In practice, decisions to disconnect ventilators are often made in concert by patient, physician, and family, not because the ventilator is burdensome, but because the patient's quality of life is so low and unlikely to improve. (If such patients do not die promptly when ventilators are removed, the universal reaction is seldom jubilation. Often, as most clinicians attest, it is discomfort and even impatience.) In such cases, what is gained by a policy that insists that physicians must never intend a patient's death—that is, never share that part of their dying patient's thinking that actually hopes that death will come soon? Sometimes the only effect such a policy has in practice is to invite physicians to be disingenuous about their own reasons for acting as they do.

Killing Versus Letting Die

Intuitively, allowing a patient to die—in particular withholding life-prolonging treatment from a patient who has refused such treatment—is one thing, and actively killing is another. At first blush the former seems morally defensible in some contexts, but the other absolutely indefensible. Moreover, there are obvious arguments supporting this intuition. On the face of it, actively killing a patient is clearly in violation of both the law and the general moral imperative never to kill an innocent person. Withholding treatment, on the other hand, can be justified on various grounds, as noted above.

On closer examination, however, this moral distinction is also subject to challenge. First, as with the previous distinction between deaths that are intended and those that are merely foreseen, there are many cases in which it is unclear whether a particular course of action should be classified as a matter of killing or of letting die. Often, for instance, what is at issue is not the withholding of a treatment that has never been undertaken, but the withdrawing of a treatment already under way. Moreover, some "treatments" (e.g., ventilation) are continuous, and their withdrawal can precipitate death. If the *conceptual* distinction is not sharp, it cannot, of course, provide the basis for a sharp criterion for distinguising between what is morally permissible and what is not. At best, it can provide a criterion that is as vague as the conceptual distinction itself.

Howard Brody argues that what happens in practice is often not that the distinction between killing and letting die guides moral judgment, but rather the other way around; that is, an initial moral judgment of a course of action is made on other grounds, and then on that basis the action is construed as either a case of killing or a case of letting die (29). Brody invites us to consider a suffering, ventilator-dependent patient who asks his physician to disconnect his ventilator. If the physician does so, this will probably be regarded as morally acceptable and seen as a matter of "letting die." However, if moments before the physician does so a homicidal enemy of the patient slips into the patient's room and performs the same act, he is surely guilty of homicide, that is, of killing. Again, some patients' deaths are hastened by respiration-suppressing painkillers such as morphine. If a terminal patient were to beg his physician to put him out of his misery with a dose of morphine sufficient to end his life, the physician would certainly be ill-advised to document that request and his compliance in the patient's chart. If, however, the physician were to administer the same dose, but no mention has been made of mercy killing, and this time declared that his intention was only to kill the pain, the patient's death will almost certainly not be construed as a morally reprehensible killing, but simply as an attempt at pain management. Moreover, the law endorses this interpretation, both by accepting the underlying medical condition as the cause of death in such cases and, in some states, by stipulating that physicians whose intention is merely to kill the pain are not liable for homicide (30).

Even if it were possible to classify a particular death as an instance of killing or of letting die independent of any moral judgment, the moral relevance of this distinction has been challenged by a number of scholars (31, 32). James Rachels, for instance, has argued that although most actual killings are morally wrong and most cases of "letting die" morally acceptable, that is not because of any intrinsic difference between the two, but rather because of accidental features (33). Most actual killings are malevolently motivated and occur without the consent of their innocent victims, who do not wish to die. When physicians let patients die, on the other hand, we usually approve because the physicians' motives are usually benevolent, and we believe that those who die (or their proxies) have consented. Rachels invites us to strip away these incidental differences. On the one hand, he asks us to consider how we would view a malevolent person about to drown someone but suddenly realizes with delight that he does not have to: he comes upon his intended victim slipping in a bathtub and sliding underwater unconscious and watches in glee as his victim drowns. Rachels believes his behavior (nonintervention) is as reprehensible as it would have been had he actively killed the person. Conversely, Rachels asks us to consider a patient from whom treatment is withheld because the quality of life is so low that it has been determined death will be a net benefit. Rachels challenges us to to show why simply withholding treatment and waiting for the patient to die—often over some period of time and after considerable suffering—is better than bringing about death, which is the outcome desired by the suffering patient, as quickly as possible by actively killing.

Rachels' position has been criticized in several ways, most of which appeal in one way or another to the notion that medicine must maintain its presumption in favor of maintaining life and resist embracing the view that hastening the death of a patient is ever desirable. Yet, this criticism would apply to the withholding or withdrawing of life-prolonging treatment as certainly as it would to intentional killing. Again, Steinbock has argued that although physicians may sometimes have to accept the withholding of a treatment, even when this results in an earlier death, they must never do anything with the intention of hastening death (34). In the same spirit, others have argued that for physicians to embrace active killing would put our society on a dangerous slippery policy slope and that it would violate the essential mission of medicine. (See the articles by Brock [35] and Arras [36] for critical surveys of such arguments.) Willard Gaylin, Leon Kass, Edmund Pellegrino, and Mark Siegler combine these arguments and insist that physicians must never kill because of the effect it would have on the integrity of the profession and the public perception of it:

> One of the first and most hallowed canons of the medical ethic [is]: doctors must not kill. . . . Western medicine has regarded the killing of patients, even on request, as a profound violation of the deepest meaning of the medical vocation. The very soul of medicine is on trial. . . . This issue touches medicine at its moral center; if this moral center collapses, if physicians become killers or are even licensed to kill, the profession—and, therewith, each physician—will never again be worthy of trust and respect as healer and comforter and protector of life in all its frailty. (37)

Double-Effect Deaths: Administration of Death-Hastening Doses of Painkillers

Do Gaylin and coauthors mean to condemn any physician who administers palliative drugs knowing this will probably hasten death? That would certainly be a logical inference from the above passage, as well as from the title of their article. A more careful reading of their article, however, suggests otherwise. Their article is laced with references to *intentional* killing. Presumably this is because they do not wish to condemn the widespread practice, alluded to earlier, of so-called double-effect deaths.

As I suggested earlier in this chapter, the conventional wisdom, embodied in both the law and medical codes, holds that physicians must never kill intentionally. At the same time, both the law and various health professional codes are quick to distinguish intentional killing, which is condemned, from such aggressive use of palliation for terminal patients that the hastening death may be foreseen. Even the AMA and the codes of the American Nurses Association, American Geriatric Society, and National Hospice Organization, cited earlier for their unequivocal condemnation of the intentional hastening of a patient's death by a healthcare worker, all quickly clarify that they do not mean to condemn such aggressive palliative treatment. (Indeed, each does so within the same paragraph.) Again, the law bolsters the conventional wisdom by treating the underlying condition as the cause of death in such cases, even though death is precipitated by administration of drugs with the intention of palliation (38).

Such "foreseen but unintended deaths" from palliative drugs are sometimes referred to as *double-effect deaths,* because scholars who defend them but still condemn intentional killing often appeal to a principle of Roman Catholic moral reasoning, the "principle of double effect." This principle holds that doing evil intentionally is never justified, but that causing evil is sometimes permissible in the course of doing good if the good that one intends outweighs the bad effects of one's action, and if the bad effects are not a *means* to the good but merely a foreseeable but unintended "side effect" (39). The argument in the present context is that death is an evil that therefore must never be caused intentionally, but that causing death may be morally permissible if it is not intended, either as a means or an end, but merely foreseen as a side effect of achieving a greater good (palliation).

Because the conventional wisdom draws (and defends) the line between the permissible and the impermissible in a way that relies on both of the distinctions we have challenged above, I suggest it represents gravely flawed moral reasoning. I argue here that the reasons usually given for a moral distinction between many double-effect deaths and mercy killing are unpersuasive, and that the step from these practices to physician-assisted suicide is smaller than many people imagine. Let us examine a range of cases.

No doubt in some double-effect deaths the hastening of death is only foreseen as a possibility: it is not clear whether the palliative dose is large enough to hasten death. Moreover, doubtless, healthcare workers sometimes try to limit palliative medication to what is absolutely necessary for pain control, anxious to avoid any suppression of respiration that might hasten death but still foreseeing that as an unfortunate possibility. In other cases, the inexorability of the dying process may have been accepted by patient, family, and healthcare providers, and postponing it is consciously and easily subordinated to the goal of "keeping the patient comfortable." In still others, as I suggested earlier, the patient (and perhaps family) are genuinely "ready for the end," and empathetic healthcare workers may well share the patient's and family's view that the sooner the death occurs, the better for everyone. Consider, finally, a case identical to this last one, except that the physician is one of many who questions the moral legitimacy of the conventional wisdom, and favors the legalization of physician-assisted suicide. Can it plausibly be maintained that this physician, who shares the patient's feelings that the sooner death occurs the better, is guilty of murder if she intends the patient's death, but is behaving completely within the law if she merely foresees the outcome that she and everyone else desires, but does not intend it?

As we move through this series of cases, the distinction between a death that is intended and one that is merely foreseen becomes murky at best and invites rationalization and outright self-deception at worst. Again, choices must be made from available alternatives in all their complexity. In some of these situations the alternatives seem to come down to either the patient's life and suffering continuing longer or the patient's suffering and life ending sooner. If a treatment option is apt to hasten a patient's death, that is a terribly important moral feature of that option—one that should not be swept under the carpet as a mere "side effect." This reasoning holds true even if in the final analysis death is the least burdensome option. In these cases, the question that is absolutely central is whether the patient is better off alive but still suffering, or not suffering but dead. If the former, then hastening the death of the patient with a painkiller is morally indefensible because it yields a net harm to the patient. If the latter, then the death of the patient is no longer an evil, but a good—that is, the best among bad options—and hence involves no evil that requires the justification that the principle of double effect was invoked to provide.

As noted above, advocates of double effect usually claim that since the death is merely foreseen and not intended, the physician does not kill the patient. This view is supported by the law, but surely not by common sense. The assumption here seems to be that before one can be said to have done something, one must intend to do it. But that would be an extraordinary claim in any other context: someone can hardly deny he damaged another's car simply by noting he did not intend to. If the law chooses to deny there is an element of killing in these cases, so the criticism goes, so much the worse for the law. One advocate concedes this final criticism: after suggesting "good doctors and wise patients often agree and plan for such a moment beforehand," he grants that "technically speaking it may be a kind of homicide" (40).

Practical problems result from the way the principle of double effect is used to draw the line between the permissible and the impermissible in connection with palliative care near the end of life. Both the line itself and the reasons for it are so unclear that different physicians may interpret it quite differently. Some physicians believe that killing a patient is wrong even when it is unintended. Skeptical of both the moral significance of the distinction between forseen and intended consequences, and the principle of double effect, these physicians may be very conservative in connection with palliative care that poses any possibility of hastening the death of a patient. Patients who happen to fall under the care of these physicians may be in for painful and protracted deaths even after they have given up any hope for recovery and just long for the end. The recent SUPPORT study (41) is only one of many suggesting that American physicians routinely fail to provide adequate palliation to their patients. Other physicians, also acting in good faith, construe the principle of double effect as an invitation to downplay the moral significance of giving dying patients palliative care in doses that may hasten their deaths. This may play out both in their own thinking and in their consultations with patients and their families. Knowing that few suffering patients would take issue with "effective pain management," and minimizing the hastening of death as a mere side effect, physicians who are uncomfortable discussing death (or who believe the patient and family may be) may ignore the need for frank and open discussion with patients and/or families about the possibly lethal consequences of palliative measures they are proposing. Thus, patients who might strenuously object to palliation that might hasten death are given no chance to object. If the right to informed consent means anything, it surely means the right of competent patients to be informed clearly and unequivocally that the course of treatment the physician is proposing may hasten their death.

Physician-Assisted Suicide

The idea of physician-assisted suicide has made tremendous advances recently in the United States. What opponents see as a betrayal of the traditional mission of medicine, much of the public sees as a logical extension of compassionate care of the dying. The winds of legal change seem to be blowing as well: initiatives for legalization were narrowly defeated in California and Washington in 1992 and 1993, respectively, and a similar initiative finally passed, in Oregon, in 1994. The Oregon initiative was originally tied up in court challenges and then sent back to the voters in 1997 in the form of a call for repeal. Supporters and opponents alike were stunned when the call for repeal was rejected 60% to 40% by the voters, thereby finally legalizing physician-assisted suicide in Oregon.

Most of the chapters in this volume suggest that if and when physician-assisted suicide is legalized, there is a central role for psychiatry to play. The most obvious issue to which psychiatric expertise is relevant involves determinations of competence of persons requesting aid in dying. Even advocates of legalization are quick to acknowledge that most actual suicides are irrational (42). Thus, at the very least, legalization will require criteria and procedures for distinguishing those requests for physician assistance in suicide that should be accommodated from those that should not. Some proposed criteria, such as the presence of a terminal condition, imply no special role for mental health professionals. However, the central requirement—namely, that the patient requesting physician-assisted suicide must be competent—clearly implies such a role. Given the further assumptions that physicians frequently underestimate the quality of life of their sickest patients (43), often fail to provide adequate pain control (44), and often fail to detect depression in their terminally ill patients (see Block and Billings, Chapter 8, this volume), and, of course, that assessments of competence require expertise (see Youngner, Chapter 2; Block and Billings, Chapter 8, this volume), the conclusion seems inescapable that if physician-assisted suicide is to be practiced responsibly, psychiatrists should be involved in assessing the competence of patients requesting it. Some advocates have gone so far as to suggest that a psychiatric evaluation be standard for any patient requesting physician-assisted suicide (45; Block and Billings, Chapter 8, this volume).

However, psychiatrists have traditionally been quite unsympathetic to the notion of rational suicide. As Thomas Szasz (46) has documented, 25 years ago conventional psychiatric wisdom held that suicide was always irrational, that anyone who would attempt suicide was mentally troubled in some way and ipso facto incompetent, and that the proper response of mental health professionals to any suicidal client was to prevent the suicide, even if this required coercive measures. This view is still reflected in our civil commitment laws and practices, as well as in various health professional codes.

Thus, legalization of physician-assisted suicide, if such occurs, will represent a special challenge for psychiatry. Psychiatrists, many of whom have viewed all suicides as irrational and seen their professional duty as requiring prevention of suicide whenever possible, may soon be recast by legalization in the alien role of gatekeepers identifying those persons whose suicides should be facilitated. Presumably, psychiatrists who are unalterably opposed to physician-assisted suicide will be able to excuse themselves from participation in competency determinations of patients who have made such requests.

Some insist there are good reasons for doing so: the most persuasive opposition to physician-assisted suicide now centers on the sort of concern advanced by Gaylin and coauthors involving the distrust of physicians this might engender (47) and/or on more general slippery slope concerns. Detailed exploration of these arguments is beyond the scope of this chapter. At the very least, however, I hope the above discussion will give pause for psychiatrists who would be inclined, on the grounds that no one in his or her right mind could wish for death, to dissociate themselves from involvement with patients seeking physician-assisted suicide. That claim seems indefensible today in light of the fact that at present most Americans die following a deliberate decision that the further preservation of life is not worth the costs—physical, emotional, and economic. Regardless of how individual psychiatrists respond, however, I believe it would be a grave disservice for psychiatry as a profession to back away from participation in practices designed to ensure that physician-assisted suicide is practiced as responsibly as possible.

References

1. Katz J: The Silent World of Doctor and Patient. New York, Macmillan, 1984
2. Katz, The Silent World, p 4; emphasis added
3. Katz, The Silent World, p 4
4. Katz J: Experimentation With Human Beings. New York, Russell Sage Foundation, 1972, p 649
5. Freud A: The doctor-patient relationship, in Moral Problems in Medicine, 2nd Edition. Edited by Gorovitz S, Macklin R, Jameton A, et al. Englewood Cliffs, NJ, Prentice-Hall, 1983, pp 108–110
6. Meisel A: The Right to Die. New York, Wiley, 1989
7. Mill JS: Utilitarianism, in The English Philosophers From Bacon to Mill. Edited by Burtt E. New York, Random House, 1939, pp 895–948
8. Jones WT: A History of Western Philosophy: Hobbes to Hume. San Diego, CA, Harcourt Brace Jovanovich, 1969, Chapter 3, pp 67–117
9. Feinberg J: The nature and value of rights, in Ethical Theory: Classical and Contemporary Readings, 2nd Edition. Edited by Pojman L. Belmont, MA, Wadsworth Publishing, 1995, pp 680–689
10. Locke J: An essay concerning the true original, extent and end of civil government (The Second Treatise of Government), in The English Philosophers From Bacon to Mill. Edited by Burtt E. New York, Random House, 1939, pp 403–503; see p 437

11. Kant I: The foundations of the metaphysic of morals, in Ethical Theory: Classical and Contemporary Readings, 2nd Edition. Edited by Pojman L. Belmont, MA, Wadsworth Publishing, 1995, pp 255–279

12. Katz, The Silent World

13. Schloendorff v NY Hospital, 221 NY 127, 129, 105 NE 92, 93 (1914)

14. Katz, The Silent World, p 59

15. President's Commission for the Study of Ethical Problems in Medicine and Biomedical and Behavioral Research: Making Health Care Decisions, Vol 1: The Ethical and Legal Implications of Informed Consent in the Patient-Practitioner Relationship. Washington, DC, U.S. Government Printing Office, 1982

16. President's Commission, Making Health Care Decisions, Vol 1, p 2

17. President's Commission for the Study of Ethical Problems in Medicine and Biomedical and Behavioral Research: Deciding to Forgo Life-Sustaining Treatment: Ethical, Medical, and Legal Issues in Treatment Decisions. Washington, DC, U.S. Government Printing Office, 1983

18. President's Commission, Deciding to Forgo Life-Sustaining Treatment, p 1

19. President's Commission, Deciding to Forgo Life-Sustaining Treatment, p 3

20. President's Commission, Deciding to Forgo Life-Sustaining Treatment, p 3

21. McCartney JJ: The development of the doctrine of ordinary and extraordinary means of preserving life in Catholic moral theology before the Karen Quinlan case. Linacre Quarterly 47:215–224, 1980; see p 216

22. Munson R: Intervention and Reflection: Basic Issues in Medical Ethics. Belmont, MA, Wadsworth Publishing, 1996

23. Steinbock B: The intentional termination of life, in Moral Problems in Medicine, 2nd Edition. Edited by Gorovitz S, Macklin R, Jameton A, et al. Englewood Cliffs, NJ, Prentice-Hall, 1983, pp 290–295

24. Steinbock, Intentional termination of life, p 290

25. American Medical Association: News release: AMA soundly reaffirms policy opposing physician-assisted suicide. Chicago, IL, American Medical Association, 1996

26. American Nurses Association: Position statement on assisted suicide. Washington, DC, American Nurses Association, 1994

27. American Geriatrics Society: Policy statement on physician-assisted suicide and voluntary active euthanasia. New York, American Geriatrics Society, 1994

28. Statement of the National Hospice Organization opposing the legalization of euthanasia and assisted suicide. Arlington, VA, National Hospice Organization, 1990

29. Brody H: Causing, intending, and assisting death. J Clin Ethics 4:112–117, 1993

30. Meisel, The Right to Die
31. Brock D: Voluntary active euthanasia. Hastings Cent Rep 22:10–22 1992
32. Arras J: The right to die on the slippery slope. Philosophical Quarterly 32:285–328, 1982
33. Rachels J: Active and passive euthanasia, in Moral Problems in Medicine, 2nd Edition. Edited by Gorovitz S, Macklin R, Jameton A, et al. Englewood Cliffs, NJ, Prentice-Hall, 1983, pp 286–289
34. Steinbock, Intentional termination of life
35. Brock, Voluntary active euthanasia
36. Arras, Right to die on the slippery slope
37. Gaylin W, Kass L, Pellegrino E, et al: Doctors must not kill. JAMA 259:2139–2140, 1988; see p 2140
38. Meisel, The Right to Die
39. Garcia J: Double effect, in Encyclopedia of Bioethics, Vol II. Edited by Reich W. New York, Macmillan, 1995, pp 636–641
40. Maltsberger J: What I think about rational suicide. Newslink (Newsletter of the American Association of Suicidology) 18:3–4, 1992
41. The SUPPORT Principal Investigators: A controlled trial to improve care for seriously ill hospitalized patients. JAMA 274:1591–1598, 1995. See also Perry S: The undermedication for pain: a psychoanalytic perspective. Bulletin of the Association for Psychoanalytic Medicine 22:77–85, 1983; Cleeland CS, Gonlin R, Hatfield AK, et al: Pain and its treatment in outpatients with metastatic cancer. N Engl J Med 330:592–596, 1994
42. Mayo D: The concept of rational suicide. Journal of Medicine and Philosophy 11:143–155, 1986
43. Uhlmann R, Pearlman R: Perceived quality of life and preferences for life-sustaining treatment in older adults. Arch Intern Med 151:495–497, 1991
44. SUPPORT Principal Investigators, A controlled trial; see also Perry, Undermedication for pain; Cleeland et al, Pain and its treatment
45. Brock, Voluntary active euthanasia
46. Szasz T: The ethics of suicide, in Suicide: The Philosophical Issues. Edited by Battin MP, Mayo D. New York, St Martin's Press, 1980, pp 185–198
47. Gaylin et al, Doctors must not kill

11

Physician-Assisted Suicide: Moral Questions

Daniel Callahan, Ph.D.

The right to control our bodies and our lives is a characteristically American claim. "Give me liberty or give me death" is a part of our history. The idea, however, that we should have the freedom to ask another, a doctor, to help us reach death is something relatively new, even for Americans, who have rarely set limits on what might be claimed in the name of liberty. It goes against some 2,500 years of Western Hippocratic medicine and against long-standing American laws and medical principles. Yet we are now in the midst of a great national debate on physician-assisted suicide (PAS).

It could well be said that the PAS movement represents the last, definitive step in gaining full individual self-determination. It seeks to reassure us we can die as we choose and to provide a technically decisive solution to our dying. However mistaken in its direction and emphasis—as I will argue it is—a turn to PAS is a perfectly understandable response to the increased difficulty of dying a peaceful death, a dying ever more ensnared in technological and moral traps. On the one hand, there are all the obstacles thrown in the way of simply allowing people to die from disease. Medicine tends to conflate the value of the sanctity of life and the technological imperative, rendering an acceptance of death morally suspect. On the other hand, with all deaths increasingly being judged to be a human responsibility, with the distinction between omission and commission erased, there is now every incentive to seek a final and decisive control over the process of dying. Euthanasia and assisted suicide present, seemingly, the perfect way to do just that.

The euthanasia-PAS movement rests on two basic claims, secondarily supported by other considerations as well. Those claims are our right to self-determination and the obligation we owe to each other to relieve suffering, but especially the obligation of the physician to do so. The deepest point of this movement might simply be understood as this: If we cannot trust disease to take our lives quickly or peacefully, and if we cannot rely on doctors to know with great precision how or when to stop treatment to allow that to happen, then we have a right to turn to more direct means. Physicians should be allowed in the name of mercy to end our lives at our voluntary request or, alternatively, permitted to put into our hands those means that will allow us to commit suicide. We will then be assured a peaceful death, one that we have fashioned for ourselves. For the peaceful death no longer (and never assuredly and perfectly) given us by nature, we must shape, by our choice, one of our own making.

This is a dangerous direction to go in the search for a peaceful death. It rests on the illusion that a society can safely put in the private hands of physicians the power directly and deliberately to take life (i.e., euthanasia) or to assist patients in taking their own life (i.e., PAS). (I see no moral difference between them—just as the law in most places would see no difference between my shooting someone and giving a gun to another so he can do it.) It threatens to add to an already sorry human history of giving one person the liberty to take the life of another still another sad chapter. It perpetuates and pushes to an extreme the very ideology of control—the goal of mastering life and death—that created the problems of modern medicine in the first place. Instead of changing the medicine generating the problem of an intolerable death, available in almost all cases by good palliative medicine, it simply treats the symptoms, all the while reinforcing, and driving us more deeply, into an ideology of control.

The fear of dying is powerful. Even more powerful sometimes is the fear of *not* dying, of being a burden on one's family, or of being forced to endure destructive pain or to live out a life of unrelieved, pointless suffering. The provocations to embrace PAS can seem compelling: prolonged agony; a sense of utter futility; pain that can only be relieved at the price of oblivion; a desperate gasping for breath that, if relieved, will be followed again and again by the same gasping; or, perhaps even worse, months or years in a nursing home. The possibilities of inhuman suffering should not be minimized, and I do not want to rest my resistance on any slighting of that kind. I can well imagine situations that could drive me to want such relief or feel driven to want it for others. The movement to legalize euthanasia and assisted suicide is a strong and, seemingly, historically inevitable response to that fear. It draws part of its strength from the failure of modern medicine to reassure us that it can manage our dying with dignity and comfort. It draws another part from the desire to be masters of our fate. Why must we endure that which need not be endured? If medicine cannot always bring us the kind of death we might like through its technical skills, why can it not use them to give us a quick and merciful release?

The Relief of Suffering: Virtues and Duties

No moral impulse seems more deeply imbedded than the need to relieve human suffering. It is a basic tenet of the great religions of the world. It has become a foundation stone for the practice of medicine, and it is at the core of the social and welfare programs of all civilized nations. Unless we have been brutalized, our feelings numbed by cruelty or systematic indifference, we cannot stand to see another person suffer. The tears of another, even a total stranger, can bring tears to our own eyes. At the heart of the virtue of compassion is the capacity to feel with, and for, another. With those closest to us, that virtue often leads us to feel the pain of another as if it were our own.

And sometimes our impulse of compassion is stronger than that: it is a source of intensified anguish that we cannot lift from another the pain we would, if we could, make our own. A parent feels that way about the suffering of a child, and a spouse or friend about the suffering of a loved one who is trapped by pain that cannot be moved from one body to another.

Yet for all the depth of our common response to suffering, our general agreement as a civilized society that it should be relieved, the scope and depth of that moral duty are not clear, especially for physicians. The problem of PAS forces us to answer a hard question: Ought the general duty of the physician to relieve suffering encompass the right to assist a patient to take his or her own life if that is desired and seems necessary? The question can be put from the patient's side as well: Is it a legitimate moral request for a patient to ask his or her doctor to assist him or her in committing suicide?

But there is an even more fundamental question that must be explored before turning to those questions: What should be done in response to such suffering? Is it simply a *nice* thing to relieve suffering if we can, a gesture of charity or kindness worthy of praise? We might say that our impulse of compassion is a good to be cultivated and expressed; that we will all be better off if we entertain that as an ideal in our lives together. Or is there more to it than that? Might it be that the relief of suffering is a moral *duty,* not just a noble ideal, to which we are obliged even if our sense of compassion is faint, and even if what is asked of us might cause some suffering on our own part? How far and in what way, that is, does our duty extend in the relief of suffering, and just what kind of suffering is encompassed within such a duty?

One common answer to questions of that kind is that we are, at the least, obliged to relieve the suffering of others when we can do so at no high cost to ourselves, and we should do so when the suffering at stake is unnecessary. But that does not tell us much that is helpful, though it is surely important to repeatedly remind ourselves and others of such obligations. The hard cases are those in which the demands on us may be morally or psychologically stressful and there is uncertainty about the significance of the suffering.

There are two burdens that it is useful to distinguish. One of them is when the demand on us is to act, to do something specifically to relieve the suffering. That may mean giving our already overcrowded time to just be with someone in pain, whose need is for companionship and for closeness; or perhaps providing otherwise needed money to improve the nursing care of a dying parent; or taking the trouble to find a better doctor, or hospital, for a spouse receiving poor care. Demands of that kind can be heavy, pressing our sense of duty to the limit; and sometimes it can be unclear just where the limit is.

The other burden is more subtle: that of knowing when suffering cannot, or should not, be wholly overcome, and when our duty may be one of accepting the suffering of another, just as the person whose suffering it is must accept it. Many legitimate moral demands, for instance, carry with them the possibility of suffering, and they should not for that reason be shirked. To take an unpopular position, to stand up for one's rights, to remain true to one's promises and commitments can all entail unavoidable suffering. A parent's commitment to the good of a child may require, and probably will at times require, that, for the sake of the child's development, the parent accept the need for the child to bear the penalties of his or her own choices and mistakes, and thereby to suffer. The same can be said of many other human relationships, such as friends and lovers, husbands and wives. As bystanders to the suffering, we have to accept its unavoidability for the sufferer. We cannot relieve that suffering. The demand in some cases is to accept the suffering that another must endure, not run from it. Patience, loyalty, steadfastness, and fortitude are called for in accompanying the person who must suffer, to help and allow them to do and be what they must, however heavy the burden on them and others. We are called on to suffer with the other and to be a supportive presence.

For just those reasons it cannot be fully correct to say that our highest moral duty to each other is the relief of suffering. More precisely, our duty is to enhance the good and the welfare of each other, and the relief of suffering will ordinarily be an important way to accomplish that. But not always. What we need to know is whether the suffering exists because, without it, some other human good cannot be accomplished; and that is exactly the case with the suffering caused by living out one's moral duties or ideals for a life.

Therein lies the ambiguity of the term "unnecessary suffering," frequently invoked as the kind of suffering PAS can obviate. Suffering will surely be "unnecessary" when it serves no purpose, when it is not an inextricable part of achieving important human goals. Unavoidable necessary suffering, by contrast, is that which is the essential means, or accompaniment, of valuable human ends; and not all suffering is. Yet the real problem here is in deciding on our goals, and the hardest choice will be in deciding whether, and how, to pursue goals that may entail suffering. If we make the avoidance or relief of suffering itself the highest goal, we run the severe risk of sacrificing, or minimizing, other human purposes. Life would then be focused on avoiding pain, minimizing risk, and craftily eyeing all possible life projects and goals in light of their likelihood of producing suffering.

If that is hardly desirable in the living of our individual lives, it is no less problematic in devising social policy. A society ought, so far as it can, to work for the relief of pain and suffering; and that is to state a simple moral principle. But a more complex principle is needed: a society should work to relieve only that suffering which is not an unavoidable part of living out its other values and aspirations. That means it must ask, on the one hand, what those values are or should be and, on the other, what policies for the relief of suffering might subvert its general values.

The most profound question we must then ask is this: If the suffering of illness and death come from the profound assault on our sense of integrity and self-direction, what is the best way we can, as those who give care and who want to do right by a person, honor that integrity? The claim of PAS proponents is that the assault of terminal illness on the self is legitimately relieved, even mercifully and honorably so, by recognizing the right to self-determination, and that what the individual wants—a deliberately chosen death assisted by another—is appropriate as a way of relieving suffering.

Yet notice what we have accepted here. It is the idea that our integrity can *only* be served by the self-determination that brings death, by the direct implication of another in our death, and by accepting the implicit assumption that the suffering is "unnecessary"—meaningless, avoidable. To accept that comes close to declaiming that life can only have meaning if marked by self-determination, a strange notion indeed, flying directly in the face of human experience. That experience shows that a noble and heroic life can be achieved by those who have little or no control over the external conditions of their lives, but have the wisdom and dignity necessary to fashion a meaningful life without it. We would also be declaring that a life not marked by self-mastery and self-determination is a meaningless one once burdened with unwanted suffering. It is not for nothing, perhaps, that modern medicine in its quest for cure has itself contributed to the harmful idea that all suffering is pointless, representing not life and its natural condition, but the failure of medicine to overcome, or relieve, that condition.

But might it not be said, in response, that a social permission for PAS would not be to take a general position at all on the meaning of life, death, and suffering, but only to empower each individual and his or her accomplice physician to make that determination themselves? Would it not be, in that sense, socially neutral? Not at all. To establish PAS as social policy is, first, to side with those who say that some suffering is meaningless and unnecessary and to be relieved as decisively as possible, and that only individuals can determine what such suffering that is; and, second, to say that such a highly variable, highly subjective matter is best left to the irrevocable judgment of doctor and patient. That is not a neutral policy at all, but one that makes a decisive judgment about what constitutes an appropriate, socially acceptable response to dying—the mutually agreed-on deliberate death of a person—and about social policy—the legitimation of PAS as a response to perceived threats of suffering and loss of self-integrity.

A great hazard of this approach is that it declares some forms of human suffering—but only those forms determined by private, variable responses—to be beyond human help and caring, and open only to death as a solution. It is, moreover, a striking break with both the medical and moral traditions of medicine to treat the desires and wishes of patients as if they alone provide legitimation of a doctor's skills. It is to make doctors artisans in the fashioning of a patient's life—and in this case a death—a role well beyond the traditional range of medicine, that of restoring or maintaining health.

There is little disagreement about the duty of the physician to relieve physical pain, even though there are some significant disputes about how far that effort should go. Of more pertinence to my concern here, however, is the extent of the duty of the physician to relieve suffering—that is, to try to relieve the psychological or spiritual condition of a person who, as a result of illness, suffers (whether in pain or not). I want to contend that the duty is important but limited.

Two levels of suffering can be distinguished. At one level, the principal problem is that of the fear, uncertainty, dread, or anguish of the sick person in coping with the illness and its meaning for the continuation of life and intact personhood—what might be called the psychological penumbra of illness. At a deeper level, the problem touches on the meaning of suffering for the meaning of life itself. The question here is more fundamental: What does my suffering tell me about the point or purpose or end of human existence, most notably my own? The questions here no longer are just psychological but encompass fundamental philosophical and religious questions.

The physician should do all in his or her power to respond, as physician, to the first level, but it is inappropriate, I contend, to attempt to solve by lethal means the problems that arise at the second level. What would that distinction mean in practice? It means that the doctor should, through counseling, pain relief, and cooperative efforts with family and friends, do everything possible to reduce the sense of dread and anxiety, of disintegration of self, in the face of a threatened death. The doctor should provide care, comfort, and compassion. But when the patient says to the doctor that life no longer has meaning, or that the suffering cannot be borne because of its perceived pointlessness, or that a loss of control is experienced as an intolerable insult to a patient's sense of self—at that point the doctor must draw a line. Those problems cannot properly be solved by medicine, and it is a mistake for it even to make an attempt to do so.

The purpose of medicine is not to relieve all the problems of human mortality, the most central and difficult of which is why we have to die at all or die in ways that seem pointless to us. It is not the purpose of medicine to give us control over our human destiny or to help us devise a life to our private specifications—and especially the specification most desired these days, that of complete control of death and its circumstances. That is not the role of medicine because it has no competence to manage the meaning of life and death, only the physical and psychological manifestations of those problems.

Medicine's role must be limited to what it can appropriately do, and it neither has expertise nor wisdom of a kind necessary to respond to the deepest and oldest human questions. What it can do is to relieve pain and to bring comfort to those who psychologically suffer because of illness. That is all, and that is enough. When physicians would use medical knowledge, designed to help with the task of relieving pain and comforting, to directly cause death as a way of solving patients' problems with life and mortality itself, they go too far, exceeding their own professional and moral rights and those of the profession to which they belong. There has been a long-standing, historical resistance to giving physicians the power to assist in suicide precisely because of the skill they could bring to that task. Their technical power to help death along must not be matched by a moral or legal authority to engage in PAS, which would open the way for a corruption of their vocation.

I do not claim that a sharp and precise line can always be found between the two levels, but only that some limits can be feasibly set to enable us to say when the physician has strayed too far into the thickets of the second level—the meaning of suffering for the meaning of life itself. For ordinary purposes, it remains appropriate to speak of the duty of the physician to "relieve pain and suffering," but only as long as it is understood that this can be done only to relieve the problems of illness, not the problems of life itself. What life itself may give us, at its end, is a death that seems, in the suffering it brings, to make no sense. That is a *terrible* problem, but it is the patient's problem, not the doctor's. The doctor can, at that point, relieve pain if that is present, make the patient as comfortable as possible, and be another human presence. Beyond that, the patient must be on his or her own. We have no resource left but ourselves at that point.

There is also another side to the issue. When PAS is requested, the doctor is being asked to act on the subjective suffering of another— variable from person to person, externally unverifiable, and always in principle reversible—but to respond with an action that will be objective and irreversible. As the human response to evil and suffering suggests, there is nothing in a particular burden of life, or in the nature of suffering itself, that *necessarily* and *inevitably* leads to a desire to be dead, much less a will to bring that about. That will and must always be a function of the patient's values and the way they are either legitimated or rejected by the culture of which that patient is a part. Suffering in and of itself is not a good clinical predictor of a desire to be dead, and this is why depression or a history of previous mental health problems is a far better predictor of a serious desire for suicide than illness, pain, or old age. If that is the case, then we have a complex, double challenge before us: to determine if, under those ambiguous circumstances, we should empower one person to help another to kill himself or herself; and if so, what the moral standard should be for the one who is to do the helping.

Physician-assisted suicide is mistakenly understood as only a personal matter of self-determination, the control of our own bodies, just a small step beyond our already available legal right to commit suicide. But, unlike unassisted suicide, an act carried out solely by the person himself or herself, PAS should be understood as of its nature a social act. It requires the assistance of someone else. Legalizing PAS would also provide an important social sanction for suicide, tacitly legitimating it, and affecting many aspects of our society beyond the immediate relief of suffering individuals.

All civilized societies have developed laws to reduce the occasions on which one person is allowed to kill another. Most have resisted the notion that private agreements can be reached allowing one person to help another take his or her life. Traditionally, three circumstances only have been acceptable for the taking of life: killing in self-defense or to protect another life, in the course of a just war, and in the case of capital punishment. With the exception perhaps of self-defense, killing both in war and by capital punishment have been opposed by some, and most successfully in the case of capital punishment, now banned in many countries, most notably in western Europe.

The proposal to legalize PAS is nothing less than a proposal to add a new category of acceptable killing to those already socially legitimated. To do so would be to reverse the long-developing trend to limit the occasions of legally sanctioned killing (most notable in the campaigns to abolish capital punishment and to limit access to handguns). Civilized societies have slowly come to understand how virtually impossible it is to control even legally sanctioned killing. Even with carefully fashioned safeguards, such killing invites abuse and corruption.

Does it not make a difference that the absolute power is given, not to subjugate another (as in slavery), but as an act of mercy, to bring relief from suffering? No. Although the motive may be more benign than in the case of slavery as usually understood, that motive is beside the point. The aim in prohibiting PAS is to avoid introducing into society the inherent corruption of legitimated private killing. "All power corrupts," Lord Acton wrote, "and absolute power corrupts absolutely." It is that profound insight—a reflection on human despotism, usually justified initially out of good, empathic motives—that should be kept in mind when we would give one person the right to kill another.

We come here to a striking pitfall of the common argument for euthanasia and assisted suicide. Once the key premises of that argument are accepted, there will remain no logical way in the future to 1) deny euthanasia to anyone who requests it for whatever reason, terminal illness or not, or to 2) deny it to suffering incompetent persons, even if they do not request it. We can erect legal safeguards and specify required procedures to keep that from happening. But over time they will provide poor protection if the logic of the moral premises on which they are based are fatally flawed. The safeguards will appear arbitrary and flimsy and will invite covert evasion or outright rejection.

Where are the flaws here? Recall that there are two classical arguments in favor of euthanasia and assisted suicide: our right of self-determination and our claim on the mercy of others, especially doctors, to relieve our suffering if they can do so. These two arguments are typically spliced together and presented as a single contention. Yet if they are considered independently—and there is no inherent reason why they must be linked—they display serious problems. Consider, first, the argument for our right of self-determination. It is said that a competent, adult person ought to have a right to PAS for the relief of suffering. But why must the person be suffering? Does not that stipulation already compromise the right of self-determination? How can self-determination have any limits? Why are not the person's desires or motives, whatever they be, sufficient? How can we justify this arbitrary limitation of self-determination? The standard arguments for PAS offer no answers to those questions.

Consider next the person who is suffering but not competent, perhaps demented or mentally retarded. The standard argument would deny euthanasia and PAS to that person. But why? If a person is suffering but not competent, then it would seem grossly unfair to deny that person relief simply because he or she lacked competence. Are the incompetent less entitled to relief from suffering than the competent? Will it only be affluent middle-class people, mentally fit and able, who can qualify? Will those who are incompetent but suffering be denied that which those who are intellectually and emotionally better off can have? Would that be fair? Do they suffer less for being incompetent? The standard argument about our duty to relieve suffering offers no response to those questions either.

Is it, however, fair to euthanasia advocates to do what I have done, to separate, and treat individually, the two customary arguments in favor of a legal right to euthanasia and PAS? The implicit reason for so joining them is no doubt the desire to avoid abuse. By a showing of suffering and terminal illness being required, the aim is to exclude perfectly healthy people from demanding that, in the name of self-determination and for their own private reasons, another person can be called on to kill them or assist them in suicide. By requiring a show of mental competence to effect self-determination, the aim is to exclude the nonvoluntary or involuntary killing of the depressed, the retarded, and the demented.

My contention is that the joining of those two requirements is perfectly arbitrary, a jerry-rigged combination if ever there was one. Each has its own logic, and each could be used to justify euthanasia and PAS. But in the nature of the case, that logic, it seems evident, offers little resistance to denying any competent person the right to be killed, sick or not; and little resistance to killing the incompetent, so long as there is good reason to believe they are suffering. There is no principled reason to reject that logic, and no reason to think it could long remain suppressed by the expedient of an arbitrary legal stipulation that both features, suffering and competence, be present.

There is a related problem worth considering. If the act of PAS, as conventionally understood, requires the uncoerced request and consent of the patient, it no less requires that the person to do the assisting have his or her own independent, moral standards for acceding to the request. The doctor must act with integrity. How can a doctor who voluntarily brings about, or is instrumental in, the death of another legitimately justify that to himself or herself? Would the mere claim of self-determination on the part of someone be sufficient: "It is my body,

doctor, and I request that you help me kill myself"? There is a historical resistance to that kind of claim, and doctors quite rightly have never
been willing to do what patients want solely because they want it. That
would reduce the doctor's role to that of an automaton, subordinating
his or her integrity to patient wishes or demands. There is surely
a legitimate fear, moreover, that if such a claim was sanctioned, there
would be no reason to forbid any two competent persons from entering
into an agreement for one to kill the other, a form of consenting-adult
killing. Perhaps also the resistance arises out of a reluctance to put
doctors in the role of taking life simply as a means of advancing patient
self-determination, quite apart from any medical reasons for doing so.

Yet the most likely reason for resistance to a pure self-determination
standard is that our culture has, traditionally, defined the appropriate
role of the physician as someone whose duty it is to promote and
restore health. It has thus been customary, even among those pressing
for euthanasia and PAS, to hang on to some part of the physician's
traditional role. That is why a mere claim of self-determination, which
requires no reference to health at all, is not enough. A doctor will not
cut off my healthy arm simply because I decide my autonomy and
well-being would thereby be enhanced.

What can we conclude from these still-viable traditions? For a doctor to justify committing an act of PAS, she must have her own independent moral standards to maintain her integrity. What should those
standards be? The doctor will not be able to use a *medical* standard.
A PAS decision is not a medical but a moral decision. Faced with
a patient reporting great suffering, a doctor cannot, therefore, justify
PAS on purely medical grounds. To maintain professional and personal
integrity, the doctor will have to justify it on her own moral grounds.
The doctor must believe that a life of subjectively experienced intense
suffering is not worth living, if she is to be justified to take the decisive
and ultimate step of killing the patient. It must be *her* moral reason to
act, not the patient's reason (even though they may coincide). But if
she believes that a life of some forms of suffering is not worth living,
then how can she deny the same relief to a person who cannot request
it, or who requests it but whose competence is in doubt? There is no
self-evident reason why the supposed duty to relieve suffering must be
limited to competent patients claiming self-determination. Or why

patients who claim death as their right under self-determination must be either suffering or dying.

There is, moreover, the possibility that what begins as a right of doctors to engage in PAS under specified conditions will soon become a duty to offer it up front to patients. On what grounds could a doctor deny a request by a competent person for PAS? It is not sufficient to just stipulate that no doctor should be required to do that which violates his or her conscience. As commonly articulated, the argument about why a doctor has a right to assist in suicide—the dual duty to respect patient self-determination and to relieve suffering—is said to be central to the vocation of being a doctor. Why should duties as weighty as those be set aside on the grounds of "conscience" or "personal values"?

These puzzles make clear that the moral situation is radically changed once our self-determination requires the participation and assistance of a doctor. It is no longer a solitary act, but a two-person, social act. It is then that doctor's moral life, that doctor's integrity, that is also and no less encompassed in the act of PAS. What, we might then ask, should be the appropriate moral standards for a person asked to help another kill himself or herself? What are the appropriate virtues and sensitivities of such a person? How should that person think of his or her own life and find, within that life, a place for PAS?

Now I could imagine someone granting the weight of the considerations against euthanasia I have advanced and yet having this response: Is not our duty to relieve suffering sufficiently strong to justify running some risks? Why should we be intimidated by the dangers in a decisive relief of suffering? Is not the present situation, where death can be slow, painful, and full of suffering, already a clear and present danger?

Our duty to relieve suffering—by no means unlimited in any case—cannot justify the introduction of new evils into society. The risk of doing just that in the legalization of PAS is too great, particularly since the number of people whose pain and suffering could not be otherwise relieved would never be a large one (as even most PAS advocates recognize). It is too great because it would take a disproportionate social change to bring it about, one with implications that extend far beyond the sick and dying, reaching into the practice of medicine and into the sphere of socially sanctioned killing. It is too great because, as the history of the twentieth century should demonstrate, killing is a contagious disease, not easy to stop once unleashed in society. It is too great a risk because it would offer medicine too convenient a way out of its hardest cases, those in which there is ample room for further, more benign reforms. We are far from exhausting the known remedies for the relief of pain (which are frequently, even routinely, underused) and a long way from providing decent psychological support for those who, not necessarily in pain, nonetheless suffer because of despair and a sense of futility in continuing life.

The legalization of PAS is, finally, too great a risk because it would lend credence to the mistaken notion that a self-chosen death is a "rational" way to deal with suffering. It is probably no coincidence that the Romans, who justified suicide on the grounds that our bodies are a form of property, also justified slavery on similar grounds, that one person may own the body of another.

Physical pain and psychological suffering in the critically ill and dying are great evils. The attempt to relieve them by the introduction of euthanasia and assisted suicide is an even greater evil. Those practices threaten the future security of the living. They no less threaten the dying themselves. Once a society allows one person to take the life of another based on their mutual private standards of a life worth living, there can be no safe or sure way to contain the deadly virus thus introduced. It will go where it will thereafter.

Index

*Page numbers printed in **boldface** type refer to tables or figures.*

Acquired immune deficiency
syndrome (AIDS), patients. *See*
AIDS patients
Acton, John E. E. Dalberg-Acton,
Lord, 293
Actual-wishes standard, 245–247
constitutionality of, 246
Adolescents
decision making, participation in,
149–151, 160, **160**
developmental characteristics,
148–149
treatment refusal by, 149, 157
Advance directives, 109. *See also*
Do-not-resuscitate orders;
Living wills; Treatment
preferences
of ALS patients, 120
of cancer patients, 120
combination directives, 251
elderly patients, 84–85
feared loss of care control and,
211
of HIV-infected patients, 120
of incompetent patients,
surrogate decision-making
role, 249–253
legal aspects, 79, 266
limitations on, 251
nonstatutory
oral, 79, 252
written, 79, 252

physicians' knowledge of laws
about, 123
physicians' knowledge of
patients', 117, 123
religious, 113
stability of preferences, 117,
120–121
Affective disorders, inability to
appreciate medication risks and
benefits, 63–64
African Americans, treatment
preferences, 96
AIDS (acquired immune deficiency
syndrome)
cancer compared, 185
death rates, 180
inevitable fatality perception,
179, 186
slow onset, 190
therapeutic options, 180
AIDS patients, 179
assisted suicide and, 198–199
decision to forgo pentamidine
mist treatments, 268
depression in, care preferences
and, 185
do-not-resuscitate orders,
121–122, 185
euthanasia rates, 194
futile treatment for, 181–182
hastened death, acceptability in
gay culture, 209

AIDS patients (*continued*)
  manner-of-dying concerns, 181
  as medical consumers, 182
  organic mental disorders, suicide
    risk factor, 216
  quality of life considerations, 80,
    185
  substance abuse in, 216
  suicidal ideation, 186–189
  suicide rates, 187, 209
  terminal care
    aggressive, 182
    palliative, 180
    preferences, 185
    willingness to discuss, 185
  wish to die, 209
Alcohol
  attempted suicide and, 189
  suicide and, 193
Alcohol abuse, in HIV-infected
  patients, 193
Alzheimer's disease
  advance directives and, 251
  depression in, medication, 62
Ambivalence, of families, toward
  addicted/abusive members,
  90–91
American Board of Internal
  Medicine, 126
American Geriatrics Society, 269,
  274
American Medical Association, 269,
  270, 274
  Council of Ethical and Judicial
    Affairs, 125
American Nurses Association, 269,
  274
American Suicide Foundation,
  198

Amyotrophic lateral sclerosis (ALS)
  patients
  CPR preferences, 120
  physician-patient
    communication, 116,
    119–120
Analgesics, withholding for
  substance abusers, 216–217
Anticonvulsants, 212
Antidepressants, 66, 215
  tricyclic, 212
Anxiety, physicians, in talking with
  dying patients, 126
Anxiety disorders
  hastened-death desire and,
    215–216
  in terminal illness, 7, 215–216
Appelbaum, P. S., 26, 27, 33, 35, 60,
  62, 64, 69
Appropriate death, 13–14
Aristotle, 262
Assisted suicide. *See also*
  Euthanasia; Hastened death;
  Physician-assisted suicide;
  Suicide
  as alternative to suffering, 207
  bungled attempts, 198–199
  constitutionality of, 254–255, 266
  as crime, 254–255
  HIV/AIDS patients and, 198
  integrity of medical profession
    and, 273, 278–279
  as last resort, 227
  marketing of, 198
  privacy rights and, 255
  psychiatrists' attitudes toward, 206
  rates, in The Netherlands, 208
  state laws, 254–255
AZT (zidovudine), 180

Beck, A. T., 61
Beck Depression Inventory, 186
Beck Scale for Suicide Ideation, 187, 189
Bedell, S. E., 100
Benzodiazepines, 49, 71, 212
Berman, S., 165
Best-interests standard, 249
Beth Israel Deaconess Medical Center (Boston), 189
Borderline personality disorder
  patient-generated pressure on caregivers, 220
  self-destructive patients, desire for physician-assisted death, 219–220
Bouvia, Elizabeth, 56, 240, 268–269
Bouvia case, 56–57, 58, 240, 268–269
Breitbart, W., 208
Brennan, T. A., 101
Brock, D. W., 23, 26, 29, 30–32, 33, 63, 149
Brody, Howard, 41, 271
Brown, G. R., 193
Buchanan, A. E., 23, 26, 29, 30–32, 33, 63
Bursztajn, H. J., 63

California, physician-assisted suicide, legalization initiative, 277
Callahan, D., 4
Canada, euthanasia choices of healthcare workers and depressed patients compared, 66
Cancer, AIDS compared, 185

Cancer patients
  advance directives, stability of preferences, 120
  depression in, 65, 185, 209
  do-not-resuscitate orders, 121–122, 185
  pain in, 212
  physician-assisted suicide acceptable by, 208
  suicidal ideation, 189
  suicide risk, 209
    pain factor, 212
    substance abuse and, 216
  terminal care, willingness to discuss, 185
Caralis, P. V., 96, 99, 112
Cardiopulmonary resuscitation (CPR). *See also* Do-not-resuscitate orders
  physician-patient communication about, 116, 119
Cardozo, Benjamin, 237, 263
Care preferences. *See* Treatment preferences
Cassel, C. K., **95**, 197
Catholic Health Association Affirmation of Life, 113
Catholics. *See* Roman Catholic Church
Chicago Multicenter AIDS Cohort Study, 186
Children
  critically ill
    awareness of prognosis, 155–156
    communicating medical information with, 154–156
    countertransference, 165–166

Children (*continued*)
  critically ill (*continued*)
    families of, 151–154
    family assessment issues, 151,
        167
    healthcare teams' ways of
        coping, 165–166
    palliative care, 167–168
    parental denial, 162–164, 166
    pediatric team characteristics,
        139–140
    physicians' guilt, 166
    psychiatric consultation,
        138–140, 158, **159**
    treatment discontinuation,
        158–160
    treatment refusal, 156–157
  death perceptions, developmental
      stage and, 143–144, 146,
      148
  decision making by, 145, 147,
      149, 156, 157–158
  decision making for, 140, 141,
      142–143, 145–146, 147, 149
  competence and, 160, **160**
  development
    childhood/preadolescence
        (7-12 years), 146–147
    early childhood (2–7 years),
        143–146
    infancy (0–2 years), 141–143
    late childhood/adolescence
        (12+ years), 146–151
  grieving for, 151, 152, 169–170
    pathological, 170–171
    physician's follow-up, 171, **172**
    by siblings, 153, 170
Childress, James F., 64
Chinese-American patients, 113–114

Chochinov, H. M., 208
Christians. *See also* Jehovah's
      Witnesses; Roman Catholic
      Church
  end-of-life treatment preferences,
      112
  fundamentalist, treatment
      preferences, 96
  sanctity of life values, 70
Cirrhosis patients,
      do-not-resuscitate orders,
      120–121
Cogen, R., **95**
Cohen-Cole, S. A., 66
Communication. *See also*
      Physician-patient
      communication
  ability, competency
      determination and, 26, 62
  bad news identified with the
      messenger, 125
  competency evaluation refusals
      and, 46
  with critically ill children,
      154–156
  in hospitals, 2
  physicians' lack of education in,
      125–126
Compassion, 285–286
Competence
  concept of, 20–21, 23–24, 63
  decision-making capacity vs.,
      20–21, 24
  fluctuation over time, 35
  incompetence vs. competence,
      25–26
  insanity vs. incompetence, 2, 25
  interpersonal dynamics and,
      35–36

legal standards, 29–30, 62
physician-assisted suicide and, 21
power and, 41
social context influence on, 35–36
suicidal ideation and, 58
Competency determination
ambivalent patients, 47–48
attitude of medical personnel
and, 23
authentication of patients'
histories, 35
burden of proof, 57, 59, 70
clinical issues in, 33–36
coping strategies and, 36, 38,
49–50
decision specificity, 24–25
decision-making attributes
required, 26–27, 62–63
decision-making capacity and,
220
decision-relative approach to,
33
depression
failure to recognize, 30, 60
natural vs. pathological, 37–38
treatment refusal and, 60–64
as dichotomous choice, 20, 24
evaluation tests, 28–32, 63
case commentaries, 30–32
evaluator's personal values and,
36–37
harmful-decision influence on, 21
in hospitals, 38
incompetence
legal concept of, 25
as mask for paternalism, 38–41
mental illness proof required
for, 25
informed consent, 49

adequacy of information for,
22–23, 35
in life-threatening emergencies,
40, 63
moral implications, 22, 49
moral vs. clinical judgment, 37,
42–43
patients' attributes
ability to express a preference,
29
ability to understand relevant
information, 26, 30, 62,
63–64
appreciation of treatment risks
and benefits, 64
communication ability, 26, 62
reasoning ability, 26–27, 30, 62
values stability, 27–28, 30–31
patients' refusals of, 46, 47
for physician-assisted suicide, 43
process defects, 30
by psychiatrists, 21, 64–65
personal values' influence, 37,
42–43
power to see the unobvious,
43–46
qualifications, 48–50
psychodynamic factors in
patients' decisions, 34
standards for, 32–33, 62–63
in treatment refusal, burden of
proof, 57, 59
treatment risk and, 33
values stability, 27–28, 30–31
depression and, 28, 30
who should evaluate, 48–50,
64–65, 220
Consultation-liaison psychiatry,
129–130

Control, patients' needs for, 7–8
Control ideology, 284–285
Coping strategies, competency assessment and, 36, 38, 49–50
Countervailing state interests, 238–240
CPR. *See* Cardiopulmonary resuscitation
Cruzan, Nancy, 79
Cruzan case, 100, 246, 253
Culture. *See also* Ethnicity grieving and, 152–153
Culver, Charles M., 63

Danis, M., **94**
"Daughter from California Syndrome," 91–92, 101, 103
Death
    appropriate, 13–14
    of children, 137–138, 171–172
    as enemy to be conquered, 4, 10, 124
    hastened. *See* Euthanasia; Hastened death
    inevitability, physician culture's denial of, 124
    intended vs. foreseen but unintended, 268–269, 275–276
    as least worst alternative, 9, 46
    peaceful, assurance of, 284
    physician-assisted. *See* Do-not-resuscitate orders; Euthanasia; Physician-assisted suicide
    as physician's personal failure, 124, 126–127, 223

Deciding to Forgo Life-Sustaining Treatment: Ethical, Medical, and Legal Issues in Treatment Decisions (President's Commission for the Study of Ethical Problems . . .), 265
Decision making. *See also* End-of-life decisions
    attributes required for, 26–28, 149
    changing milieu of, 78–81
    family-centered model, 96
    patient autonomy model, 96
Decision-making capacity
    of adolescents, 149
    competence vs., 2, 20–21, 24
    competency determination and, 220
    depression and, 28
    hastened-death desires and, 220
    standards for, 62–63
Delirium, from benzodiazepine withdrawal, 49
Demographics
    advance directives, stability of preferences, 121
    end-of-life decisions, 3, 111–112
    physician-assisted suicide and, 3
    physicians, euthanasia attitudes, 3
    suicide risk, 192
    treatment choices, 3
Denial
    family guilt and, 91–92
    about one's illness, 115
    in parents of terminally ill children, 162–164, 166
Denmark, suicide rates, 209

Depression
    ability to make rational end-
        of-life decisions and, 184
    biological markers, 67
    in cancer patients, 65, 185, 209
    diagnosis, 66–67
        criteria compared, 67
    do-not-resuscitate orders and, 61
    effect on values, 28, 30
    in elderly patients, life-sustaining
        preferences, 61–62
    failure to recognize, 30, 60
    grief and, 168–169
    hastened-death desires and, 9–10
    life-sustaining preferences,
        elderly patients, 61–62
    in the medically ill, 65
        diagnosis difficulty, 66–67, 214
        perceived as normal, 215
    medications for, 62, 66, 215
    natural vs. pathological, in
        competency
        determinations, 37–38, 62
    palliative care for, 71
    in palliative care patients
        diagnostic criteria, 67
        rates, 67
    patient autonomy compromised
        by, 60–61
    patients' treatment decisions and,
        61–62
    psychotherapy efficacy, 66
    as reasonable response to illness,
        37, 65–66
    suicide risk and, 192–193
    in terminal illness, 67, 71,
        213–215
    treatment, in the medically ill,
        61–62, 66, 71

    as treatment refusal cause, 27–28,
        60
Desmond, B., 113, 114
Dexamethasone suppression test, 67
Dextroamphetamine, 66, 215
Diagnosis
    do-not-resuscitate orders and,
        121–122
    hospice care and, 122
Diagnostic strategies, for depression,
    in the medically ill, 66–67
DNR orders. *See* Do-not-resuscitate
    orders
Do-not-resuscitate orders, 2, 10. *See
    also* Cardiopulmonary
    resuscitation (CPR)
    AIDS patients, 121–122, 185
    cancer patients, 121–122, 185
    consent for, in futile cases, 125
    "Daughter from California
        Syndrome," 91–92, 101, 103
    from depressed psychiatric
        patients, 61
    diagnosis influence on,
        121–122
    physician-patient communication
        about, 122
    Roman Catholics' acceptance of,
        96
Double-effect deaths, 266, 272,
    273–277
    legal aspects, 274
    moral reasoning
        flawed, 275–277
        Roman Catholic, 274
Drane, J. F., 63
Drugs. *See* Medications; *specific
    drugs or types of drugs*
Duckworth, K., 65

Dying
  emotional aspects, 5
    physicians' discomfort with, 4
  fear of, 285
  fear of not dying, 285
  manner of, 284
  patients' control over, 7–8
Dysthymia, as reasonable response
    to illness, 66

Economic pressures, 3, 89–90,
    96–97, 221
Elderly patients
  advance directives, 84–85
  chronic depression seen as
    reasonable in, 66
  family decision making and, 85
  life-sustaining preferences,
    depression and, 61–62
  treatment preferences, ethnicity
    and, 96
Electroconvulsive therapy (ECT), 66
  do-not-resuscitate orders and, 61
Emanuel, L., 120
End-of-life decisions. *See also*
    Decision making;
    Physician-patient
    communication
  by/for adolescents, 149–151, 160,
    160
  ambivalence in, 47–48
  for children, 140, 141, 142–143,
    145–146, 147, 149,
    158–160, **160**
    psychiatric consultant's role,
      161–164
  chronic-illness factors, 116
  contradictory choices, 48, 117
  cultural factors, 113–115

demographic factors, 3, 111–112
  ethical changes and, 265
  ethics consultation, 5–6
  family dynamics, 45
  family pressures, 7, 79–80
  financial coercion, 221
  illness variables, 97
  for incompetent patients,
    241–242
    actual-wishes standard,
      245–247
    best-interests standard, 249
    dispute resolution, 244
    family consensus, 244
    judicial involvement, 242–243
    legal standards, 244–249
    probable-wishes standard,
      247–248
  inconsistency with advance
    directives, 117
  inconsistent choices, 117
  intention criterion, 58–59
  legal consensus on, 236–241,
    244–245
  legal tradition in, 4
  managed care cost concerns, 3
  medical technology and, 5
  patient autonomy, 1–2, 4
  patient-physician relationship
    and, 8
  personality disorders and,
    115–116
  presumption in favor of
    sustaining life, 265
  psychiatrists' involvement in, 4,
    5–6
  psychological factors, 115
  rationality, depression and,
    184–185

religious factors, 112–113
shared decision making, 1–2
surrogate decision makers, 2, 22,
243–244
treatment burden vs. benefit,
267–271
End-of-life-decisions, for children,
child's participation in, 145,
147, 149, 157–158
Endicott, J., 67
Epicurus, 262
Ethics
acceptance of others' suffering,
287
changes in, regarding treatment
termination, 265–266
concurrent medical and mental
illnesses, 58
consultation on, 5–6
control ideology, 284–285
double-effect deaths, 266,
273–277
of dying, 235, 259–260
euthanasia, 265–266
denial of, 224, 293
pre-1975, 235
informed consent doctrine,
21–22, 64, 70,
237–238
philosophical roots,
261–264
intended vs. foreseen death,
267–271, 275–276
killing, legally sanctioned
circumstances, 292
killing vs. letting die, 128, 253,
266, 271–273
medical, patient's right to refuse
treatment and, 239–240

physician-assisted suicide
movement, 283–285, 288,
289
purpose of medicine, 290–291
relief of suffering, 284, 286–287,
295
sanctity of life, 284
self-determination, 262–263,
288, 292
treatment burden vs. benefits,
267–268
treatment termination decisions,
265–266
unnecessary suffering, 287–288
Ethics committees, 102, 130–131,
156–157
Ethnicity. See also Culture
decision-making models and, 96
minority status, distrust of
treatment team, 93, 96
treatment preferences and, 96
Euthanasia, 256. See also Assisted
suicide; Hastened death;
Physician-assisted suicide;
Treatment limitation;
Treatment refusal
active
legalization of, 256
moral considerations, 268–270
vs. passive, 195, 253, 266,
271–273
as alternative to suffering, 206,
213, 285
artificial nutrition/hydration
withdrawal, 59, 246
for children, 158–160
choices, depressed patients and
healthcare workers
compared, 66

Euthanasia (*continued*)
  criminal liability, 237
  denied, 224, 293
    incompetence and, 293–294
  ethics, pre-1975, 235
  family acceptance of, 10, 96
  killing vs. letting die, 128, 253,
    266, 271–273
  as last resort, 227
  moral considerations, treatment
    burden vs. benefit, 267–271
  passive
    legalization of, 55, 79, 100,
      236, 237, 239, 255
    moral considerations, 268–270
    vs. active, 195, 253, 266,
      271–273
  physician-assisted suicide vs.,
    10–11
  physicians' attitudes toward,
    demographic factors, 3
  pregnancy and, 251
  public opinion, 194–195
  suicide vs., legal determination,
    239, 253–254
  withholding vs. withdrawing
    treatment, 127–128

Families
  acceptance of euthanasia by,
    10
  ambivalence of hospital staff
    toward, 77–78
  cohesion, 85–86
  cover-up of secrets, 87
  of critically ill children, 151–154
  "Daughter from California
    Syndrome," 91–92, 101,
    103
  decision making by
    anniversaries/special events
      and, 97
    authority of members, 87–88
    patient's age and, 84–85
    patient's family role and, 84
    developmental stage, 84–85
  "difficult," 154
  disagreements with treatment
    team, 99–101
    interventions, 101–102
  distrust of public institutions,
    89–90
  dysfunctional, ambivalence
    toward patient, 90–91
  end-of-life decisions, influence
    on, 45, 79–80, 83
  euthanasia discussions with,
    97–99
  financial concerns, 3, 89–90,
    96–97, 221
  gay/lesbian partners, 86–87
  guilt, 91, 98
  influence of family
    myths/traditions, 89
  information withholding, to
    protect secrets, 87
  medical sophistication, 93
  next-of-kin hierarchy, 81, 86
  patient-physician communi-
    cation, involvement in, 118
  presence in treatment settings,
    77–78
  protection needs, 88, 89
  psychopathology within, 91
  responses to patients' decisions,
    81–83
  as surrogate decision-makers,
    244

suspicions of withheld
entitlements, 89–90
treatment choices, demographic
factors in, 3
Family dynamics
in end-of-life decision making, 45
hastened-death desires and, 221
research issues, 103–104
Family size, 85
Family structure, 80–81, 86–87
closed system, 87
decision-making authority, 87–88
extended, 85
Final Exit, 209
Florida, assisted suicide,
constitutional right of privacy
and, 255
Florida District Court of Appeals,
Perlmutter case, 238–239, 240
Fogel, B. S., 185
Freud, Anna, 261
Freud, Sigmund, 169
Freyer, D. R., 160, **160**
Futile treatment, 181
for AIDS patients, 181–182
patient/family disagreement,
anticipated, 125
patients' motivation for, 4–5, 6,
10
physicians' denial of, 6, 102, 125
prolonged ventilation, acceding
to family desire for, 99

Gaylin, Willard, 273, 278
Gert, Bernard, 63
Goldstone, I., 182
Gonda, T. A., 102
Grief, 168–169
cultural aspects, 152–153

depression and, 168–169
pathological, 170–171
patients', 213
psychotherapy for, 213
patterns of, 152
religious aspects, 152–153
for terminally ill children,
169–170, 171
physician's follow-up, 171,
172
by siblings, 153, 170
Grisso, T., 26, 27, 62
Gruman, G. J., 4
Guardians. *See* Surrogate
decision-makers
Guilt
of family members, 91–92
hastened-death desires and,
222
Gutheil, T. G., 65

Hackett, T. P., 13
Hackler, J. C., 98
Halpern, J., 46–47
Hare, J., **95**
Harm
competency determination and,
21
informed consent and, 22
Hastened death. *See also* Assisted
suicide; Euthanasia;
Physician-assisted suicide
acceptability in gay culture, for
AIDS patients, 209
desire for, 9–11
anxiety disorders and, 215–216
borderline personality disorder
and, 219–220
care setting and, 210

Hastened death (continued)
  desire for (continued)
    clinical evaluation
        considerations, 211
    contradictory hopes, 223
    contributing factors, 207–208
    depression and, 9–10, 214–215
    hospice programs and, 210
    lability of, 7
    narcissistic personality
        disorder and, 218–219
    with nonterminal illness,
        57
    OCPD and, 218–219
    occasional vs. serious, 185
    organic mental disorders and,
        216
    pain relief and, 212
    personality disorders and,
        218–220
    personality style and, 217–218
    rationality of, 9, 184–185
    social suffering and, 220–221
    spiritual despair and, 222
    substance abuse and, 215–216
    suffering and, 8, 207, 213
  physician-patient relationship
        and, 222–224
  requests
    clinical approach to, 210–211
    frequency of, 208–209
    persistent, 224–226
    physicians' responses to,
        223–224
    psychiatric assessment
        functions, 226, 227
    sustained, 211
    to test family love and/or
        commitment, 221

validating, 199
  by respiration-suppressing
        painkillers, 272
Healthcare organizations. See also
    specific organizations by name
  physician-assisted suicide,
        opposition to, 3, 269
Healthcare powers of attorney. See
    Proxy directives
Healthcare proxies. See Proxy
    directives; Surrogate
    decision-makers
Heart failure, do-not-resuscitate
    orders, 121–122
Helplessness
  fear of dying in hospitals and, 7
  need for control and, 7–8
Hendin, Herbert, 198
Hiller, F. C., 98
Hippocrates, 235, 260
Hispanic Americans, treatment
    preferences, 96
HIV testing
  psychological distress, 186
  suicidal ideation and, 186
HIV-infected patients. See also AIDS
    patients
  advance directives, stability of
        preferences, 120
  alcohol abuse, 193
  combination treatment efficacy,
        180–181
  interest in physician-assisted
        suicide, 9–10
  organic mental disorders, suicide
        risk, 193–194
HIV/AIDS. See AIDS
Holland. See The Netherlands
Hopelessness, suicide risk and, 192

Hospice care. *See also* Palliative care
  depression and, 71
  diagnosis influence on, 122
  hastened-death desire and,
    210
Hospitals
  administrators' legal/publicity
    concerns, 128
  communication difficulties in, 2,
    80
  competency evaluation requests
    in, 38
  ethics committees, 102, 130–131,
    156–157
  families' distrust of public
    institutions, 89–90
  patients' fear of helplessness, 7
  physician-patient communication
    in, 122–123
  religious affiliation, end-of-life
    care alternatives, 113
Human immunodeficiency virus.
  See AIDS; HIV testing;
  HIV-infected patients
Huntington's disease
  slow onset, 190
  suicide rates, 190

Illich, Ivan, 198
Incompetence. *See also* Surrogate
  decision-makers; Surrogate
  decision making
  determining the threshold for,
    36–38
  euthanasia denial and, 293–294
  insanity compared, 25
  paternalism and, 38–41, 63
  proof of mental illness required
    for, 25

Informed consent
  adequacy of information
    provided, 22–23, 35
  communication impediments, 23
  competency evaluation and, 49
  patient autonomy and, 22
  patient understanding of
    information, 23
  right to medical information, 237
  right to privacy and, 237–238
  voluntariness of the decision, 22,
    23
Informed-consent doctrine, 21–22,
  64, 70, 237–238
  philosophical roots, 261–264
Insanity, incompetence compared,
  25
Insanity compared, incompetence, 25
International Conference on AIDS
  (Vancouver, 1996), 180

Jacobson, J. A., 209
Jefferson, Thomas, 262
Jehovah's Witnesses, blood
  transfusion refusals, 238, 239,
  240–241, 266
Jellinek, M. S., 158, **159**
Jewish Health Care Proxy of
  Agudath Israel of America, 113
Jews
  advance directives, 113
  end-of-life treatment preferences,
    112, 113
  views on death, 96
Joseph, J. G., 186

Kant, Immanuel, 263
Kass, Leon, 273
Katz, J., 260, 263, 264

Kevorkian, Murad "Jack," 207, 253
Kolata, Gina, 199
Korean-Americans, treatment preferences, 96

Lee, D. K. P., 98
Legal norms, withholding vs. withdrawing treatment, 127–128
Legal system
  end-of-life decisions, consensus on, 236–241, 244–245
  patients' medical decisions, validity criteria, 22–23
  standards for end-of-life decisions, 244–249
  treatment refusal, countervailing state interests, 238–240
Leikin, S., 149, 157
Lidz, C. W., 22, 33, 69
Lindemann, E., 168
Living wills, 79, 250
  actual-wishes standard and, 250
  as evidence of stable values, 70
  physicians' knowledgeability about, 123
  probable-wishes standard and, 248
  suicide intentions and, 58, 59
Locke, John, 262
Los Angeles Multicenter AIDS Cohort Study, 186
Loss of control, suffering and, 221

Maine, substituted judgment standard, rejection of, 247

Making Health Care Decisions: The Ethical and Legal Implications of Informed Consent in the Patient-Practitioner Relationship, 60, 264
Martin case, 246–247
Marzuk, P. M., 190
Massachusetts Supreme Judicial Court
  countervailing state interests, 239
  judicial involvement in end-of-life decisions, 243
  treatment refusal based on religious principles, 241
McKegney, F. P., 187
Medical Outcomes Study, 65
Medications
  antipsychotic, patient refusal, 57–58
  for depression, 62, 66, 215
    inappropriate choices, 215
  hastened death from, 272
  inability to appreciate risks and benefits of, 63–64
  intravenous drug use, suicide risk, 193
  symptom control, in terminal illness, 212
Medicine
  denial of death's inevitability in, 124
  purpose of, 290
Meier, D., 197
Meisel, Alan, 22, 33, 56, 57, 59, 63, 69
Mental disorders. *See* Organic mental disorders; *specific disorders by name*

Mental disturbances, recognizing
psychological vs. organic, 49
Mental health professionals. *See*
Psychiatrists
Mental illness
proof required for incompetence
declaration, 25
suicidal ideation as evidence of,
58, 61
treatment refusal for, 57
Mercy killing. *See* Physician-assisted
suicide
Methylphenidate, 66
Mexican American patients,
114
Mexican Americans, treatment
preferences, 96
Michigan, substituted judgment
standard, rejection of,
247
Miles, S. H., 97, 182
Mill, John Stuart, 262
Mini-Mental State Exam, 29
Missouri, substituted judgment
standard, rejection of, 247
Missouri Court of Appeals, *Warren*
case, 246
Missouri Supreme Court
actual-wishes standard, 246
Cruzan case, 246
Molloy, D. W., 101
Mood disorders, suicide risk and,
193
Mor, U., 185
Moral considerations. *See* Ethics
Morphine, 272
Mount, B. M., 167, **167**
Muller, J., 113, 114
Muslims, views on death, 96

Narcissistic personality disorder,
hastened-death desire and,
217–219
National Hospice Organization, 269,
274
The Netherlands
AIDS patients, euthanasia rates,
194
assisted-suicide rates, 208–209
euthanasia in, 59, 194
hastened-death requests, pain
relief and, 212
physician-assisted suicide in,
12–13
voluntary euthanasia rates,
208–209
New Jersey Supreme Court, 182
judicial involvement in
end-of-life decisions, 242
Quinlan case, 56, 79, 100, 236,
237, 255
New York Court of Appeals,
Schloendorff case, 237
New York State
assisted suicide, criminal law, 254
substituted judgment standard,
rejection of, 247
New York Times, assisted suicide
reports, 198
Next-of-kin, as surrogate
decision-makers, 244
Nursing home placement, patients'
refusals, 19, 39
Nutrition/hydration withdrawal, 59,
246

Obsessive-compulsive personality
disorder, hastened-death desire
and, 217–219

O'Dowd, M. A., 187
Ogden, Russel, 198, 199
Oliver, R. C., 171
On Liberty (Mill), 263
Oncology patients. *See* Cancer
  patients
Opioids, 216
Oregon
  physician-assisted suicide,
    legalization, 3, 13, 226,
    228, 253, 254, 277
  psychiatrists' attitudes toward
    assisted suicide, 206
Oregon Death with Dignity Act,
  206
Organic mental disorders
  hastened-death desire and, 216
  suicide risk, 193–194
  in terminal illness, 216
Ouslander, J., 94

Pain. *See also* Suffering
  in cancer patients, 212
  as determinant of treatment
    choices, 8
  undertreatment of, 212, 216
Pain management. *See also*
    Double-effect deaths
  addiction concerns, 212
  substance abuse complications,
    212, 216–217
Palliative care. *See also* Hospice care
  for children, 167–168
  constitutional right to, 206
  for depression, 71
  need for enhanced services, 206
  physicians' education in, 126
  psychosocial aspects, psychiatric
    involvement, 226–228

Palliative care patients. *See* Terminal
  illness
Parkes, C. M., 168
Paternalism (medical)
  historical tradition of, 260–261
  incompetency as mask for, 38–41
  repudiation of, 260, 261
Patient autonomy, 78–79
  compromised by depression,
    60–61
  end-of-life decisions and, 1–2, 4
  inappropriate treatment requests
    and, 182
  informed consent and, 22
  omniscient psychiatrist vs., 61
  power of healthcare personnel
    and, 42
  psychiatric disorders and, 6–7
  states' interests and, 240
Patient rights, right to refuse
    treatment, 266
Patient Self-Determination Act
  (1990), 79, 252–253, 266
Patient surrogates. *See* Surrogate
  decision-makers
Patient-physician relationship. *See*
  Physician-patient relationship
Patients
  attributes required for decision
    making, 26–27
  benefit vs. burden assessments in
    care choices, 8–9
  confusion, fluctuations in, 49
  control needs, 7–8
  feared loss of care control,
    alleviated by preference
    discussions, 211
  grief for anticipated losses, 213
  helplessness fears, 7–8

medical decisions by, legal
validity criteria, 22–23
quality-of-life, physicians'
underestimate, 69
values, competency and, 27–28,
30
Patients' rights
to create advance directives, 253
to determine, 186
to medical information, 237, 261,
263
to palliative care, 206
right to die, 55–56
court decisions, 56–57,
253–255
societal emphasis on, 4, 6
treatment refusal, 236–237
absoluteness of, 241
medical ethics and, 239–240
Pellegrino, Edmund, 273
Perlmutter case, 238–239, 240
Perry, S., 186
Personality disorders
end-of-life decisions and,
115–116
hastened-death desire and,
218–220
Personality style, hastened-death
desire and, 217–218
Physician-assisted suicide. *See also*
Assisted suicide; Euthanasia;
Hastened death; Suicide
acceptability
by cancer patients, 208
patient burden on family and,
208
competence and, 21
competency determination for,
43

constitutional rights and, 2–3,
205–206, 254–255
court rulings, 254–256
demographic aspects, 3
desire for autonomy and, 8
disease variables, 8
distrust of medical profession
and, 278–279
euthanasia vs., 10–11
feared loss of control over care
and, 210–211
healthcare organizations'
opposition, 3
HIV patients' interest in, 9–10
increased interest in, 209
legalization of, 2–3, 256, 277, 297
mandatory psychiatric evaluation
issues, 12–13, 43, 46,
206–207
mental health clinicians' roles,
207
in The Netherlands, 12–13
personality disorders and, 8
physicians' integrity
compromised by, 294–295
physicians' support for, 2
psychiatrists' assessment
capabilities for, 206, 228
psychiatrists' role in, 278
public support for, 2
self-determination and, 283–285,
288, 292
as social policy, 283–285, 288,
289, 292, 297
suicidal ideation and, 10
Physician-patient communication.
See also Communication
about advance directives, 117
ALS patients, 119, 120

Physician-patient communication
(*continued*)
about cardiopulmonary
resuscitation, 119,
122–123, 124
critically ill children, 154–156
cross-cultural difficulties in,
113–115
about DNR orders, 122
about end-of-life care, 133
medical-legal concerns,
127–123
patients' emotional reactions,
119–120
patients' reluctance to discuss,
115, 116
physicians' avoidance of,
123–128
physicians' denial of death's
inevitability and, 124
physicians' feelings of
vulnerability and,
126–127
physicians' vulnerability and,
126–127
psychiatrists' role, 128–129
recommendations for
facilitating, 131–133
about euthanasia, 97–99
family involvement in, 118
full disclosure, American cultural
insistence on, 115
about futile treatment,
anticipated disagreement,
125
honesty in, 118–119
in hospital settings, 2, 122–123
about impending death, 125
informed consent and, 23

language barriers, 23, 113–114
medical-legal concerns,
administrative aspects, 128
physicians' fear of being
bad-news bearers, 124–125
physicians' fear of causing pain,
123
timeliness of, 109–111, 118
Physician-patient relationship
ambivalence in death
discussions, 222–223
dysfunction in, hastened-death
desires and, 222–224
fragmentation of medical care
and, 80, 124
influence on end-of-life
decisions, 8
misunderstanding of medical
information, 222
power in, 41–42
Physicians
advance directives, knowledge
about, 117, 123
communication skills, education
lacking, 125–126
countertransference, terminally
ill children and, 165–166
deaths as personal failures, 124,
126–127, 223
demographic factors and,
euthanasia attitudes, 3
denial of death's inevitability, 124
depression unrecognized by, 30,
60
DNR orders, diagnosis influence
on, 121–122
emotional aspects of dying and, 4
end-of-life discussion avoidance,
reasons for, 123–128

euthanasia attitudes, 3
fear of death, 126–127
hastened-death refusals,
    emotional aspects, 224
hastened-death requests,
    emotional responses to,
    223–224
inappropriate treatment requests
    and, 182
obligation to relief suffering, 284,
    286–297, 295
organic mental disorders
    unrecognized by, 216
palliative-care education, 126
paternalism, 38–41
patients' quality-of-life
    underestimated by, 69
pseudo-empathy with patients,
    36, 37, 65–66
suicide assistance, integrity
    compromised by, 295
vulnerability, terminal illness
    and, 126–127
Power, 292–293
bureaucratic, 42–43
competency and, 41
in physician-patient relationship,
    41–42
psychiatrists', in competency
    determinations, 43–46
Power of attorney (healthcare). *See*
    Proxy directives
Pregnancy, euthanasia decisions
    and, 251
President's Commission for the
    Study of Ethical Problems in
    Medicine and Biomedical and
    Behavioral Research, 60, 264,
    265, 267

Privacy rights
    assisted suicide and, 255
    informed-consent doctrine and,
        237
Probable-wishes standard, 79,
    247–248
    decision factors in, 248
Prognosis, perceptions of, illness
    and, 97
Protease inhibitors, 180, 181
Protestants, end-of-life treatment
    preferences, 112
Proxies. *See* Surrogate
    decision-makers
Proxy directives, 250–251
    feared loss of care control and,
        211
Psychiatrists
    attitudes toward assisted suicide,
        206, 278
    bureaucratic power, 42–43
    clinical hunches, 45–46
    competency determination
        qualifications for, 48–50
    role in, 21, 51, 64–65
    consultation
        for children, 138–140
        with children's parents, 158,
        159
    as consultation liaisons, 129–130
    end-of-life consultation, 4, 11–13
    on ethics committees, 130
    hastened-death requests, collegial
        role in, 224–227
    as informed-consent technicians,
        65
    moral judgments on suicide, 37,
        43
    omniscience, 61

Psychiatrists *(continued)*
  physician-assisted suicide,
    mandatory consultation
    issues, 13–14, 43, 46,
    206–207
  physician-patient communication
    role, 128–129
  power to see the unobvious, in
    competency
    determinations, 43–46
  stability of patient's values, in
    competency assessment,
    27–28, 30–31
  treatment-limitation
    consultation, 11–12
  treatment-refusal consultation,
    64–65
Psychological tests, for competency
  evaluation, 29
Psychostimulants, 66, 67, 212, 215
Psychotherapy
  efficacy for depression, 66
  for grief, in the terminally ill, 213
Psychotropic drugs, 216

Quill, T. E., 195, 197, 198, 253
Quill v. Vacco, 254
Quinlan, Karen Ann, 56, 235,
  255–256
Quinlan case, 56, 79, 100, 236, 237,
  239, 255
  significance of, 236, 255

Rabkin, J., 186
Rachels, James, 272–273
Rationality, in competency
  determination, 27
Religion
  advance directives and, 113

grieving and, 152–153
Right to die, 55–56
  court decisions, 56–57, 253–255
  nonterminal illness and, 57
Roman Catholic Church. *See also*
  Christians
  advance directives, 113
  do-not-resuscitate orders, 96
  double-effect deaths, moral
    reasoning on, 274
  treatment withholding, moral
    reasoning on, 267–268, 274
  Vatican Declaration on
    Euthanasia, 112
Roth, L. H., 22, 33, 35, 60, 64
Ruark, J. E., 99, 102
Rundell, J. R., 189

Saikewicz case, 239–240
Sanctity of life, religious and
    philosophical traditions of, 70,
    112
Scalia, Antonin, 253
Schaffner, Kenneth F., 59
Schloendorff case, 237
Schneiderman, L., 117
Seckler, A. B., 94
Selective serotonin reuptake
    inhibitors (SSRIs), 215
Self-determination, 262–263, 283
    physician-assisted suicide and,
    283–285, 288, 292
  suffering and, 289, 293
Seneca, 70
Sertraline, 62
Siegel, K., 197
Siegler, Mark, 273
Slavin, L. A., 156
Smedira, N. G., 97, 100

SSRIs (selective serotonin reuptake
inhibitors), 215
State laws, assisted suicide
constitutionality, 254–255
Steinbock, Bonnie, 269, 273
Stone, Alan A., 47, 61
Study to Understand Prognoses and
Preferences for Outcomes and
Risks of Treatment. *See*
SUPPORT study
Substance abuse
AIDS patients, 216
cancer patients, 216
family ambivalence toward
abusing members, 90–91
hastened-death requests and,
215–216
pain management and, 212,
216–217
suicide, by drug overdose, 190
Substituted-judgment standard. *See*
Probable-wishes standard
Suffering. *See also* Pain
acceptance of, 287
assisted suicide as alternative to,
207
as determinant of treatment
choices, 8, 9
euthanasia as alternative to, 207,
213, 285
existential/spiritual, 221–222
as failure of medicine, 289
fear of, 285
grief, 213
human response to, 285–286
obligation to relieve, 284,
286–297, 295
psychological/spiritual, 213–220,
289–290

self-determination and, 289, 293
social, in terminal illness,
220–221
subjectivity of, 291–292
treatment refusal and, 238, 239
unnecessary, 287–288
values and, 291
Suicidal ideation
AIDS vs. cancer patients, 189
competence and, 58
friendship with HIV/AIDS
patients and, 187
in gay men, 186
HIV testing and, 186
in HIV/AIDS patients, 186–189
making preparations without
acting, comfort from,
188–189
physician-assisted suicide interest
and, 10
psychopathology and, 189
Suicide. *See also* Assisted suicide;
Physician-assisted suicide
artificial nutrition/hydration
withdrawal as, 59
by asphyxiation, 209
attempted
alcohol use and, 189
impulsivity of, 189–190
living wills and, 58
need for coping skills and, 190
causation criterion, 58–59
euthanasia vs., legal
determination, 239,
253–254
as evidence of mental disorder,
58, 61
hopelessness, as predictor of, 61
intention criterion, 58–59

Suicide (*continued*)
  living wills and, 58, 59
  by medication overdose, 190
  psychiatrists' moral judgments
      about, 37, 43
  rates
    cancer patients, 209
    in Denmark, 209
    HIV/AIDS patients, 187,
      209
    Huntington's disease, 190
  rational, 196–198
  risk factors
    demographic, 192
    depression, 192–193
    HIV/AIDS patients, 192–194,
      216
    hopelessness, 192
    intravenous drug use, 193
    mood disorders, 193
    organic mental disorders and,
      193–194, 216
    psychopathology, 192–193
    substance abuse, 193, 216
  treatment refusal vs., 58, 184
Sullivan, M. D., 184, 199
SUPPORT study, 112, 116, 117,
  220, 276
Surgery, right to refuse, and legal
  rights, 263–264
Surrogate decision-makers, 2, 22,
  243–244
  for adolescents, 160
  discordance between patients and
    proxies, 92–93, **94–95**
  family members as, 244
  patient control over care and, 211
Surrogate decision making, 241–242
  actual-wishes standard, 245–247

advance directives, role in,
  249–253
best-interests standard, 249
for children, 140, 141, 142–143,
  145–146, 147, 149
judicial involvement, 242–243,
  244
probable-wishes standard, 79,
  247–248
procedural aspects, 242–244
substantive aspects, 244–249
Szasz, Thomas, 278

Technology
  end-of-life decisions and, 5, 9,
    259, 267
  right to die and, 55–56
Terminal illness
  anxiety disorders in, 7, 215–216
  care choices, 8, 9
  coping strategies, 36, 38, 49–50
  depression in, 67, 71, 213–215
  emotional reactions to, 36
  fear of helplessness in, 7–8
  grief in, 213
  ICD-9 classification proposal for,
    12
  organic mental disorders and, 216
  physician vulnerability, 126–127
  social suffering in, 220–221
  substance abuse disorders and,
    212
  suicidal thoughts in, 58
  symptom control
    behavioral treatments, 212–213
    medications for, 212
Tertiary-amine tricyclics, 215
Thanatology, 5
Todres, I. D., 171, **172**

Torian, L. V., 93
Treatment, life-sustaining. *See also*
Futile treatment
against the patient's will, 40–41
emotional impact, 4–5
for neonates, 142
options, understanding vs.
appreciating, 64
patients' decisions, depression
and, 61–62
religious aspects, 113–114
Treatment choices, pain tolerance
and, 8
Treatment limitation, psychiatric
consultation for, 11
Treatment preferences. *See also*
Advance directives
ALS patients, 120
cultural factors, 113–115
depression and
AIDS patients, 185
elderly patients, 61–62
ethnicity and, 96
HIV/AIDS patients, 120, 185
physician-patient communication
about, 109–111, 211
religious factors, 112–113
stability of, 117, 120–121
Treatment refusal. *See also*
Euthanasia
age and, 182–183
antipsychotic medication, 57–58
based on religious principles, 241
caused by depression, 27–28, 60
competency, 24–25
burden of proof, 57, 59, 70
case examples, 19, 27–28
decision-making attributes
required, 26–28

countervailing state interests,
238–240
critically ill children, 156–157
ethical changes and, 265–266
intention criterion, 58–59
by Jehovah's Witnesses, 238, 239,
240–241, 268
leading to death, legal aspects,
58–59, 238
for mental illness, 57–58
involuntary hospitalization
and, 58
in nonterminal illness, legal
aspects, 56–57, 182–183,
240
patients' rights, 236–237
absoluteness of, 241
medical ethics and, 239–240
physical power and, 41–42
psychiatric consultation, 64–65
reasons, physicians' reluctance to
explore, 69–70
suffering and, 238
suicide vs., 58
surgery, and legal rights,
263–264
Treatment risk, competency
determination and, 33
Treatment withholding/withdrawal.
See Euthanasia

Uhlmann, R. F., 94
Understanding, as inherent ability,
26
U.S. Air Force
HIV-seropositive personnel
alcohol abuse, 193
mood disorders, 193
suicide attempts, 189

U.S. Supreme Court
  assisted-suicide rulings, 2–3, 209,
      254–255, 266
    state laws and, 254
  Cruzan case, 246
  physician-assisted suicide ruling,
      2–3
  right-to-die rulings, 246, 253–255
Utilitarians, 262

Values
  Christian, sanctity of life, 70
  depression's effect on, 28, 30, 70
  patients'
    as basis for medical decisions,
        263
    different from physicians', 43,
        64, 263
  psychiatrists', in competency
      assessments, 37, 42
  sanctity of life, 70
  stability of, 27–28, 30–31
    in competency determination,
        27–28, 30–31, 70–71
    living wills as evidence of,
        70–71

suffering and, 291
Vatican Declaration on Euthanasia,
    112
Villarreal, S., 165

Wachter, R. M., 181, 185
Warren case, 246
Washington (Natural Death) Act, 59
Washington State
  assisted suicide, criminal law, 254
  physician-assisted suicide,
      legalization initiative,
      277
  state courts, judicial involvement
      in end-of-life decisions, 243
Weisman, A. D., 13
Wenger, N. S., 46–47
Wisconsin, substituted judgment
    standard, rejection of, 247
Woolley, H., 165

Youngner, S. J., 184, 199

Zidovudine (AZT), 180
Zweibel, N. R., 95

DATE

A-L-A